R. H. STETSON'S MOTOR PHONETICS
A RETROSPECTIVE EDITION

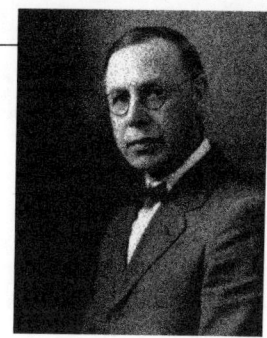

R. H. STETSON'S MOTOR PHONETICS
A RETROSPECTIVE EDITION

Edited by

J. A. S. Kelso, Ph.D.
Professor of Psychology
Director of the Center
for Complex Systems
Florida Atlantic University
Boca Raton, Florida

K. G. Munhall, Ph.D.
Assistant Professor
of Psychology
York University
North York, Ontario
Canada

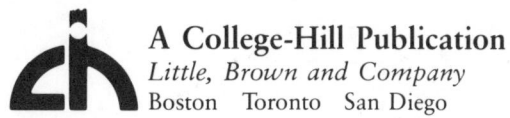

A College-Hill Publication
Little, Brown and Company
Boston Toronto San Diego

College-Hill Press
A Division of Little, Brown and Company (Inc.)
34 Beacon Street
Boston, Massachusetts 02108

© 1988 by Little, Brown and Company (Inc.)

All rights, including that of translation, reserved. No part of this publication may be reproduced, stored in a retrieval system, or transmitted in any form or by any means, electronic, mechanical, recording, or otherwise, without the prior written permission of the publisher.

Library of Congress Cataloging in Publication Data
Main entry under title:

Stetson, R. H. (Raymond Herbert), 1872–1950.
  R.H. Stetson's motor phonetics.

  "A College-Hill publication."
  Reprint. Originally published: Motor phonetics / R.H. Stetson. 2nd. ed. 1951. With editor's remarks.
  "Bibliography of published works by R.H. Stetson"
  Includes index.
  1. Phonetics. I. Kelso, J. A. Scott. II. Munhall, Kevin G., 1954–   . III. Title. IV. Title: Motor phonetics. [DNLM: 1. Speech—physiology. 2. Voice. WV 501 S841m 1951a]
  QP306.S69   1988   612'.78   87-33896

ISBN 0-316-48702-3

Printed in the United States of America

CONTENTS

Preface to the Retrospective Edition		vii
Stetson: A Biographical Sketch, by Louis D. Hartson		1
Recollections of R. H. Stetson, by Robert Galambos		9
Recollections of R. H. Stetson, by Roger Sperry		12
Personal Impressions of R. H. Stetson, by J. M. Pickett		15
Preface to the Second Edition		23
CHAPTER I.	The Basic Conceptions of Phonology Editors' Remarks	25
CHAPTER II.	Methods and Apparatus in Experimental Phonetics Editors' Remarks Suggested Readings (Editors' Addition)	34
CHAPTER III.	Coordination of the Movements of Speech Editors' Remarks	52
CHAPTER IV.	Influence of the Phonetic Units on Each Other Editors' Remarks	83
CHAPTER V.	Classification of Phonemes Editors' Remarks	113
Editors' Remarks to Chapters VI, VII, and VIII		118
CHAPTER VI.	Stress and Rate and Their Relation to the Syllable and to the Breath Group	119
CHAPTER VII.	The Breath Group in English Dependent on the Stress Pattern of the Words	130
CHAPTER VIII.	Rhythm and the Characteristic Utterance of a Language	147
Appendices		149
References		212
Glossary of Motor Phonetic Terms		215
Bibliography of Published Works by R. H. Stetson		225
Author Index		227
Subject Index		229

PREFACE TO THE RETROSPECTIVE EDITION

When people speak, the movements of their articulators—at respiratory, laryngeal, and supralaryngeal levels—must be precisely ordered in space and time. It is, after all, the coordinated workings of the vocal tract that structure sound for a listener. This problem of understanding how a very complex system—capable of transporting meaningful information from one individual to another—is coordinated has become a central one in contemporary science. It has grabbed the attention of scientists and engineers alike, taking on multiple forms in many disciplines, including neuroscience, cognitive science, computer science, speech science, and movement science (or kinesiology) itself. Understanding how a complex, multivariable system is controlled and coordinated may also hold a key to successful applications in, for instance, robotics, prosthetics, computer architectures, and pattern recognition devices. A better appreciation of disorders and how to treat them seems a logical spinoff. As we approach the second millenium, such applications and implications are no longer pipe dreams. Yet it is worth remembering (if only to temper one's hubris) that it was not until the early sixteenth century that Kepler (1571–1630) formulated the laws governing the motion of heavenly bodies. The laws governing the coordination of earthly bodies still elude us.

In the motor systems field, we have been fortunate that such problems have inspired and fueled the genius of some great scientists. In this century, the Soviet physiologist and biomechanician, Nicolai Bernstein, and the German behavioral biologist, Erich von Holst, can certainly be counted among them. This book is about another, Raymond Herbert Stetson, an American who formulated a field that he called *motor phonetics*. Motor phonetics, as Stetson himself defined it, is the study of *skilled movements* involved in the process of handling articulatory signals. It deals with the organization of speech articulators, tailored as they are to linguistic function.

In some sense, Stetson posed himself an even more daunting task than many of his contemporaries, that of actually observing and measuring motions of the (rather inaccessible) vocal tract. This monograph attests to the fact that the effort was worthwhile. Stetson eschewed the linguistic approaches of his contemporaries. (e.g., Martin Joos) that reduced articulatory movements to the logistic symbols of a phonemic alphabet and then proceeded in a formal fashion. For him, the posited layers of linguistic structure that interpenetrate, the segmentation (often accompanied by what he called neural "assumptions"), and so on would "straighten out" once speech movements were subjected to the same treatment as any system of skilled movement. The phoneme *qua* symbol belonged to *La Langue*, whereas the *signal*, the articulation itself, formed the system of *La Parole*. The basic mystery remains, however: although utterances can be described as sequences of discrete linguistic units, it is far from clear how this type of representation is related to the continuous flow of articulatory and acoustic events that constitutes speaking. The problem appears in particularly striking form in attempts to describe disordered speech, where phonetic transcription fails miserably in capturing those perceptually salient characteristics that give speech its deviant quality. Here again, Stetson looked to articulation as the source of speech disorders. His whole image of the scientific investigation of speech and language can be summed up in one eloquent phrase: "Speech is rather a set of movements made audible than a set of sounds produced by movements" (orig version, p. 33; this edition, p. 58).

As technology advances and as the problems of understanding that uniquely human function known as speech become ever more scientifically significant, R. H. Stetson's work grows in importance. Yet, the Second Edition of *Motor Phonetics*, which is reproduced here in its entirety, was last published in 1951 for Oberlin College, where Stetson spent his entire scientific and academic career. Stetson, in fact, did not live to see it appear. We thought a great deal about editing the Second edition; each time we tried, however, something of the work's flavor was lost. As we tampered with pieces of the manuscript, we became acutely aware that we were tampering with a little bit of history. Moreover, our main goal was simply to make the book available again to the scientific community–especially to those interested in speech and hearing. Stetson's book is a landmark in the study of movement and speech and has been out of print for too long. Even apart from its enduring qualities (and flaws), we believe that serious study of Stetson's work will suggest new directions for research in the field, and a better appreciation of the issues. Not only do many gaps in Stetson's program remain to be filled, but there is a springboard here for further discovery.

As editors, therefore, we have inhibited a tendency to interfere with Stetson's prose–some of the repetitious statements and discussions of no longer burning issues–and instead have simply provided brief guiding remarks at the beginning of most chapters. We took one further, somewhat unusual, step: In our curiosity about Stetson the person–what was he like?—it became apparent, through inquiries and some historical research, that he was, for want of better words, "a real character", literally a legend in his own time. Not only that, but Stetson's students constituted a prestigious list indeed. In an attempt to convey something of the human side of this man of science, we have included—in addition to a brief bibliography of his publications—recollections of some by his former students and one of his late colleagues, Louis D. Hartson, Professor Emeritus of Psychology at Oberlin College. In fact, an abbreviated version of Professor Hartson's comments was published as an obituary to R. H. Stetson in the *American Journal of Psychology* (1951, 64, 276–280), but we preferred the longer, more personal account included here. We were fortunate to obtain such through the kindness of Dr. J. M. Pickett, a former student of Stetson's and Director of Gallaudet Research Institute's Center for Auditory and Speech Sciences. Indeed, Dr. Pickett deserves our gratitude for the many ways in which he helped us bring this project to fruition.

We would like to further express our thanks to Professors R. W. Sperry, R. Galambos, and J. M. Pickett for kindly sharing their impressions and recollections of Stetson; in particular, the impact he had on their academic careers–each impressive in its own right. Mr. W. E. Bigglestone, former archivist at Oberlin College, was very helpful in providing biographical material about Stetson. The Stetson letters and other papers occupy somewhat more than one linear foot, according to Mr. Bigglestone, in Oberlin College's archives. The generosity and kindness of Mrs. Ruth Hudgins, whose late husband, Dr. C. V. Hudgins, played a major role in completing the second edition of *Motor Phonetics* in 1951, is much appreciated. We are extremely grateful to Dr. Sadanand Singh of College-Hill Press, whose enthusiasm and encouragement at the early stages of the project provided the necessary impetus, and to Marie Linvill, also of College-Hill Press, for her constant but gentle prodding to finish it.

Motor Phonetics was first published in the Archives Neerlandaises de Phonetique Experimental in 1928. It is a demonstration of the power of movement analysis to understanding speech processes. Surely, it is a fitting tribute to its author, Raymond Herbert Stetson, that this work retains its freshness now, sixty years after it was first published.

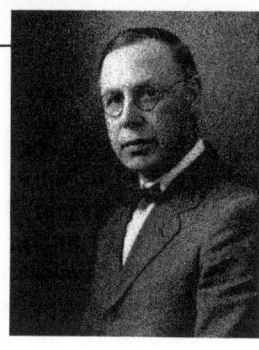

STETSON: A BIOGRAPHICAL SKETCH
Louis D. Hartson*

Raymond Herbert Stetson was born March 1, 1872, a third generation Western Reserve farm boy whose intellectual curiosity drove him from his earliest boyhood to acquire all manner of things and find out what could be done with them. In the machine shop of his grandfather's farm he soon developed a mechanical knack. Repeatedly, his hopeful elders would teach him some useful process such as harness mending, thinking that his help would be valuable, only to find that his interest was not in the needed harness, but in the process itself. He taught himself to play the piano chiefly to be able to write down the melodies and harmonies that came to his mind. He puttered with oil paints, not in order to express a great artistic talent, but that he might find out what could be done with oils. And in this he would have nothing to do with "store paints," sold in neat tubes, but rather must grind his own colors in oil using the native ochre and hematite. Funds for a learned career were not readily forthcoming from the family exchequer. A sympathetic and understanding aunt supplied the first funds, and it was characteristic of Stetson that he returned the debt manyfold even into that good woman's advanced old age.

There being no chemistry laboratory at Elyria High School, Stetson and Ray Cogswell, who later took the first photographs of a trip down the Grand Canyon of the Colorado, set up their own laboratory, and they insisted on writing and balancing all equations before they attempted an experiment. When Stetson came to Oberlin as a freshman in 1890, having completed the Elyria High School course in two and two-thirds years, he had only enough money to pay for three years in college. Accordingly, he went to Professor Jewett, the head of the chemistry department, and asked permission to shorten the course by taking an examination. Jewett was skeptical, but at Stetson's insistence, made out an examination. At this point, the Stetson-Cogswell Laboratory proved its worth. Balanced equations were asked for and were given, and when Jewett asked for a description of the compounds of chromium and their properties, it surfaced that the two experimenters had specialized in chromium. In 1893 Stetson was graduated from Oberlin, having done his pricipal work in chemistriy. The following year he continued as graduate assistant in chemistry.

The foregoing passage is quoted from an

---

*Professor Emeritus of Psychology, Chairman, 1939–1947, Oberlin College.

article written by Donald M. Love, now Emeritus Secretary of Oberlin College (Love, 1951).

Stetson remained as a student at Oberlin until 1896, when he received a master's degree in zoology, thus laying a foundation in the sciences which he was ever afterwards to recommend to students. With the exception of his earliest papers, his publications were based upon his experimental studies. His first paper, published in 1896, was entitled "Types of Imagination" (Stetson, 1896).

In 1897, there appeared a paper, "Piano Tone-Color from a Physical and Psychological Standpoint" (Stetson, 1897), which decried the current theories of piano playing, and stated that there is no tone variation without dynamic variation, and that most of the effects ascribed to tone color (or tone effects, as he preferred to call them) are due to self-deception. This was but the first of several papers he was to publish in musical journals.

From 1896 until 1899 Stetson served as Professor of Biology at Tabor College, Iowa. There he built up a zoology laboratory, accumulating a slide collection by exchanging with the University and Medical centers slides which he made of turtle blood cells fixed in osmic acid. In Tabor he also took up the study of hypnosis. During this period he picked up an excellent command of spoken French by residing, for two summers, in an Icarian French community nearby.

These years in the laboratory were excellent preparation for graduate work at Harvard, which Stetson entered in 1899. There he worked with Royce on logic and concepts, with Santayana on ethics and aesthetics, and with James, who had just returned from delivering the Edinburgh Lectures on the Psychology of Religion. These lectures constituted the points of departure for courses in aesthetics and religion which he was to give in later years. He also worked in the laboratory with Munsterberg, and he often said it had been difficult to make the choice between Royce and Munsterberg when it came to the preparation of a dissertation. But Munsterberg provided the stronger attraction, partly because Stetson was able to capitalize on Munsterberg's interest in motor activity in perception. In a dissertation in which he developed a "Motor Theory of Rhythm and Discreet Succession," he obtained his Ph.D. in 1906. (His was the twelfth Harvard doctorate in psychology.)

Stetson accepted a position at Beloit College, teaching first in the Academy, later as Professor of Philosophy and Psychology. There he continued his work on the motor theory of rhythm (Stetson, 1903), and substantiated the classification of movements made by Beaunis (1885) and by Richet (1895) (Stetson, 1905). From the Beloit days comes the background for one of the favorite Oberlin sayings about Stetson, that he could teach any class in college on 10 minutes' notice. As his friend Donald Love tells the story: "A certain lad at Beloit, whom we may call Scott, sought to turn over a new leaf at the middle of his course and become a student. He found, however, that such a procedure would be considered desertion by his fraternity brothers. In this predicament he went to Stetson announcing his decision to leave Beloit and go to another college where he could make a record as a student without incurring social stigma. It was of no avail to point out that there was a studious group in the same fraternity with which it would be possible to affiliate. The youth was certain that the only solution was to leave the college. A few days later Stetson met some of Scott's fraternity brothers who asked whether he knew that he was the cause of Scott's intended departure. Somewhat puzzled, Stetson asked for an explanation and received it in these terms: 'Well, Scott is saying that he had English, Mathematics, Chemistry, and Latin with you in the Academy, has had French, English Composition, and Psychology with you in College and if he stays here another year he'll have to take Logic and Philosophy with you, and that's why he is leaving.'"

In 1908 Stetson was chosen as head of the newly created Department of Psychology at Oberlin College, from which position he retired in 1939. He has been cited as the best representative, among Oberlin teachers, of the transition from the period when teachers were marked by general competence to the age of narrow specialization. It was this versatility to which President Wilkins was to refer in 1942, when Stetson was cited for the degree of Sc.D., with the words: "Leonardo at last turned psychologist." His interest in the arts was not limited to music. In the summer of 1922, when Louis Lord, Director of the Bureau of University Travel, needed a conductor for a tour of English cathedrals, he persuaded Stetson to take the assignment. Although conversant with the history of the fine arts, he had not been abroad. On this occasion his "10 minutes' preparation" consisted of an early morning preview of the church. On the eve of their departure for the continent, Lord again insisted that Stetson act as a conductor, although this also included the museums. According to another of these guides, Stetson was an exceptionally good conductor, even if he occasionally had difficulty in locating the paintings.

The skill and ingenuity that Stetson was able to employ in his research was well manifested in the series of experiments he conducted during the years from 1910 to 1915. These were concerned with the determination of the role of the hair follicle in cutaneous sensitivity (Stetson, 1923). This involved removing a hair and its follicle through a tiny incision, snipping off the follicle, and replacing the hair. This required instruments finer than any available in the surgical supply sources. So he constructed tiny hooks, knives honed razor sharp, and pincers, using #8 steel needles. His collaborator, C. C. W. Nicol, wrote: "With these tiny instruments many hundreds of hairs and follicles were operated. There was only one serious catch. We had great difficulty getting subjects because the operation was sharply painful, as no anesthetic was used." A decade later Stetson counseled a student all the way through from senior year to doctorate in the study of thermal sensitivity. With reference to Stetson's contribution to the theory of cutaneous sensitivity, Karl P. Heiser said: "I doubt if anyone antedated his hunch that the character of sensation is determined by patterning of neural impulses, and that in cutaneous temperature sensations this pattern would be dependent upon sense organ or nerve-ending temperature, the rate of change of this temperature due to whatever stimuli were used, the character of the blood supply to this area, and other important features which could be measured, and, possibly, controlled." His was, from the outset, an organismic, rather than an atomistic, approach to an explanation of psychological processes.

Stetson's own research soon became concentrated upon a study of skilled movements. Although he gave credit for prior discovery of the existence of the ballistic movement to Beaunis and Richet, he was the first American to call attention to the fact that there are two types of skilled muscular contraction: that which is under continuous control and the thrown, ballistic type. It was in the laboratory that he developed in Oberlin that methods were perfected and recordings made of a variety of athletic skills, of locomotion, singing, piano playing, eye movements, and the details of the complicated processes involved in speech.

He had been interested in the structure of language from childhood. While other boys were making stamp collections he was collecting alphabets. But it was not until the years 1922 to 1923, spent in Paris with the Abbé Rousselot, that his research became focused upon the analysis of the motor processes involved in vocalization. During the following 20 years he expended thousands of dollars of his own money building a laboratory and, most of the time, paying the salaries of technical assistants. He requested no aid from foundations or the government, and, at first, not even from the college.

If one were to draw conclusions merely from an examination of Stetson's publications, one might assume that he had been interested only in a limited area of applied physiology. Actually, his was a much more fundamental interest. His basic purpose was to obtain experimental evidence to support the hypothesis that the motor adjustment and its feedback into the brain provides a more illuminating approach to an understanding of the intellectual processes than a study of stimulus patterns or subjective states. He held that "the eyes that see are moving eyes, the ears that hear are moving ears, the hands that feel are moving hands. We cannot, therefore, count a man to be a man merely because he sees, hears or feels, for such a procedure would fail to cover such remarkable cases as Beethoven and Helen Keller. We cannot think of Psychology as the science of the sense organs alone, but rather as the science of movements which are essential to the functioning of these organs. Nor can we use the central nervous system to explain these movements because no satisfactory experimental techniques are available for work in this area. Any experimentally induced lesion does an act of violence to the organism and seriously affects, if it does not vitiate, the results of such experimentation when applied to the intact organism. Movements, on the other hand, can be recorded and controlled, thus controlling the kinesthetic stimuli which are always with us and which can never be eliminated." (Quoted from a statement prepared by Love and Back at the time of Stetson's retirement in 1939.)

This basic concept has been elaborated by Roger W. Sperry, one of Stetson's students, in a paper from which the following excerpts, based on lecture notes and conversations, are quoted: "The interrelation of motor and mental activity is one of cyclic and reciprocal interdependence.... Temporally as well as spatially the mental and the motor patterns must interact, mesh, and interlock.... Perception is basically an implicit preparation for response.... Essentially, thinking is implicit symbolic preparatory adjustment. Significance and meaning in overt adjustment. Significance and meaning in brain function do not derive from the intrinsic protoplasmic or other analytic aspects of neural excitation, but rather from their higher-order functional and operational effects as these work upon successive brain states, upon the motor system, and thereby into the environment, and back into the brain" (Sperry, 1952). Hence, the importance of language as furnishing the symbols for mental operations.

For the purpose of obtaining an integrated picture of the motor processes involved in human skills, and particularly of speech, Stetson, aided by the inventive genius of James H. Snodgrass, H. D. Bouman, and Paul F. Brown, developed the electromyograph, which applies action-current recording to direct measurement of muscle contractions (Stetson & Bouman, 1935). With the assistance of C. V. Hudgins, he perfected pneumographic and electrographic techniques, combined with the sound spectrograph, for recording simultaneous contractions of as many as nine groups of muscle systems (Stetson, 1951, 1954; Stetson & Hudgins, 1930). K. U. Smith, in a personal communication, stated: "This work stands as a model of research on movement-produced feedback in hearing and speech production. No modern cybernetic concept of speech would be possible without the type of neuromotor and sensory analysis which was carried out by Stetson and his students. His work was the first to show that language behavior is necessarily productive and generative and not passive. These dynamic, productive features of movement generation are not accounted for by standard research on verbal learning or by informational psycholinguistics. In this area, as in the recording domain, Stetson anticipated critical problems by several decades." Smith added: "Stetson's demonstration of the difference between ballistic movements and the continuously controlled movement, supported by a flexible posture, led to a concept of multi-dimensionality of response, and constituted the first realistic appreciation of what psychologists refer to as 'behavior in process.'"

It is Smith's judgment that "Stetson is one of the giants of modern science, whose technical excellence so far outdistanced the efforts of his contemporaries in psychology, physiology, and psycholinguistics that his work never was recognized by more than a limited few. Stetson worked two generations ahead of his time. His scientific image suffered from the fact that he dealt with real times and real aspects of behavior and physiology in a day when most psychologists were juggling hidden mediating drive states, gestalts and the abstract factors of learning theory. Stetson's memorial should read that he was one of the first control theorists of modern science who rose above the theoretical fads of his contemporaries.... Stetson studied and defined some of the diversified mechanisms of response control decades before the concepts of cybernetics and feedback were spelled out.... He was psychology's first systematic psychologist in the area of behavior and language control."

Referring to the mind as substantive, Stetson said: "I believe in total abstinence. I wouldn't be caught dead with a mind." His was a molar behaviorism which considered the postural set not only as basic to skilled movements but as an integral part of the mechanism of the intellectual processes. He maintained that the residual traces of symbolic processes also involve "fields" so extensive that they cannot be confined to any definite set of sense organs, or nerve cells, or muscle fibers, nor definite combination of them. "Pangram," he said, would be a better term than "engram" to represent the memory trace.

A distinguishing characteristic of Stetson's research was that so much of it was done in collaboration with his students, a practice rather unique in undergraduate colleges. One of his older colleagues used to say to him: "There you go, always towing a lot of old derelicts and shooting at every legitimate craft in sight." A rather large percentage of these "derelicts" must have been carrying valuable cargo, for, during the period from 1910 to 1939, while the number of major students in psychology averaged but 3.4, more than 30 of those who worked with him later earned the Ph.D. To quote Karl F. Heiser: "Acceptance by Stetson as a major was something like joining the priesthood or an elite order. One sort of took a vow of poverty and chastity, in that he started with a poverty of knowledge and had to work damned hard for what he got, and he was certainly protected against seduction by popular, comfortable ideas and theories. But the rewards were great, and the greatest was to hear: 'Very fair, Herr _____'. One knew that he belonged to the inner circle if he was called 'Herr.'"

"Stetson turned me loose in the shop and lab with no doubts in my mind that I would become *the authority* on cutaneous temperature sensation. I had at least an hour a week with Stetson in which he patiently probed my reading and thinking and revealed to me my shallowness and ignorance. I've never known another teacher so able to stimulate and lead a student's intellectual development. But no matter what gem of obscure knowledge I might dig up in the library with which to impress Stetson, I would find that he already knew it and could treat it as a scholar. Our reading might take us far beyond the accepted bounds of psychology."

In 1931, Albert E. Lumley, at that time an instructor in physical education at Oberlin, recorded the muscular contractions of breathing during running on a treadmill. His findings indicated that an essential difference between successful runners and poor runners is that the former coordinate their breathing with the contractions of the limbs. Lumley continued his contacts with Stetson after moving to Amherst, and when, as Major Lumley during World War II, he became Chief of Rehabilitation, in the Third Service Command, U.S. Army, he called upon Stetson for advice. He now writes that it was Stetson who set up the program of rehabilitation for this command, and that it was widely copied in the other commands. In his letters to Lumley, Stetson said that the first problem is that of dealing "with the Army MD for whom 'psychology' means the handling of men recovering from what they will call 'psychic shock', and waiting for them to get out of it. For this 'psychic shock' the first thing to do is to drive hard the idea that THESE MEN ARE NORMAL. Their discouragement, or sporting nerve to meet the thing, dislike of meeting friends, hatred of drool and pity, their daze because they don't know what they'll do, or how to act, and even the business of lying down, throw up sponge, complete dejection, is exactly what normal men do *in these circumstances*."

He then continued: "But when it comes to re-education after operation because of numbness, scar tissue, et al., et al., that is all physiological, and not 'Psychology', as the MDs and psychiatrists see it. As for re-education there is too much reliance on the men finding their own ways-to-do-it." After citing experience with paretics, cleft-palate, and laryngectomy, Stetson made the following suggestions: "(1) Be alert to the chance success with the movement; nail it for the patient right then and there. (2) Movements ought to be got into light, ballistic form, with a flexible posture. I don't think your psychiatrists or your psychologists will see anything in this prescription but a kind of high-grade folderol."

Stetson treated all forms of "abnormal" behavior as an exacerbation of the normal. As summarized by Lloyd H. Beck: "A person will be judged abnormal either if his behavior has changed from his own norms as judged by his associates or if it is socially or culturally deviant. Neuroses are learned forms of behavior and can be unlearned. For example, he treated stammering by speech re-education, after first diagnosing the 'specific stumbling block', paying little attention to its emotional background." Arthur L. Benton said: "Stetson was scornful of psychoanalytic theory and critical of the then prevailing psychoanalytic practice of getting the patient to focus on past events." He often referred to writer's cramp as the prototype of neurasthenia, which he thought of as a prolongation of tension movements. He grouped the psychoses into (1) the toxic, of which the archtype is alcoholism, with its manic-depressive inclinations, and (2) the organic, typified by dementia praecox involving postulated microscopic cellular cortical lesions.

H. D. Bouman, who had come from Amsterdam during 1931 to 1932 to work with him, wrote, at the time of his death, of his appreciation of "the privilege it had been to have been one of Stetson's students," declaring, "Much of the work I have done in later years, and am continuing to do (as Professor of Physical Medicine at the University of Wisconsin Medical School) on muscular coordination in clinical medicine, particularly in relation to poliomyelitis, got its start during the year that I spent in the Oberlin Psychology Department." Lumley said: "I found that Stetson knew more about anatomy, physiology and bone structure than anyone I have ever known. When he put this together with his psychological knowledge the results were fantastic. When I am asked, 'Who is the greatest physical education man?' I always put R. H. Stetson at the top. He had no peer in the realm of skilled movements or in his insight into an individual problem with skilled movements."

Stetson's gift of time, and frequently, of money, was not limited to students in pursuit of a degree. He never accepted a fee. After diagnosing a subject's disability ("piano arm," congenital spasticity, cleft palate, constant twitching of the gastronemius muscle, stammering, etc.), he asked that the fee be paid to the student who would conduct the therapeutic exercises. J. M. Pickett wrote: "Stetson's interest in clinical problems, such as stammering or laryngectomy, was that they were important to him because of their potentiality for theoretical purposes. His approach to the treatment was strictly physiological and depended on his theory, or 'model' as we say now, of speech production. Thus in my therapeutic sessions with one stutterer, one nasality case, and one laryngectomy, he would encourage me to train the patient in the correct movements and not worry about the 'functional' etiology. At that time it was common practice for laryngologists to give a little bedside instruction in oesophageal speech, but to leave the rest to the patient. Stetson was interested in oesophageal speech because he felt that the best speakers demonstrated the necessity of syllabic air-pulse productions for normal-sounding speech. In contrast to a large reservoir of air under a steady general pressure, as in the belch from the stomach, the best speakers manipulated a small amount of air in and out of the tip of the oesophagus. Ten years later there began to be professional oesophageal teachers, who apparently now have a good press."

One recalls an amusing incident. A woman from Dayton, whose larynx had been removed, came for assistance in the use of an artificial larynx. After responding successfully to instruction, being habitually very loquacious, she fairly exploded in her enthusiasm at being once more able to talk. She insisted on phoning home immediately. However, her new larynx had a baritone pitch, and when she identified herself, the response that came from the incredulous housekeeper was a loud "Oh yeah!"

One may ask why Stetson's work was not more widely recognized during his lifetime; why, in fact, he obtained wider recognition abroad than in America. One reason is that most of his basic research work was published in Amsterdam. This was due, in the first place, to the fact that he felt a closer kinship with the Europeans than with his fellow workers in this country. Responding to a request for reprints from Karl Buhler, which the writer transmitted from Vienna in 1933, Stetson wrote: "It is pleasant to know that one's work has been heard of abroad—It's usually Madrid or Amsterdam, Hamburg or Paris, etc., rather than near at home." And as late as 1950, at the time he was about to publish his last book, he wrote: "The majority of the people interested are still Europeans." He was more attracted to international congresses in Copenhagen, Paris, London, or Amsterdam than to one in New Haven. The choice of an Amsterdam publisher may have been influenced, in part, by his association with I. Vorkink, a Dutch publisher who had taken up residence in Oberlin.

Evidence that his students and departmental colleagues appreciated the distinctive nature of Stetson's work is attested by the "Festschrift" of papers written on the occasion of his retirement, which constitutes a full number of *The Journal of General Psychology* (1939). His work had become to such an extent the center of his life that it was natural, after his formal retirement, for him to be deeply disappointed when it seemed impossible for an expanding department to continue making his project the core of its experimental activities.

As a personality, to quote from The Minute adopted by the Oberlin Faculty at the time of Stetson's death: "Although shy and diffident, he was a warm-hearted, friendly man.... He was generous to a fault in his dealings with those who were unfortunate. He was as patient and understanding with a child who stammered as he was exacting and particular with a colleague in a matter of educational policy. He was as zealous in securing fair consideration of a fellow teacher as he was in solving a scientific problem." That his colleagues trusted his evaluation of candidates for appointment or promotion is evidenced by his frequent re-election to the Committee on Appointments. Former students express appreciation of his insightful counsel. One who had become certain that he was destined to remain a slow reader was taught, as Stetson phrased it, "Rapid reading is not fast reading but selective reading." He persuaded another student, who was about to discontinue his program of preparation for the practice of medicine because he bled easily, that this should not prevent his becoming a surgeon. He subsequently became a successful physician. Students of piano who developed a "piano arm" were advised to divide their practice time into shorter periods to avoid fatigue, and were taught a flexible posture. He had become familiar years earlier with the technique employed in Leschetizky (1830–1915) in instructing such artists as Paderewski, Gabrilowitsch, and Leginska. Karl W. Gehrkens, who, as a member of the faculty of the Oberlin Conservatory of Music and founder of the first Department of School Music, took several advanced courses with Dr. Stetson, wrote that he "spent many hours in the laboratory in the investigation of musical rhythm, and learned many things which the majority of musicians have never even dreamed of. It was he who advised me to submit my first large manuscript to the Graduate Committee as a thesis (for the M.A.), and to have it published as a book." And after 40 years Professor Gehrkens is still receiving some royalties for his "Music Notation and Terminology," which started with this thesis.

His judgment as to the potentialities of students may be illustrated by the contrast between the two following cases. One student was recommended by Stetson, at the time he left Oberlin, "as a man of very unusual ability and possibilities, the sort whom you expect to go far in a scientific career. He has unusual insight and reaches out for new things, the spirit who makes the good research man, and the integrity, independence and resourcefulness which makes a scholar." When, years later, this student was appointed to a professorship in the Graduate School of Yale University, the Dean described him as "a distinguished scientist." Of the other youth, Stetson said in a personal letter: "He would wheedle his father in setting him up in a filling station, which is his *Fach, metier, niveau: Damme Junge, Taugennichts, Schemil ist er!*"

J. F. Dashiell, who was a member of the Oberlin staff from 1919 to 1921, wrote: "Stetson seemed at times to be a man of pure intellect. Certainly any demonstration of emotion was restricted. Once he remarked that he was so inhibited as to feelings or anything the least bit demonstrative that he experienced difficulty in completing his letters with the 'Yours truly'." (Letters to this writer began with "Herr Hartson" and usually concluded simply with a typed R. H. S.) Karl F. Heiser wrote: "Never have I known a person with such incisive, smooth and deliberate control over his emotions." Dashiell added: "One of Stetson's students had the effrontery to refer to him as 'such a clam'. That he never was. I think much conversation was of a level and kind which bored him; and yet I recall his describing with delight how conversations in French groupings and families sparkled with many a quick and clever turn of phrase." He was himself an insightful impersonator, witty and given to aphorisms. Seeing a squirrel scampering across the road before the approaching car, he might remark: "There are two kinds of squirrel, the quick and the dead."

One of Stetson's idiosyncracies was his manner of dress. During his winter in Paris he was known as "Le Monsieur sans Monteau," because he never wore an overcoat. His one concession to cold weather was a kid glove on the left hand, in which he carried its mate. He always wore the same style of black hat, gray, hard-worsted suits, black shoes, and string-tie. When charged with wearing a uniform, he retorted: "It's not a uniform: it's a habit." This was no mere pun, for he recognized that this habit saved him the effort of deciding each morning what to wear. He always carried a $20.00 bill in his wallet, which he never spent. Other money he spent with great liberality.

He was a prolific letter writer. To H. J. Haskell, an intimate friend since the middle 1890s, he wrote twice a week; to Professor Richardson, a former Beloit colleague, every other week. The letter might consist of a single paragraph, at times it was four pages long. Of one letter which he was writing to me, while I was on sabbatical leave in Vienna, his housemate inquired: "Is this letter to be bound, or is it to be sent loose-leaf?" His typewriter had elite type, he used single space, and employed his peculiar shorthand. A citation from one of the five pages written during one semester to a student preparing a thesis in kinesthesiology will illustrate this shorthand and also indicate how deeply he identified himself with a student's research. "Th questn's nev. been settld wheth. th hum. muscles *could* contract fast nuf to exert a contin. force on th movg limb; th rate wh th musc. wd hv to continue to bulge, up to point where head of golf club comes in contact w. ball wd. be *high* and also continuously increasg. Fact is tt th rapid contractns of musc.s don't show any such curves of contracts; and of course th musc. wd hv to be und. powerfl tensn durg th bal. phase of mvt—and there is simp. no evdce of tht, eith. by pneumat. bulge meth.s nor by ac. cur. meth.s." These letters cite historical background, related work done elsewhere, bibliographical references, and counsel as to tactful methods of dealing with a skeptical advisor, and contain moral support of a substantive character, completely devoid of coddling. One is not surprised when this student writes: "You ask what Stetson has contributed to me. I will say this: He has been the dominant influence in my life."

Stetson never married. Until 1922 he made his home with his aunt, and after that he provided for her separate support. Beginning in 1924, he shared living quarters with Professor Artz, another bachelor. In 1934 he became aware of the onset of intermittent claudication in one of his lower extremities. It was in that year that Artz built his own residence and provided ground floor accommodations for his housemate. Stetson had an elevator installed in Peters Hall on the campus, initially at his own expense, purchased a car, and engaged a student driver.

In 1948 one leg was amputated above the knee, but only after instruction to have the skin cut far enough below the former to make it possible to study the recovery of cutaneous sensitivity. He intended to take no time off for convalescence. Shortly after the amputation he wrote: "Have got Motor Phonetics revisn out of way—few more things to do; but it's now in shape so tt some one else cd easily put thro press and that's relief. Workg just now in Siamese phonology and couple of oth. phonetics pprs, and shall then go to work on a sort of 'Motor Psychology'." After being fitted with a prosthesis, he wrote to another friend: "Am learning to handle this artificial LEG: thts a new and unexpcted game; but on the whole I prefer it to golf—some sense to it." He did not live to write his Motor Psychology for he died on December 4, 1950. He had no fear of death, and realizing that it was imminent, the day before it came he said calmly: "Between you and me and the gate-post, Herr Love, this is serious." And thus, to the very end was manifested his dedication to high purpose and stoicism in the face of the ultimate.

REFERENCES

The Journal of General Psychology. (1939). Papers by some of his former students, presented to Raymond Herbert Stetson, on the occasion of his retirement, June, 1939. 20, 263–517. [Also published separately.]

Love, D. M. (1951, January). Scientist, scholar, friend. *The Oberlin Alumni Magazine*, p. 9.

Sperry, R. W. (1952). Neurology and the Mind-Brain Problem. *Amer. Scientist*, 40, 291–312.

Stetson, R. H. (1896). Types of imagination. *Psychol. Rev.*, 3, 398–411.

Stetson, R. H. (1897). Piano tone-color from a physical and psychological standpoint. *Music*, 11, 713–717.

Stetson, R. H. (1903). Rhythm and rhyme. *Psychol. Rev. Monogr.*, 4, 413–466.

Stetson, R. H. (1905). A motor theory of rhythm and discreet succession. *Psychol. Rev.*, 12, 250–270; 293–350.

Stetson, R. H. (1923). The hair follicle and the sense of pressure. *Psychol. Monogr.*, 32, 1–17.

Stetson, R. H. (1937). Esophageal speech for any laryngectomized patient. *Arch. Otolaryng.*, 26, 132–142.

Stetson, R. H. (1951). Motor phonetics: A study of speech movements in action. (2nd ed.) North Holland Publishing Co.

Stetson, R. H. (1954). *Bases of phonology.* Oberlin College.

Stetson, R. H. & Bouman, H. D. (1935). The coordination of simple skilled movements. *Arch. neerl. Physiol.*, 20, 179–254.

Stetson, R. H. & Hudgins, C. V. (1930). Functions of the breathing movements in the mechanism of speech. *Arch. neerl. Phon. exp.*, 5, 1–30.

R. H. Stetson

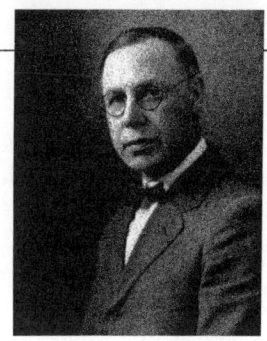

RECOLLECTIONS OF R. H. STETSON
by Robert Galambos*
March, 1987

I first came to know Mr. Stetson (which is what we always called him) during my senior year (1934–5) through the Abnormal Psychology seminar he taught. After that I spent much of my time in his laboratory between June, 1935 and August, 1937, summers included, apprenticed to such people as James M. Snodgrass, Stetson's chief technician. It was Jim, for instance, who designed and watched me build the DC-coupled physiological amplifier I then used to measure action potentials in earthworm body wall muscles (my master's thesis submitted to the biology department in 1936).

Stetson was a campus legend at that time—6 feet tall, slim, erect, rarely smiling. He invariably dressed himself in a black suit, white shirt (with detachable starched collar), black bow tie (that narrow type with limp ends that droop downwards a few inches), black socks, and black oxford shoes. Three widely circulated stories about him come to mind:

- Many years earlier he had brought back from Europe a full bolt of the cloth from which his tailor cut him a new suit every four years;
- He used his monthly salary checks as bookmarks, cashing one from time to time as needed;
- He could teach any course offered in the Oberlin College catalogue, and whenever those who did so needed help, they consulted him.

He was a dazzling figure to this undergraduate who had just been bitten by the research bug: unmarried—and hence free of all distractions—he had himself put together the most modern and best-equipped research lab on the campus; in it he conducted his own research, and to it each summer he attracted famous experimenters from throughout the world. Despite his austere and formal manner he was known to be approachable, and even a novice with few credentials beyond a burning desire could realistically aspire to enter the select group with which he surrounded himself.

In my senior year, lacking the money to go to medical school, I did approach him, with a plan to get a master's degree in the biology department, the research to be done under his guidance. He took me on, and during the next two years

---

*Former Professor of Neuroscience at University of California, San Diego. Now at Children's Hospital Research Center, San Diego, California (Eds.).

I learned all the fundamentals—how to formulate a research problem, plan the work, get it done, write it up, get it published, and finally, how to teach what you know about all this to others. During my years at both Yale and UCSD I followed his model, working throughout the summer teaching young people also just recently bitten by the research bug.

In 1934 or 1935 he found walking increasingly painful, and told us the diagnosis was intermittent claudications (Reynaud's disease, a sympathetic nervous system disorder causing abnormal constriction of the leg arteries). When it became difficult for him to walk the several blocks from his apartment to work, he first hired taxis, then bought a car and hired students (of whom Roger Sperry held the longest tenure, I think) to drive him; when it took too long to climb steps to the fourth floor of Peters Hall, where the lab (Room 48) was located, he had an elevator installed (using his own money, it was said, which must have required cashing in a fairly large number of those bookmarks); and in order to spare his legs as much unnecessary work as possible, he dieted and slimmed off another 20 pounds or so. From his example we learned the man of science handles both scientific and personal problems in the same way; you identify the problem exactly, and after analyzing it (accepting whatever of it you must) you do whatever seems reasonable and necessary to solve it.

The only research enterprise of his I became involved in is the one related to speech production by people without a larynx. He had collected for study a small stable of these laryngectomees, some of whom spoke with the help of a small box containing a reed caused to vibrate by air conducted to it through a tube connected to the hole where the larynx used to be. He was interested in both the chest muscle activity that drove the air into the box, and in the mouth and tongue movements that made speech out of the sounds conducted by a second tube from the box to the inside of the mouth. But other laryngectomees did not use this prosthesis; they had developed esophageal speech, which is the art of swallowing air and returning it in what might be called a protracted, smoothly controlled belch while one moves the mouth and tongue to make words. I have no recollection of how I acquired the skill, but once Stetson heard my esophageal speech he added me to this stable.

One day he stated his need to discover the dynamics of the storage and return of the swallowed air, and in particular, whether it actually reached the stomach. "Mister Man (he used either this term, Herr, or my last name), the way to answer these questions is to go to Cleveland (some 30 miles away) where Dr. Somebody has agreed to make the series of X-ray exposures we need for the analysis. We will take two sets of pictures, one from someone-else, who has no larynx, the other from you, who will be our control. Meet me for breakfast next Saturday at the apartment, and we will leave from there." I remember three things about that breakfast: it took place on a beautiful spring morning; the coffee was prepared by the drip method, and was very strong (a Stetson trademark); and he poured sherry over the fresh fruit.

I suppose I drove the car to Cleveland, because Stetson did not know how, and I connect neither Sperry nor Snodgrass with this expedition. I clearly remember the X-rays, however, and Stetson's satisfaction with the entire enterprise. It turns out that the swallowed air never reaches the stomach; it forms a little spindle in the esophagus that decreases in size with each utterance (if that is the correct term) and disappears when an experienced speaker (?) reaches the end of his sentence or when an *in*experienced one simply runs out of gas. The dynamics of spindle formation and decay appeared to be similar in all major respects for both Mr. Someone-Else and me, as I recall, but his word count per eructation was much higher than mine. We concluded that this was because he had had more practice.

When I left Oberlin in the fall of 1937, I saw Mr. Stetson for the last time. We exchanged a few letters, but none of them has survived. Jim Snodgrass has uncovered one, however, as always, typed, and in Stetson's unique shorthand, and from it we extract two paragraphs that perhaps will have particular interest for the readers of this volume.

"157 N. Professor st.,Oberlin,O. IX-7-'50

Herr Snodgrass:

[Two paragraphs omitted]

Hudgins was here, and we drove to mtgs,Ann Arbor;

read ppr,wh went all very well. Came back and got up ppr for final sec.of appendix of Mot.Phon revised. And sent it to Amsterdam;and hv signed contract for publicatn: 1500 cop.s, half of 'em cloth-bound, ca.$ 3000.; or I may hv it stereotyped,w.and ed.nof 1000. So tht's def.undrway. And 'twill come out: for money's on deposit in Holland, and Miss Z. and Hudgins cd read proof and look aft. distributn in U.S. Ca.500 cop.s 'll be used for subscribers of Arch.neerl.de phon.exper, and for oth.s who can hrdly afford th thng,espec. in Europe.

Now Hudgins and I will get to work on a "Motor Phonetics for th Deaf": and I shall pay good share,or all, of cost of prting,and turn it ov.to th Volta BU. to mk wht they can of th distributn: they want some bks of th sort, and did get out an Am.ed.of Haycok's bk,wh it went out of print in Eng. Tht will be good way of distributg it."

[Eight paragraphs (70 lines of news and opinion) omitted]

R.H.S."

In 1942 I sent Mr. Stetson four reprints, each originally a chapter in my Ph.D thesis, which I had had bound together in a small volume for him, and which he acknowledged; and that was my last contact with him. I could not attend his funeral because I first heard of his death many months after it happened.

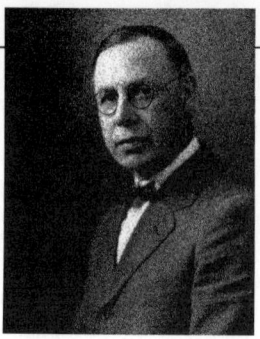

RECOLLECTIONS OF R. H. STETSON
by Roger Sperry*

Professor Raymond Stetson had a major influence in the launching of my scientific career, something for which I have always felt extremely fortunate. Given the chance, I would go the same route over again, starting in psychology under Stetson after an undergraduate major at Oberlin in English, then switching later to neuroscience and neuropsychology. I was extremely lucky as a student to have had other fine mentors, including Paul Weiss, Karl Lashley, and in class work, other scientific giants of the 1930s and 1940s, but no one else ever impressed me as quite measuring up to Raymond Stetson in sheer depth and breadth of intellect. Certainly no one else had so much impact on my professional outlook.

Stetson once volunteered, when the conversation had turned to things people live for, such as wealth, power, friends, and happiness, that he and always lived for "*ideas*, to collect ideas." Even the way he walked and moved seemed to affirm this, that everything else that was part of him was there to carry and sustain his brain.

I first met Stetson when I signed up for his course in introductory psychology because it happened to be given at an hour that fit the rest of my schedule. After little more than 10 minutes into his first lecture, it became apparent that this would not be an ordinary college course. He was already toying with original perspectives on behavior and philosophy beyond anything I'd come across thus far. We had a textbook as a formality, but the substance of the course was in Stetson's lectures. The psychology he presented was a very brain-oriented, experimental, and philosophic sort, not clinical, and much influenced by William James while Stetson was at Harvard.

One day I stopped to question him after class, thinking actually I should set him straight on something he had touched on about "follow-through," or lack of it, as in a golf swing. I don't recall specifics or who was right or wrong, but I do recall quite clearly that in a situation where many professors might well take offense, his eyes merely twinkled amusedly as he tried to explain very kindly to this misguided young muscle man that the muscular contractions in many common

---
*Professor of Neurobiology, California Institute of Technology. In 1981 Professor Sperry received the Nobel Prize in Physiology and Medicine (Eds.).

movements, as shown by physical records in the laboratory, are very different from what one would expect from one's subjective impression.

The details of muscle action during different types of movement were important in Stetson's thinking. He reasoned that essentially *all* behavior, including speech and writing, is constituted of muscle contraction patterns. Activating the musculature in correct contraction patterns is what brains are mainly designed to do and the primitive function for which they evolved originally. Later stages in brain evolution had to be developed out of and imposed upon this preceding basic design. To understand brain function, therefore, it seemed important to Stetson to have a working conception of the underlying patterns and principles of the brain's motor output.

It was in this context that I had been prompted to question his treatment of follow-through. Later I was to learn, after seeing Stetson in other debates and confrontations, that he typically handled all these in a similar manner. Instead of getting angry, heated, or raising his voice, he would kindly and patiently, with varying degrees of amusement, explain what he thought the other party needed to know.

As the lectures in his course progressed, I began to realize that this subject of brain function, and the great mind-brain riddle with its intrinsic interest and central tie-ins to age-old questions of crucial concern, was something in which I could become genuinely interested as a choice for my life's work, something I had not been able to settle on up to this point.

On mentioning this to Stetson, he encouraged me to stay at Oberlin for a master's degree in psychology. I completed this in two years, then stayed an additional year as a "student at large" to pick up biology and physics courses prerequisite for doctoral work in neurobiology at the University of Chicago. Here again, Stetson had been very helpful and the prime influence in obtaining my acceptance in Chicago.

During the years at Oberlin I took all the courses Stetson offered—psychology of aesthetics, abnormal psychology, and phonetics, along with the departmental faculty-student seminar. In all these, Stetson continued to open new vistas in personal insights and associations that went far beyond the subject matter of the textbooks into realms of his own advanced and unique (but unpublished) perspectives.

Perhaps as much or more than the benefits from this formal coursework were those I was privileged to share while working as Stetson's chauffeur when I replaced his regular driver, James Snodgrass, who went East for graduate work. Part of the advantage of this "driver" job was eating meals at the Faculty Club with Stetson and other members of the faculty. With my small town nonacademic upbringing and after having spent most of my spare time as a youth in outdoor pursuits, athletic fields, gymnasiums, etc., the conversational interchanges among and with the faculty over meals were to me an education in itself. Stetson's reputation for being able to teach any course on campus, given 10 minutes notice, became all the more believable after hearing him expound on the inner intricacies of issues in the widely diverse specialities of different faculty members—from the conservatory of music, department of art, languages, any of the sciences, history, or whatever. It would be difficult to pin Stetson down with a label. He was deeply versed in the humanities as well as being a scientist. One might say he specialized in being a generalist who qualified as a specialist in many varied disciplines.

It was Stetson's philosophy that most interested me and how he tied it in with psychology, brain function, art, and practical living. I took formal courses in the department of philosophy, but these seemed dead and out of touch compared to Stetson's treatment, which brought the issues down to everyday living and made them come alive. Stetson was able to make great intellectual figures of history seem like acquaintances of his who were striving to find answers like the rest of us. More than once he described philosophy as "the progressive history of human error." A spinoff of his down-to-earth analyses of what the great philosophies were trying to say was a lasting disenchantment on my part with any appeal to authority, any dependence on specialized jargon or on academic formalities, plus a lasting skepticism of accepted doctrine I probably never otherwise would have had.

The philosophic perspectives I gained in give-and-takes with Stetson during those years were to carry through the rest of my life. Although I was to change rather radically some of my own specific positions on certain issues, I never have had any feeling of having outgrown the general perspectives I absorbed from Stetson during those years at Oberlin. More than this, I have always since had a sense of having an advantage over my colleagues in science who had come up entirely within science. I still have the feeling of having been exposed to rare intellectual realms and insights that few others are privileged to see, and which ever since have continued to enrich my science, values, and life outlook.

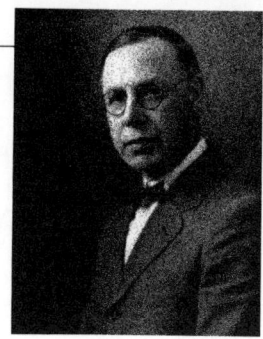

PERSONAL IMPRESSIONS OF R. H. STETSON
by J. M. Pickett*

In 1941, I was an Oberlin sophomore who wanted to be a scientist but had only a D in chemistry, then a C in economics, a serious illness, and some highly interesting catch-up courses in phonetics during the summer at Kent State. My high school debating coach had emphasized physiology in his speech course, so I decided I wanted to be a sort of physiological phonetician. Oberlin was too good a school to leave, but Vivian Turner, the Kent State professor, said psychology would be a good background major for graduate study in phonetics. That fall, when I registered as a junior and was counseled about the major by Professor Louis Hartson, he asked me why I wanted to be a psychology major. When I told him I really wanted to be a phonetician he said the department did have a well-known emeritus but active phonetician, and so I might be able to take some special courses. He took me back to an old laboratory area, knocked on a door in a wall of glassed-in temporary offices, and introduced me to an elderly professor seated at his portable on a small wood typing table surrounded by papers and books on lab benches. R. H. Stetson wore a black bow tie and a dark gray hard-worsted suit. He looked at me with kindly, probing brown eyes and that was the start of the most important association of my academic life.

It turned out that I became an especially close student/house/car companion of Stetson because his regular "driver," an older graduate psychology student, was soon called into the war and I was the only male student remaining around the department. Stetson could not walk more than a few hundred yards, so the driver's job was to come to the house for breakfast, drive Stetson to his lab, take him to lunch and dinner, and in the summers, when his housemate F. B. Artz, a history professor, was often traveling, to stay in the house "just in case." I was the driver from 1942 to 1944 and 1946 to 1947; there were quite a number of drivers, but I was the only one in phonetics. The ostensible pay of the driver was meals and summer lodging. The driver was invited to all dining and social functions of the household and to any others that Stetson attended. So the true rewards were the companionship of Stetson and participation in the scintillating, intellectual life of his colleagues.

Stetson was an intensely student-oriented scientist and, through his interest in me, I eventually

---

*Center for Auditory and Speech Science, Gallaudet Research Institute, Gallaudet University.

made some contributions to speech science that reflect some of his ideas. I was his last student to into speech; there were two others: Louis DiCarlo and Clarence V. Hudgins; all three of us concerned ourselves to some degree with clinical speech problems.

CHARACTERISTIC ATTITUDES

Although Stetson was a thoroughly hard-minded basic scientist, he believed that applied problems and their solutions could serve as critical tests of fundamental theoretical models. As an experimental phonetician, he considered speech disorders as experiments. To take three examples: Stuttering was a test bed for exploring speech gestural coordination. Teaching the deaf-mute to speak fluently demonstrated the necessity of correct syllable timing before consonant articulations could be correct, thus putting the theoretical emphasis on the syllable rather than the phoneme. For the laryngectomee, the routine, rapid attainment of good speech intelligibility with a passive artificial larynx showed that the glottal control for the voiced/unvoiced distinction was not as important as the coordination between supraglottal and subglottal factors.

As a motor behaviorist, Stetson also promoted students' research interest in sports; for example, in studies of running where the coordination of breathing movements with arm and leg movements was important, or of baseball batting where rapid perception of the pitched ball had to guide a complex adjustable, but powerful, ballistic swinging of the bat. He seemed to have no interest in the competitive or recreational aspects of sports, and felt that their promoters were not to be taken very seriously. One of his sports research students heard that Stetson owned some shares in the modest little Oberlin Golf Club and asked him why; he said, "I hoped it would be a good place to keep those people." However, Stetson was not a nasty or noisy critic and this story is the most harsh I ever heard attributed.

Stetson's knowledge was broad and deep, covering sciences, arts, and humanities. Legend had it that he could teach any course in the college upon 10 minutes' notice, and he had. Another story is told that two of his faculty colleagues read up in the encyclopedia on certain oriental rugs, and then proceeded at lunch to discuss a subject about which Stetson would know little. After enthralling the group for several minutes, they finally stopped, but Stetson carried on the discussion, adding some important points and developing some new ones, ending with: "You see, I wrote the encyclopedia article." However, Stetson told me this story really refers to a Professor William Martin, a renowned previous teacher at Oberlin in art history, who started the art department. Stetson was always extremely modest and gentle, so I doubt whether anyone would want to try such a trick on him. The story, though, proves the importance of both these intense men to their fields of study and education.

STETSON'S PHONETIC THEORIES

In psychology, Stetson espoused a motor theory of perception that I trace back to the Chicago "Functionalist" school of psychology and philosophy (James R. Angell, Harvey Carr, and John Dewey). In *Motor Phonetics* (1951, pp. 137–149), Stetson sketched his motor-behavioral theory of speech communication. A current motor theory of speech perception (Liberman & Mattingly, 1985) is tangentially related to Stetson's thinking. Alvin Liberman had many discussions on motor theory with Stetson when he spent a summer teaching psychology at Oberlin, and often took dinner with Stetson and me at a restaurant. However, Liberman's theory did not evolve directly from Stetson and rests on auditory phoneme perception evidence rather than motor studies. Soviet workers, L. Chistovich and V. Kozhevnikov, a wife-husband team at the Pavlov Institute of Physiology, Leningrad, independently proposed a syllabic-oriented motor theory of speech perception that was more similar to Stetson's (Kozhevnikov & Chistovich, 1965).

Stetson felt that the stampede of phoneticians from 1935 to 1945 to embrace the phonemic theory of speech as a sequence of phoneme units would be devastating to progress toward a deep understanding of the speech code via the powerful new electronic methods which became available after World War II for the combined study of the acoustic and motor patterns. He saw phonemic studies proceeding to elaborate logistic criteria for defining and classifying phonemes with little regard for their physiological embodiment in rhythmic patterns of syllables, or in naturally paced (as opposed to citation-style) speech. He formulated these criticisms in his *Bases of Phonology*, which he published himself in 1945.

As examples of his later thoughts, I quote from two letters he wrote in 1947 and 1948, commenting to Hudgins on Potter, Kopp, and Green's *Visible Speech* (1947) and Joos's monograph *Acoustic Phonetics* (1947). He expected the invention of the sound spectrograph to be a great boon to achieving a more phonetics-oriented phonology. First, he comments on *Visible Speech* and a letter from Joos:

> I sent a copy of my review of *Visible Speech* to Joos, who worked on speech analysis during the war with the Bell spectrograph, and has his own ideas, and built one model. He recognizes the need of a loudness indication, and says that his spectrograph, which belongs to the Army, did read in decibels—and if the response is fast enough it should help. But I should prefer the envelope of the syllables to numerical readings because you need to have the thing before you as a pattern.
>
> Joos says "...when I get a new spectrograph next year I hope to make records from which I can learn the acoustic results of chest-pulses among other things. For the present we must content ourselves with records that tell far more about glottal and supraglottal phenomena than they do about the infraglottal field. As you may have heard, I am writing a book under the title *Acoustic Phonetics*, to be published in 1948. The viewpoint will be entirely different from that of *Visible Speech*. Those people are interested most of all in the problem of reading the records—finding out what the speaker said. Now a linguist arrives ultimately at his own sort of statement of what was said, but he arrives there as late as possible; he examines the minutest details, establishes the patterns among them, and then states in terms of those patterns what was said. Kopp wants to get at the text-identification as swiftly as possible. As he ought to. But it keeps him from doing anything that will contribute toward linguistic analysis. There will be very little overlap between my book and that one.... Anybody who has never worked a spectrograph will, I fear, be badly misled by some of the spectrogram patterns in *Visible Speech*. There are few of them that represent natural speech throughout. The definite article is often spoken *thee*, and the indefinite is usually /e/ or /aen/ etc."

> There is no question that the speaking style used in *Visible Speech* is slow, citation style, as can be seen in the pauses, the separation of abutting consonants, and in the actual rate where the rate is shown. It's obvious that Joos is impatient with Kopp and Green. He might have added that one reason why Kopp won't find anything new is because he's a commonplace man loaded to start with, with this phonemics stuff. You note that Joos speaks of 'the acoustic results of chest-pulses...' and that he notes the 'infraglottal field'; those are hopeful signs. I think Joos is several laps ahead of Kopp-Green. R. H. S. xi–21–'47.

In a later letter to Hudgins:

> Another version of the *Visible Speech* stuff comes out in Joos' *Acoustic Phonetics*, as a Language Monograph; Joos got some limited data while working during the war: and he has some notions on the engineering side—though it's often a mixture of old-fashioned notions and modern engineering of sound. He tries to get back to the Fourier analysis, although in many cases—all, in fact—the white noise notion would fit better. And he works in the vowel rectangle with tongue positions: "high-mid-low; front-central-back" is his system of vowel articulation.
>
> Joos finds himself forced into the articulatory field, though he works acoustic data. And his handling of movements is as wild as they make them. He can't consent to a mere mechanical handling of speech organs; he's sure that inertia would make overshoot, &c., and recordings show that their movements are smooth. Therefore the movement patterns must be handled in the 'speech center' of the brain (i.e., cerebral cortex) and possibly it's timed in the cerebellum; and he has 'static patterns' of phonemes which are stored in the brain; it's curious brain-control, and engram psychology.
>
> Joos is very learned as to 'the indeterminacy' of perception; he finds 'smear' of 50 to 60 ms. Of course, that's also the limit for one-half cycle of the maximum rate of simple ballistic movement at ca. 10 to 12 cycles per second. Kinesthetic perception has the same maximum rate, of course; visual perception is even slower, and so on. Joos hangs it on the general conditions of auditory perception, instead of generalizing. He doesn't note the fact that there's another type of movement, and perception, the multiple ballistic coordination with two or more members active, in piano, violin, and wood-wind playing in which the maximum is up to 16–18 cycles per second with "smear", then, of about 25+ ms. He doesn't recognize the syllable—as the Bell engineers do—and doesn't have any way of distinguishing a basic movement unit.

The equivalent of 'syllable' in Joos' articulatory scheme is a 'slur', using the term borrowed from music; it's the build-up and decay of a vowel-centered event, which is smooth, and the consonant and vowel phases overlap and interpenetrate. It's the one place where Joos feels forced to handle a unit composed of other units. Put in plain terms, consonants and the vowel so overlap and interpenetrate in the syllable that you'll have to count that the unit.

The whole thing's a hopeless mess. Potter, Steinberg, et al. have made their way further into the problem of speech; and they write indefinitely more clearly. Joos tries to simplify the acoustic material, and I can't tell how clearly he grasps just what the spectrograph does to the acoustic output. Probably he does better than Kopp in that regard—but I don't know how much. He manages to keep orthodox, considers Pike's 'physiological' phonetics the best yet; he pays respects to Bloch's 'postulates for phoneme analysis', though he 'disagrees in some ways', and he has no grasp of the work of Marichelle, Rousselot, nor of course Stetson. He's forced into the field of speech movements, but he won't take the trouble to get up the literature. Can't remember if he is Iowa trained, but he has the earmarks of ignoring all previous work; however, Cowan's the only Iowa man he quotes.

The one point for me is his SLUR = syllable; he recognizes that you can't possibly take the consonants and the vowel apart. This shows that *that* result of *Visible Speech* has soaked in. This provides one unit which includes others, i.e., aspects of the syllable factors (phonemes), and that syllable factors are incorporated in the unit of the syllable ('slur'). You can point out that traits of the syllable and thus of the phoneme, will be modified in turn by their incorporation in the foot and breath group, and that the breath group is a unit because phonemes, and syllables, may drop out and be restored within that unit, at varying rates and depending on the stress pattern of the breath group unit.

It looks to me as if the main things I must try to get home, in this article I'm working on, and in the *Motor Phonetics* revision, are the facts that:
THE PHONEME SYSTEM MUST INVOLVE A HIERARCHY OF UNITS, citing the *Visible Speech* evidence on the syllable, and THE PHYSIOLOGY SYSTEM OF MOVEMENTS MUST BE A HIERARCHY OF MOVEMENTS, as shown by the motor phonetic data already observed. And finally the job of the article is to base the phoneme system on the system of speech movements.

Joos is no exception to the trend of the phonemicists to unchecked speculation; he has some acoustic facts, but he runs wild in the field of movements, and in brain psychology. They've always got to speculate, somewhere, somehow. They make such an utter mess of facts, and fancy, that I don't see much chance. They have their dogmatic schemes, and they twist a few 'facts', especially popular new facts, and they mean to support the old dogma with the new 'facts'; and they set up such an ink-screen that they get away with it, at least among their own general bunch; they all feel vindicated. And they go on with their fuzzy, incoherent stuff. R. H. S. vii–2–48.

Another part of the 1947 letter to Hudgins illustrates Stetson's impatience with loose psychology and his pride in Sperry's fundamental approach to brain function:

From your drafts I see that you're really working up the Oberlin analysis of movements and the literature. But it's about all that's really available in English. I hope that "Fritz" Hubbard and Slater-Hammel add to it; and think they will. And I'm glad to know that we're an exceptional group in psychology. They're always touting some special brand of psychology—ink blot, or topology, for example—in which there can be no well-defined experimenting. They count it an experimental confirmation if a formulation according to their scheme seems all-told an adequate description. My student-driver comes near pulling that sort of thing, talking about "reasoning" in animals; says that their behavior follows the type of problem solving which is defined generally as reasoning. When I ask why the dog doesn't do simple reasoning, if he "has everything needed"—generalization, delayed response and so on—he finally says that well, if you took time enough with dogs you could probably teach them to reason. The parrot and the talking dog are stumbling blocks, for they seem to have all that these animal people demand for reasoning. And of course many of the texts blur the difference between human reasoning and animal problem solving, and imply that there is no real gap.

Have I written you that Roger Sperry's been doing a critical bit of work on this business of cortical centers? In monkeys he's made lateral slices in the arm-hand Rolandic area, first through grey matter, and then through white matter also; checking the behavior and capacity for learning before and after. There goes Pavlov's brain physiology—which depended on lateral diffusion; and there goes Kohler's isomorphism, which also assumes a lateral organization of the cortex. Meantime, K. U. Smith reports on cases of severance of the hemispheres (corpus callosum) and finds that it has little effect on movement coordination. Putting the two together, negligible results of both slicing in Rolandic area and severing the hemispheres, a plentiful amount of localization and brain-center stuff goes by the board. The severing of the hemispheres puts an end to the cerebral dominance theory of stuttering of S. T. Orton Travis, et al.; the hemispheres don't seem to act as unified centers of control. But of course the brain control people can go another step down; I don't suppose real counter evidence will interfere much with doctrinaire assumptions as to the brain.

In the field of phonetics, Stetson's ideas and previous work on the study of speech movements were not extensively followed up until about 1960, when a strong resurgence of interest in experimental phonetics occurred. This revival was due I think mainly to the availability of new transducing, amplifying, and recording equipment which was far superior in performance and much easier to keep running than anything Stetson might have dreamed of. Another factor was availability of government support both for basic research on speech production and applied research toward recognition of speech by computers.

One of Stetson's major tenets, the physiological, production existence of the syllable as a basic, delimitable chest-movement, has been clearly demonstrated only for utterance rates up to about four syllables per second (see Figure 57, p. 96). The grouping of syllables into rhythmic stress patterns is now recognized as having extremely important effects on the smaller articulatory "gestures," as they are now called, for the consonants and vowels.

Stetson's work has been well noted and he is often mentioned as a pioneer. Somehow, though, his influence in his time was not equal to his quality. In my opinion there are four reasons: (1) he refused to politic in speech-phonetic circles; (2) his writing was too condensed and somewhat cryptic (in contrast to his infinite patience with students); (3) he tended to overgeneralize from his data; (4) his housemate, Artz, claimed that Stetson spent too much time on "problem"students, not picking and carefully grooming only the best to carry on his work.

STETSON'S STUDENTS

Two of the physiological students became very prominent; Robert Galambos, in auditory physiology, did a master's thesis under Stetson on the mode of muscle action for the crawling movements of earthworms. Hallowel Davis, at Harvard, also had a great effect on Galambos's career.

Roger Sperry, in neurology of behavior, did his master's thesis under Stetson on the phases of action of the arm muscles in performing circular movements of different types. Paul Weiss at the University of Chicago mainly formed his career and Sperry recently received a Nobel Prize in Physiology and Medicine.

Clarence V. Hudgins, Louis DiCarlo, and myself are the only students who made careers in the field of speech communication. DiCarlo's work was not as prominent as Hudgins's; they were both older than Sperry and Galambos, who were older than me. The work of the latter three of us has been very heavily supported by U.S. government programs.

I have contributed to knowledge about speech communication in noise and new speech aids for the deaf, and I published a textbook, *The Sounds of Speech Communication*, which is a basic book on the subject for students in speech and hearing, for audiologists, therapists, and some educators of the deaf; also the book is an introduction for linguists, psychologists, and engineers. The book is a direct outgrowth of Stetson's insistence on a thorough scientific grounding for education of the deaf and for speech therapy of all kinds.

STUDIES IN THE LATE YEARS OF THE LABORATORY

Stetson's only research associate when I arrived in 1941 was James N. Snodgrass, an early expert in biopotential recording and analysis. He and Stetson, usually with Stetson's own funds, had built a research facility called the Oscillograph Laboratory. It was not long before Snodgrass had to leave for military research for the Navy in the field of underwater sound. The Oscillograph Laboratory was on hold throughout the remainder of Stetson's career, but there was still much to be learned about speech movements using the well-established, classic kymographic recording technique for speech events, here carried to its peak of accuracy and flexibility over the 20-year period after Stetson worked with it in Rousselot's laboratory in Paris. Looking back over speech instrumentation since then, wave-event recording did not greatly improve in convenience over the kymograph until the advent of the easy-to-use, relatively inexpensive ink-recorder, the Mingograph, which I first encountered in G. Fant's laboratory in 1960.

A modicum of manual skill was necessary for using kymographic methods but, once these were in hand, an experiment was often very rapid and easy to monitor, change, adjust, or abandon, because each record, even though relatively lengthy, could be available to measure within the few minutes needed to take the record from the drum, pass it through a fixing bath, and dry it. Only recently, with the advent of digital methods, such as ILS (Interactive Laboratory System), has it become easier than with the kymograph or the later ink-writer to record and examine speech movement data. The kymograph's accuracy of representation was dependent on mechanical and pneumatic conditions, but with due care for physical analyses and adjustment of these transducers, high performance was obtained. Stetson and Hudgins estimated that the accuracy of measuring event times was to be about 10 ms. Lags in the course of pressure falls could be compensated in the measurements but this was much more problematic and it will be noted that *Motor Phonetics* is largely an analysis of consonant articulatory on-off events rather than of pressure values. The incorporation of extensive, accurate pressure recordings was planned via the Oscillograph Laboratory facility, but in *Motor Phonetics* only Figures 15 and 18–21 include such data.

The pressure contours labeled A (intraoral pressure) and CT (tracheal pressure) in these figures were recorded with a small phosphor-bronze, 2-element bellows (pneumodeik) as the transducer. The onset of a pressure-rise was recorded with negligible delay (see p. 48); however, there was probably a total of about 10 ms lag over the course of the rise and fall portions of these curves because the bellows is a volume-to-length transducer (Hudgins & Stetson, 1932).

The most important of the recording conditions for the reader of these contours are the circular recording arcs due to the fixed-length recording lever movement about a fixed axis. These are shown as dashed segments of circles for the pressure tracings of Figures 18 and 20. When these curves are used to correct the pressure changes, the rises and falls are considerably steepened and rectified. For example, in Figure 20, the rises in the [p] consonants to maximum occurs in less than 40 ms instead of what appears to be about 200 ms in Figure 20.

The two studies that I carried out (using the kymographic techniques) may be cited as examples of Stetson's research approaches. They were the last phonetic studies conducted in the laboratory. The first study developed from a question posed by Mary Haas, a California linguist specializing in Thai in the mid-1940s. She wrote Stetson about the voicing of obstruents in Thai: they sounded both voiced and unvoiced; can you make some recordings to tell us? Stetson was immediately interested because, in his theory of consonant voicing, the vocal folds played only a passive role, their vibration being controlled by nonglottal, movement factors which affected the relation between the supra- and subglottal air pressure (*Motor Phonetics*, p. 74 and reference 56). Thai consonant voicing looked like a very interesting test. He found there was a Thai consulate nearby in Cleveland; I soon had some Thai people to record (lip and tongue contact events together with intraoral air pressure) while they were saying their wonderful "polite word" *krab(p)* and some others in suitable phrases. Within half a day we could see that there was no true voicing during the occlusions, but there was a low intraoral pressure, short preceding vowel, and no release. And a letter was on the way back to Professor Haas.

The second of my studies was designed around Stetson's concept of the syllable. The goal was to develop data on the question of how single-syllable words were organized as sequences of movements functioning to release, carry, and arrest the syllable unit. The critical question was how would syllable duration increase as a function of the number of phonemes. If the syllable is a powerful organizing unit, then its duration should be a shallow negatively accelerated function of the number of phonemes. Phrases were prepared with a reference test syllable that could be expanded by adding more sounds; for example, one series of syllables was "pin, print, spin, sprint, sprints." The syllable duration functions versus number of phonemes were indeed shallow and negatively accelerated. Thus, it was concluded that the articulation of these compound consonants was organized around one primary syllable-releasing consonant and one primary arresting consonant with the "auxiliary" consonants compressed closely in time because they were riding on the two main consonant gestures of the syllable. The only exceptions seemed to be the unvoiced fricatives as "auxiliaries" to stops.

LEGACY IN PHONETICS

Clarence V. Hudgins, Stetson's student and collaborator in the 1930s, carried out some important experiments on laryngeal movements for voicing and some early recordings of muscle action potentials coordinated with curves of the resulting movements of body members (Stetson & Bouman, 1935; Stetson & Hudgins, 1930); this technique was intensively applied to the study of speech movements, rhythmic movements, and sports coordinations in Stetson's lab. Hudgins was a stammerer, but had learned to control it, partly with Stetson's help. He took his psychology doctorate at Clark University under W. S. Hunter, the early arch-behaviorist student of learning processes. In 1936 he was appointed Director of the Barron Research Department at Clarke School for the Deaf, the first such position and department in an institution for the deaf. Together with one of the Clarke teachers, F. C. Numbers, Hudgins carried out the first modern, intensive studies of the nature of speech produced by deaf children (Hudgins, 1934; Hudgins & Numbers, 1942). Hudgins worked at the Harvard Psychoacoustics Laboratory during World War II, developing basic speech tests for assessing military voice circuits, and then applied some of these methods to communication training of deaf children (Hudgins, 1953).

Hudgins and Stetson were intensively interested in fostering applications of speech science for the deaf; they drafted a long outline of a book entitled "Motor Phonetics for the Deaf," intended for speech therapists and teachers. This project never came to fruition as Stetson died and Hudgins developed a heart condition that cut down his activities. I kept these ideas in mind and soon came into this field myself.

At first I worked on the neurology of learning (under Hunter's influence from Brown) at the University of Connecticut from 1950 to 1952. Then, I married another Brown psychologist and it was against Connecticut rules for us both to teach there. I started in speech communication research in 1952, working on speech-in-noise problems for the Air Force in a Washington laboratory, where I learned the careful Harvard psychoacoustics methods under Karl D. Kryter and Irvin Pollack. But I wanted to learn more about speech production and managed to get an NIH Fellowship in 1961 to Gunnar Fant's laboratory in Stockholm, under the guise that I would study the use of their tactile vocoder for the deaf. This I did and also fulfilled the real reason I went there. I applied to Gallaudet University, but there was no opening until 1964. Then Gallaudet and NIH launched me in my second career, on speech science for the deaf. I taught acoustic phonetics to student teachers and audiologists, saved my notes, wrote them up in trial chapters, for readings, and finally published my text, aimed at students who would be working with the deaf and hearing impaired (Pickett, 1980). Thus, Stetson and Hudgins's book came out, informed by the 30 years of great advances in speech sciences that we have seen since Stetson's death.

REFERENCES

Hudgins, C. V. (1934). A comparative study of the speech coordinations of deaf and normal subjects. *J. Genetic Psychology, 44,* 3–48.

Hudgins, C. V. (1953). The response of profoundly deaf children to auditory training. *J. Speech and Hearing Disorders, 18,* 273–288.

Hudgins, C. V., & Numbers, F. C. (1942). An investigation of the intelligibility of the speech of the deaf. *Genetic Psychology Monographs, 25,* 289–392.

Hudgins, C. V., & Stetson, R. H. (1932). A unit for kymograph recording. *Science, 76,* 59–60.

Liberman, A. M., & Mattingly, I. G. (1985). The motor theory of speech perception revised. *Cognition, 21,* 1–36.

Pickett, J. M. (1980). *The sounds of speech communication: A primer of acoustic phonetics and speech perception*. PRO-ED, Austin, TX: University Park Press.

Stetson, R. H., & Bouman, H. D. (1935). The coordination of simple skilled movements. *Arch. Neerl. Physiol.*, 20, 177–254.

Stetson, R. H., & Hudgins, C. V. (1930). Functions of the breathing movements in the mechanism of speech. *Arch. Neerl. Phon. Exp.*, 5, 1–30.

PREFACE
To the 2nd Edition

The analysis of skilled movements has been employed in the explanation of making and perceiving rhythms; it has been applied to various skilled movements including writing and piano playing. The present study has grown out of the application of this analysis of skilled movements to the processes of speech.

A phonetics based on movements is primarily concerned with the train of syllables. The vowels and consonants characterize the syllable; they do not occur alone, but only in the syllable. Since a syllable with its factors may constitute a foot of one syllable, a breath group of one foot, and a phrase of one breath group, the syllable is the simplest utterance possible. The five fundamental, simultaneous, inclusive units, syllable factor, syllable, foot, breath group, phrase, occur in every utterance; the syllable may represent them all. The syllable may or may not embody phonemes, which are significant aspects of the syllable factors.

The normal person controls the movements of speech by the sounds produced and he perceives speech by the ear. It is obvious, however, that the movements of speech, the articulations, are the primary things. The congenital deaf are able to produce speech by kinesthetic stimuli from the articulations, and to perceive speech by the eye; the deaf-blind are able to produce, and to palpate speech.

Varying the stress and the rate of utterance of a train of syllables has been the method of study in nearly all phases of motor phonetics. Full use has been made of the well determined limits of skilled movements.

For the first edition, 1928, kymograph tracings of the movements of speech were employed. The new thing added was the careful study of the air pressures in the vocal canal and especially of the syllable pulses and their grouping in the chest and abdomen.

Since 1928, oscillograph methods have been employed to record the muscular contractions of the speech apparatus, including the thoracic and abdominal movements. Oscillographic apparatus has made it possible to analyze and synthesize various acoustic aspects of the vowels and sonant consonants.

Various theoretical questions have been discussed in *Bases of Phonology*, 1945.

Fields like metrics and phonetics invite statistical treatment because measurements are possible, but the quantities measured vary constantly within limits. The large number of cases necessary is a disadvantage; but on the other hand it is impossible to get quantitative data of value in phonetics from a mere handful of cases. The statistical methods used are simple, and every effort has been made to secure accuracy. The measurements have been carefully checked; two persons have gone over all computations. Composite distribution curves have been checked by comparing the forms of the sum of the percentage curves of the various sub-groups with the curve resulting from the distribution of all the readings without reference to the sub-groups.

Objections are often made to the use of artificial combinations. But the fact is that the processes of ordinary speech are far too elaborate for unaided analysis. For many years much study has been devoted to detailed recordings of actual speech, but little has resulted for phonetic theory. In other sciences it is necessary to simplify material, to delimit problems, to work under artificial conditions. So in phonetics, experiments must be made with simple combinations under carefully controlled conditions before we can hope to attack the extremely complicated phenomena of ordinary speech.

The larger obligations of the author, especially to the great pioneer and leader in experimental phonetics, are apparent in the text. M. Henri Dupré and Mme. E. M. Guth furnished material for the comparison of the enunciation of French and English. L. E. Cole and H. E. Weaver of the Oberlin laboratory were of valuable assistance in securing the tracings used in the first edition. Later work owes everything to the expert collaboration of J. M. Snodgrass, C. V. Hudgins, and H. D. Bouman.

The present text has benefited from the work of C. V. Hudgins, J. M. Pickett, and Miss Hermina Zortz.

R. H. STETSON

May, 1950
Oscillograph Laboratory
Oberlin College
Oberlin, Ohio

Chapter I

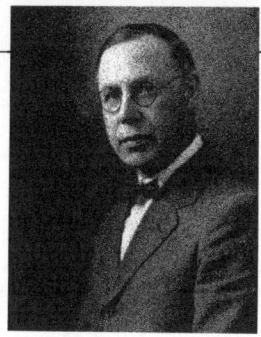

THE BASIC CONCEPTIONS OF PHONOLOGY

Editors' Remarks

In Chapter 1, Stetson expresses the rudimentary aspects of his approach and some of the central themes that run throughout the monograph. These are:

1. Motor phonetics is, fundamentally, the study of skilled movement in the service of linguistic function.

2. An (armchair) analysis of speech that relies solely on segmentation is basically flawed. Segments, as he says later, cannot be translated into movements.

3. The syllable is the basic "unit" of speech whose physiological correlate is called the "chest pulse." These are often seen as small perturbations in records of expiratory air pressure during speech. Or, as Stetson remarks metaphorically, as little ripples on the larger expiratory wave.

4. Vowels and consonants are distinguishable subunits of a syllable that are differentiated by their function—one to shape the vocal tract for the chest pulse, the other to delimit the chest pulse of the syllable.

Although themes 3 and 4 are, and have been, the subject of some empirical scrutiny and debate, themes 1 and 2, for us, stand out as a unique contribution of Stetson's, anticipating the current and quite intense interest of speech motor control researchers, phoneticians, psychologists, and linguists alike (see e.g., the special issue of *J. Phonetics*, 1986, *14*[1]). On the one hand, many are studying the "patterns and connections of articulatory movements," namely, how the vocal tract articulators are coordinated and controlled. How are the very many articulatory degrees of freedom "compressed" or constrained during the production of words? The production of even a simple syllable requires cooperation among multiple interacting articulators, and even more muscles, operating on different levels of description—supralaryngeal, laryngeal, and respiratory. Does the nervous system control these individually? A more likely alternative supported by recent data is that the many potentially independent components are flexibly assembled into a single, coherent unit for speech tasks. The essential properties of such coordinative structures are under much investigation at the moment. The nature of the task-specific patterns themselves and how they are assembled from the individual components are open questions, but crucial to the realization of the program Stetson started.

Similarly, the status of vowels and consonants as candidate units in a theory of speech production and perception, and *their* coordination in natural speech is also the subject of much current analysis. Discrete segments, as Stetson emphasizes, are never seen by perpendicular cuts of the physical records—be they acoustic, kinematic, or physiological—along the axis of time. Perhaps segments are "convenient abstractions," as Stetson says (reminiscent of Sherrington's remark that reflexes *qua* units of action are convenient fictions). This has not prevented people proceeding from the assumption that segments are physically real, no more than Sherrington's comment stopped people studying reflexes as real. Certain recent theorizing aims to characterize—in a Stetson-like fashion—the articulation of phonetic segments as overlapping sets of coordinated gestures with each set conforming to a phonetic segment. In such theories, the reality of the segment is assumed. It would appear, however, that the language to describe skilled movement coordination and the language to describe segments needs to be commensurate if a theoretical impasse is to be avoided.

THE SYLLABLE AS THE BASIC UNIT

For motor phonetics the primary concern is the train of movements of speech: the articulations and the larger movement units which incorporate the articulations. Speech can be indicated for a native by a row of signs in a line, but the signs give no hint of the pattern and connections of the articulatory movements (Note 1).

One fundamental contrast has survived all forms of notation and all sorts of theories, the contrast between the vowel and the consonant. There have been occasional efforts to whittle down the contrast or to be rid of it; but the very people who try to ignore the contrast use the distinction at every turn. One common pair of terms, "syllabic and non-syllabic" recognizes the function of the vowel (and vowel substitutes) in the syllable.

It has seemed to some phonologists that a row of "phonemes" is easier to handle than a train of syllables. But the syllable is always to be considered; it embodies the syllabic and the non-syllabic; it is the unit for the word- and the sentence-stress; it is the unit for the 'tones' of the tone languages; it is the stressed and unstressed unit of the feet of patterned verse. The syllable is the unit which incorporates the syllable factors, and in turn is incorporated in the units of the foot and breath group.

The mechanism of speech is often compared to the action of an organ: the chest is the bellows, furnishing air under pressure to the vocal folds which functions as the vibrating reed; the throat- and mouth-cavities constitute the resonating pipe, and the glottis or the consonant constriction acts as the palate (valve) to start and stop the flow of air through the vocal folds.

Careful observation shows that the action of an organ, bellows, reed, pipe, must be radically modified to fit the mechanism of speech. When the chest is slightly inflated for speaking, the air is not under pressure; like a hand bellows for blowing the fire, the volume is increased, but the nozzle is open and there is no flow of air; so the mouth and the glottis may be open as in whispering, but there is no flow of air from the inflated chest.

If one makes quick strokes of the hands while holding the inflated hand bellows, the nozzle emits little pulses of air; as the quick strokes are repeated the air pulses reduce the volume of air, and the arm muscles must bring the boards of the bellows closer and closer to accommodate for the loss of air. There has been no valve action; no palate has started or stopped the flow of air.

If the hand bellows is connected with the reed of an artificial larynx, the reed will sound for each air pulse from the nozzle; it is the quick movements of the hands which release and arrest the air pulse voiced by the reed.

In much the same way the vocal apparatus makes a series of vowel syllables, "*Oh, Oh, Oh. . . .*" The chest is inflated by the larger muscles, the quick strokes for each air pulse are made by the short muscles between the ribs, and as the chest volume gets less and less, the larger outside muscles and the abdominal muscles accommodate the walls and floor of the chest to the changing volume.

The muscles between the ribs (intercostals) produce the syllables "*Oh, Oh, Oh*. . . ." as units included in the slower movement of the breath group which is made by the larger muscles of chest and abdomen. The rapid muscle contractions are like ripples on the wave of the expiratory movement of the breath group.

No air pulse from the nozzle of the hand bellows can be made without inflating the bellows and maintaining the position of the boards of the bellows while the hands make the little strokes for the air pulse. No syllable can be uttered without inflating the chest and maintaining the chest-abdomen position while the rib muscles (intercostals) make the quick strokes of the syllable. In other words a single syllable, "Oh" must be part of the movement of a breath group. The air pulse for the syllable "Oh" is released and arrested by the rib muscles, but the supporting coordination involves the large ribcage muscles, the diaphragm, and the abdominal muscles for this one-syllable breath group.

The hand bellows connected to an artificial larynx is not fitted with anything to correspond to the constriction of a consonant in the syllable. What happens when "*beau, ope, pope*" are uttered? Experiment shows that in uttering "*beau, pope*" the lips close with the contraction of the rib muscles for the syllable pulse, and open to release the syllable pulse and the air flow sets the glottal folds in action for the vowel. In uttering "*ope, pope*" the lips close at the end of the syllable, arresting the pulse of the syllable and stopping the air flow through the glottis.

The types of syllable prove to be:

OVO a vowel syllable released and arrested by the chest muscles.

CVO a syllable released by a consonant, and arrested by the chest muscles.

OVC a syllable released by the chest muscles, and arrested by a consonant.

CVC a syllable released by a consonant, and arrested by a consonant.

Careful experimentation with all the types of syllables and consonants makes it certain that every syllable has its chest pulse delimited by the chest muscles (intercostals) or by the constriction (complete or partial) of the consonant, or by both.

The syllable pulse, like any rapid movement, consists of two strokes, a beat stroke and a back stroke; the beat stroke releases the pulse with or without the auxiliary consonant movement; the back stroke arrests the syllable pulse with or without the auxiliary consonant movement. (Note 2)

The consonant movement is always an auxiliary movement. The consonant functions only in a syllable. Recordings show that demonstrators and teachers who believe that they are producing isolated "sounds" are actually producing syllables. A chest pulse is necessary; there is either a silent vowel which the supposedly isolated consonant actually releases or arrests, or a continuant that provides the vocal-canal shape through which the pulse is emitted.

It is impossible of course to make a given vowel without releasing and arresting a pulse from the chest; shaping the vowel canal prepares for the syllable pulse of the vowel but the pulse must occur if there is to be a vowel. The lips or tongue may be in position to make the releasing or arresting stroke of a given consonant but that does not constitute a consonant; the consonant is produced when the stroke releases or arrests the air pressure of the syllable pulse. The vowel is an articulation which has the function of shaping the vocal canal for the chest pulse; the consonant is an articulation which has the function of delimiting the chest pulse of the syllable. It is only in the coordination of the syllable pulse that they act as vowel and consonant. They may be named as if separate, but that is merely a convenient abstraction. A vowel is a specific quality of a syllable when uttered through a specific vocal-canal shape; a consonant is a specific way of releasing or of arresting a syllable. Details of the processes involved come later.

The syllable proves to have three invariable factors:

The releasing factor: rib muscles or consonant movement, O- or C- ("*ope, beau*").
OVC CVO

The vowel shaping factor: muscles of tongue, pharynx, jaw, lips, -V- ("*ope, pope*").
OVC CVC

The arresting factor: chest muscles or consonant movement, -0 or -C ("*beau, pope*").
CVO CVC

Any one of these syllable factors may be characterized by one or several significant aspects; these are the phonemes. A syllable may have no significant aspect, no phoneme, or it may have as many as seven significant aspects of the syllable factors phonemes. There are compound consonants of two or three aspects, and there are compound vowels, diphthongs (and a few triphthongs). Details of the characteristics and processes involved in compound syllable factors come later (Cf. Appendix II: Artificial Larynx; Appendix III: Historical Aspects of the Syllables).

THE FOOT AND BREATH GROUP AS RELATED TO THE SYLLABLE

Often the phoneme has been considered without reference to the syllable; and often the syllable has been considered without reference to the foot, breath group and phrase in which the syllable is always incorporated. The syllable, the foot, the breath group, and the phrase, are elaborations of the movements of expiration. They must be audible; if the expiration is to be widely audible it must be through the mouth, and nasal outflow will be secondary along with the minor noises of articulation.

It is rather common but false to assume that the consonants and vowels float on the continuous pressure of the breath group. The chest is mistakenly thought of as the wind chest of an organ maintaining a steady flow under pressure throughout the breath group, interrupted by the constrictions (partial or complete) of the consonants, and colored by the shaping of the vowels; the working of the artificial larynx controverts such a notion.

Experimental study of the speech mechanism shows on the contrary that the chest does not maintain a steady pressure throughout the breath group. Instead, the chest muscles (intercostals) produce a separate pulse of pressure for each syllable; the pressure falls between the syllable pulses. The chest retains an overall posture which maintains its volume of air, but the minute contractions of the short muscles between the ribs (intercostals) force out little pulses of air which constitute the separate syllables. Even in a language like Hottentot in which suction "clicks" are prominent, there occur the usual chest pulses of the syllables grouped in the usual breath group (Note 3).

A slight pressure is generally maintained during the breath group, at least in English utterance, but the chest pulses of the syllables rise from this level. Between the breath groups the pressure goes to zero although the over-all posture and the chest volume are maintained; if there is an intake between breath groups, the pressure becomes negative.

Careful experimentation proves the breath group to be due to an abdominal movement with its culminations which mark the stresses of the constituent feet. One of these stresses constitutes the main stress of the breath group, while the syllable pulses are produced by the intercostal muscles of the rib cage.

The "foot" is the smallest unit group incorporating the syllables; it is due to an abdominal pulse which integrates a single stressed syllable or a few syllables grouped about a single stressed syllable.

After each movement of expiration for the breath group an intake may or may not occur; but there is always a readjustment to the slight change in volume of the chest. As the capacity of the chest decreases, the rib cage descends slightly and the abdominal muscles raise the diaphragm slightly to compensate for the outgo of air (Cf. Figs. 50, 57).

Any utterance however simple has all the essential movement units: the syllable is an integration of the three syllable factors; the syllable or syllables are components of a foot; the foot or feet are components of a breath group; the breath group or breath groups compose a phrase. Thus the simplest utterance will be a phrase of one breath group consisting of a monosyllabic foot. The experimental study of speech movements shows that all these units are actually present in the utterance of a single syllable, and of any group of syllables.

Movement Units in Speech

There has been some general recognition of the articulation as the fundamental event in phonology, rather than the acoustic pattern.

These articulatory events which figure as signals and symbols in speech must be classified and handled with reference to their actual function, in the processes of utterance. The various lists and classifications which prove useful in phonology are derived from the functions of consonants and vowels in the syllables of speech.

Articulate language involves the two phases: 1) A universal apparatus for speech common to all speakers; and 2) A specific, acquired language mechanism peculiar to the given language. The experience in learning foreign languages shows that the apparatus for speech is universal; any child learns any language or pair of languages with the same ease. The program of a general phonemics based on comparative phonetics proposed by Trubetzkoy (Anleitung, 1935) (98) and the project of a universal auxiliary language assume that all speakers have a common apparatus for speech. But there are also the peculiar characteristics of the specific native language which are apparent in the "accent" of the adult foreigner.

The "acquired language mechanism" of a specific language is evidently something more than a row of special "sounds". The practical teaching of language as well as the needs of linguistic analysis have led to the consideration of larger and larger units.

It is impossible to teach the "separate sounds" of a language. The sounds cannot be separated, and then assembled into syllables (syllables are not assemblies), and the proper stresses, pauses, and "intonation" added (they are not additions but basic over-all traits). Everyone realizes that "word stress", "phrase and sentence stress", "intonation" all involve units of articulation larger than the supposed "sound", or the syllable. And everyone realizes that the smallest units of articulation are parts of the larger system of utterance; everything hangs together. Concepts like "base d'articulation", "Mundstellung" grow out of the fact that the "accent" of a language involves the whole language mechanism.

Every utterance is a movement consisting of the phrase which is the larger, inclusive unit of which the breath group, foot, and syllable are organic parts. For this movement, the posture is the adjustment of the abdomen-diaphragm and external chest muscles for regulated expiration; the movements of the breath group, and of the feet within the breath group are due to the abdomen-diaphragm movements of expiration. The series of small expiratory movements, the breath groups, constitute the phrase. The phrase is followed in the breathing cycle by a rapid inhalation. Although the utterance may consist of only one or two syllables, all the fundamental movement units are present.

The feet and the breath groups are long enough to have varying culminations in the stresses and grouping for the "word accent", and for the breath-group stress. The syllable however is a single ballistic movement; it is impossible to have two stresses within one syllable (Note 4).

The various boundary markers ("Grenzsignale"), stress and intonation patterns which have been noted, are not independent traits, appearing isolated as members of a series of symbols; they are rather cues to these basic coordinated movement units which make up connected articulate speech (Note 5).

Summary of the Movement Units of a Motor Phonetics

The movement units and their coordinations may be schematized as follows:

1. OVO, CVO, OVC, CVC

    The underscoring indicates the syllable unit; chest release and chest arrest are indicated by O; consonant release and consonant arrest are indicated by C; vowel shaping is indicated by V. (Syllables occur only in the larger units of 2 and 3.)

2. OVO, CVO, CVC, OVC, CVO, OVO, CCVC

    Breath group of three feet; organization indicated by the lines below the syllables. CCVC indicates a syllable released by a compound consonant, e.g. "*trade*".

3. OVO, CVO, CVC, OVC, CVO, OVO, CCVC

    Phrase of two breath groups; the phrasing movement, and the incorporation of the two breath groups are indicated by the double lines. CCVC indicates a syllable released by a compound consonant, e.g. "*trade*".

Even though the utterance consists of only one syllable, it constitutes a foot of a single syllable, a breath group of a single foot, and a phrase of a single breath group; the posture and the abdomen-diaphragm movements, as well as the articulations of the single syllable all actually occur, as observations of boundary markers, stresses, etc., and laboratory tracings from the speech apparatus, demonstrate. (Note 6) (Cf. Appendix V: Conditioning and the units of speech; Appendix IV: Earlier stages of modern phonetics; Appendix VI: Reduction of a language to phonemes).

PHONETICS AND PHONEMICS

Since the concepts of the "phoneme" and of aspects of speech which are "phonemic" are current, it is important to contrast "phonetics" and "phonemics" ("phonologie" on the Continent).

The phonemic method of analysis is an important method and often applicable, but it is an analysis of speech to determine the signals (symbols) and not the process by which signals are produced. Language has to do primarily with meanings; the syllables are primarily meaningful syllables. They are products of the system of habitual movements of speech in a given language. The articulations and their organization for expressing meanings in the given language constitute the "language mechanism".

Therefore the signals with meaning are primary; the syllables are the minimal units. "Phonemic" means that a given articulatory change of the syllable affects the meaning. The type of change and the amount of change necessary to affect the meaning of a syllable depend on the language. The users of a language may sense a very small change as significant, or they may be indifferent to a very extensive change; and this differs from language to language, because the changes and their significance are learned with the language.

It is sometimes said that a phoneme is not an entity, but that it stands for a class; which is true of any concept in science; the phoneme stands for a class of syllables which are released in a given way, or are arrested in a given way, or have the vowel canal shaped in a given way. And again the term phoneme is very convenient as a name for the group of variants which the characterized syllable factor (phonemic signal) undergoes with the changes of syllable rate and stress. The given way of releasing, arresting, or shaping a syllable changes with rate and stress, and when the original rate and stress are restored, these variations revert to the slow careful form by which the phoneme is identified. The slow, careful forms of the units in "apart" and "opinion" make the first syllables unlike; at a rapid rate both the "o" and the "a" approach shwa. "*Telegraph*" and "*teleg'raphy*", "*monotone*" and "*monotonous*" show changes due to shifting stress. To distinguish the forms "*an icehouse*" from "*a nice house*" requires a change in grouping of the foot, $\_\_\perp\_$ for "*a nice house*", and $\_\perp / \perp\_$ for "*an icehouse*".

The phonemic method of reducing a language to its units is an obvious method; but it is not to be assumed that reference to the meanings embodied is the only way of reducing language to its units. The cryptographer deciphering an intercepted and recorded oral communication in an unknown vernacular obviously cannot depend on *meanings*. The units must be isolated and assembled to determine the language and find the meaning. The paleographer dealing with an undeciphered inscription is in the same case; the syllables and/or their factors may be determined while the meaning remains unknown; so Etruscan and Minoan.

The terms "phonetic", "sound", "articulation" refer to articulate processes of speech without regard to meaning. The articulations and their variations and combinations when identified in a given vernacular constitute the basis for phonetics. The habits of utterance of the language constitute an organized system of skilled movements which may produce meaningful syllables, or may produce nonsense syllables of the same type.

The purposes of phonemics and phonetics are often quite unlike. It is convenient to distinguish the phoneme by a trait or traits which will be differential. For taxonomic purposes diagnostic items are important. The context in which the differentiating traits are perceived and which is essential to their production and perception may be ignored. In phonemics identification and classification are usually primary; and the movement complex producing the significant trait is hardly considered or is ostentatiously ignored, although it is obvious that uttering the phonemes is quite as important as perceiving the phonemes in this the most important form of social communication.

A breath group can often be recognized by only a few distinguishing items in the pattern context of the breath group with its stress and rhythm. If these distinguishing items, however, were somehow presented alone (sometimes possible with proper apparatus), even though properly timed, they could not be perceived. And as for producing such significant items, that is impossible except as indivisible aspects of syllables in the overall rhythmic pattern of the breath group.

It may be enough for the classification of significant traits or for an orthography intended for native use, to isolate and indicate the significant items or groups of items simultaneous and successive. But for understanding the synchronous changes and the process of producing the significant traits and their combinations, and for controlling the learning of a language, the working of the language mechanism is essential.

Motor phonetics is the study of the skilled movements involved in the process of handling articulatory signals. Motor phonetics deals with the organized series of actual syllables or nonsense syllables shaped by the language mechanism. "Phonetic" refers to such physiological processes in the study of the signals of a language independent of the meanings of the signals. The signals are physiological; they are uttered and perceived by kinesthetic cues from the vocal organs, and by auditory cues; but they may be uttered and perceived by kinesthetic and visual cues in the case of the deaf; the "sounds" are not essentially auditory. A phonetic change is a mechanical change which occurs in the syllable due to context and to change of rate and stress in the utterance. Since these coordinated movements of articulation are the medium for the signals of an articulate language, the mechanical, physiological changes are important and affect the phonemes. Phonologists have often resorted to nonsense syllables for convenience in observation and experiment: F. de Saussure "*appa, apta*"; Rousselot "*afa, af-fa*"; Sievers "*alla, ar-a*"; recent writers "*pup, aftpa, faf, vav, gug*", etc.

When the language signals of different languages are compared, the discussion must strictly be phonetic. There are no consistent meanings and the syllables compared are in effect nonsense syllables treated as physiological processes. The syllables must be handled independent of the meanings, although meanings gave rise to the syllables in each language in question. Comparative phonemics becomes comparative phonetics.

Since phonetic change occurs as a phase of the acquired language mechanism, it is observable by the users of a language though the change may have no meaning. Phonemic change on the other hand is a matter of conditioning and may be so slight as to tax phonetic discrimination, or so extensive as to be very obvious—if it does not affect the meaning, however, it is negligible as a phonemic change.

Phonetic change is physiological, and occurs within the acquired language mechanism. Phonemic change is significant; it always involves the conditioned meaning of the signal (Cf. Appendix VII: Segmentation. Appendix VIII: Reduction of Trubetzkoy's Phonologie to Motor Terms. Appendix IX: American Version of Phonemics [Phonologie]).

NOTES

Note (1)

The requirements for handling the problems of phonetics and of the related problems of phonology are exacting. No single investigator can hope to be directly familiar with the details of the fields which prove essential. Collaboration will help and is important. But at least one of the collaborators must know the possibilities of all the supporting treatments and be able to judge how they are to be brought to bear.

On the one hand philological training is essential, including the phonological development of at least one historical language and, if possible, of at least one language outside the Indo-European group. There must be some first-hand acquaintance with the fundamentals of symbolic logic and the theory of symbols, and a grounding in psychology and especially in the psychology of language.

On the other hand there must be an understanding

of the processes of speech which demands special apparatus and laboratory equipment and a physiological and physical training for experimental work; there must be some first-hand experience with the problems of acoustics and especially of audition.

There is no dodging either side of the requirements of the problems. A groundwork of linguistics is essential; a mere smattering of modern logic will not do; and the psychology of language can't be improvised from the chance dicta of linguists. It is impossible to unravel the movements of speech by watching one's own processes, even with the help of "a small mirror"; the articulations are far too complicated and far too quick for that; the only result will be "a heap of spare parts" and it is impossible to settle how they work by mere speculation.

Note (2)

The functions of the syllable factors called "releasing" and "arresting":

Syllables like "*a, Ah, I,*" are released by the chest; the rapid rise of pressure of the syllable is generated by the intercostal muscles of the chest. The pulse is arrested by the intercostal muscles which take up the momentum of the pulse.

Syllables like "*pay, bay, die,*" are released by a consonant, and the process is more elaborate. The intercostals act as before, but the consonant constriction occurs at the same time, so that the air pressure develops behind the consonant closure; the syllable pulse is released when the consonant opens. Thus the "release" is always due to the combined action of intercostals and articulation.

Syllables like "*ape, Abe, ice, ire,*" are arrested by the consonant constriction which blocks the air flow and raises the pressure in the trachea and so takes up the momentum of the pulse. Thus the "arrest" may be due to the action of the articulation alone.

In spite of this difference in function, the same consonant when releasing or arresting is essentially the same articulation: it is a commonplace for an arresting articulation to become a releasing articulation, e.g. "*up, up*" becomes "*u' pup*"; "*eat, eat*" said faster and faster becomes "*tea, tea*".

Note (3)

Beach, D. M., Phonetics of the Hottentot Language, Cambridge, 1938.

The breath-groups are discussed, p. 47/48; syllables p. 53ff. The types of syllables are discussed, p. 54. The suction "clicks" occur only as part of the syllable release, i.e. as "syllable initial". The stress is noted as fairly uniform on the syllables, p. 141, in this resembling French.

The chest-pulses can be read from the kymograms, pp. 37, 38.

Note (4)

The syllable may in some cases be prolonged into a slow, "controlled" form, if the syllable is "open" or if the syllable is arrested by a voiced continuant like "*m, n, l, r,* etc." In beating time so that the baton describes a "figure-eight" the movement may be prolonged after the pulse of the beat; in the same way the beat stroke of the syllable may be arrested by a backstroke process which continues the course of the movement in a slow, "controlled" form. Movements of this sort, which begin with a ballistic pulse and are continued as a controlled movement are very common in all fields. They occur frequently in singing when the arrest is of the chest muscles and the pressure is continued in a prolonged note. In unusual cases a vocal movement of the controlled type begins perhaps in the utterance of a fricative, and is finally merged into a ballistic pulse. It is after this fashion that the preliminary slow movement of the conductor merges into the entering beat stroke of the movement (Cf. Motor Phonetics, 1928, p. 32).

Note (5)

The 1) initiation, 2) culmination, 3) termination are apparent in various movements:

Like the syllable, the golf- and tennis-strokes, the step, the leap, tapping- and keyboard strokes can culminate only in the arresting process.

The longer movement like that of the breath group is exemplified by the lateral movement of the arm which supports and organizes keyboard passage work, scales, arpeggios; the bowing movement patterns the violin phrase. The lateral arm movement carries the hand and fingers through the word in writing.

In the animal's locomotion the limb movements are subordinated to the main trunk movements. The squirrel makes his way through the leafy branches, catch as catch can, by a series of irregular initiations, culminations, and terminations. Like human speech, the birds' songs (canary, mocking bird, parrot) are all phrased by the expiration of air.

Note (6)

Articulate language is one of three forms of temporal expression. Articulate language belongs to a set of complex, coordinated systems of expression: 1) articulate language, 2) music, and 3) dramatic dancing. For these three the basic principle of organization is the grouping of basic units in larger, inclusive units by stress and time relations; it is the principle of organization of rhythmic movements.

There are also movement coordinations in the crafts, metal work, weaving, needlework, but they do not constitute organized hierarchies of signals and symbols primarily for expression as do articulate language, music, and dancing.

Picture writing, mathematics, and mechanical drawing constitute other means of expression and coordination. They are spatial, not temporal, and the organized patterns are not the result of stresses and durations.

Articulate language is the most elaborate of the three forms of temporal expression and is used primarily for the expression of intellectual matters, while music and dramatic dancing are used primarily for the expression of emotion.

The method of expression common to articulate language, music, and dancing involves specific, individualized units which are constituents of larger, inclusive units:

Articulate language	Music	Dancing
syllable	note	step

These are the basic, individualized units which are always elements in larger, inclusive units:

foot	figure	group of steps
breath group	motif	evolution
phrase	phrase	expressive pattern

There are various fusions of these rhythmic systems of expression:

1. The song and choral works (articulate language and music).
2. The ballet (music and dancing).
3. The opera, and primitive dance rites (articulate language, music, and dancing).

These fusions are possible because the method of organization is one and the same in the hierarchical coordination of rhythmic movement. All three have the traits of complex coordinated movements organized into a temporal pattern; the inclusive units are set off by pauses or by culminating stresses. In contrast to signals and symbols on paper (in one dimension) the temporal and the dynamic aspects (variations of duration, stress) are essential.

The stable, individualized, basic unit (syllable, note, step) is often complex:

The syllable must be released by the chest muscles or by a consonant, must be uttered through a definite vowel shape, and must be arrested by the chest muscles or by a consonant.

The note has its inception (attack), pitch, quality, and termination; it may be legato or staccato. These are aspects of the note which cannot of course occur alone.

The step of the dance must have a take-off, a lateral movement (stride) and a landing, but none of these phases of the step can occur alone.

Since these signals are used for 1) communication, for 2) manipulation and invention, for 3) record, a notation is important in one- or two-dimensional terms, i.e. on paper, and has been developed for articulate language and for music; but the spatial symbols merely indicate movement processes.

The identity of the syllable is not lost in the breath group. And in actual utterance it cannot be reduced to lower terms. The syllable factors are definite, stereotyped, but they must always function in a syllable to which they are essential.

Although the word has no phonetic individualization it does determine the sequences of syllables and in many languages the word determines the syllables to be stressed and unstressed. The varied groupings and connections prescribed by the sense are indicated in the larger, more inclusive units, from Sapir's simplest syntactical unit, a syllable group with a culminating stress, to the complex of elaborate phrases in a periodic sentence.

The movements of syllable factors, syllables, feet, breath groups are all due to precise, controllable muscular contractions; any significant, audible change must be due to a precise, controlled muscular contraction.

Thus the pattern prescribed by the meaning is built up in slow, careful utterance. But changes of rate and stress bring mechanical changes in the series of signals which are not subject to control, and are therefore ignored. The identity of the series of symbols is maintained though the signals of the series undergo mechanical change. The identity of the symbol is verified by the reversion of the signal to the slow, careful form when the original rate and stress are restored.

If certain phonetic collocations are counted essential to avoid ambiguity (in English, "an aim" vs. " a name", e.g.), the rate and stresses must be adjusted to conserve these aspects.

Chapter II

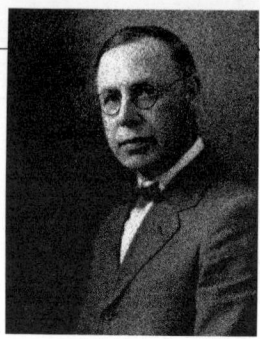

METHODS AND APPARATUS IN EXPERIMENTAL PHONETICS

Editors' Remarks

As someone once said, the fact that speech production research requires one to observe a dynamic and rather inaccessible region of the human anatomy (the vocal tract) is either a gross misfortune or a principal challenge. For Stetson, it was the *only* way to pursue his motor phonetics. "Articulate language in action," after all, needs a concrete medium from which quantifiable and reproducible observations can be made. Phonemes, he remarks elsewhere, are symbols as opposed to the *signal* which lies in articulation.

Stetson's ingenious techniques for recording movement (developed, we understand, with Mr. James Snodgrass) stand here as an historical monument, much in the same way as those of E. J. Marey and Eadweard Muybridge for the case of animal motion, in general. The modern speech researcher is confronted with many of the same kinds of technical and methodological problems as Stetson was 60 years ago, and thus, will appreciate Stetson's efforts here. Also, future chapters contain many recordings from the devices described in this chapter, and it is important to appreciate from whence these recordings originated.

Today, a chief task in speech science is to relate simultaneously recorded measures in order to understand how sound is structured by a moving vocal tract. Like Stetson, these measures fall into three categories: electromyographic records of the neuromuscular activation of articulators; kinematic (displacement and its derivatives, velocity and acceleration over time) records of the movements themselves; and aerodynamic and acoustic records of the consequences of movement. In a brief appendix we present a representative sample of "modern" techniques (some rather similar to Stetson's) for speech production research.

All the theories of phonemics and phonetics assume articulate language as the medium to be considered. Even the basic phonemic distinction of "la langue et la parole" was made within the domain of articulate language. "Ce qu'on s'imagine prononcer", "ce qu'on prononce en réalité" both assume the process of pronouncing, either in physiological or mental terms. The practical phonemicists handle "transcriptions". One of the last papers of Trubetzkoy deals with a list of universal "phonemes" for the utterance of an international, auxiliary language. Since mentalism has been abandoned in the main in phonology, articulate language in action is the concrete medium for observation and for experimentation which can be repeated.

There are two general approaches to the problem of phonetic analysis: a) the physiological and b) the acoustic. Both methods have been employed in obtaining the materials presented in this book. The primary emphasis, however, is upon the physiological analysis of the speech mechanism in action. The physiological aspects of speech may be inferred from the data obtained in an acoustical analysis of the speech sounds, but such inferences have often led to serious error with regard to the functioning of the several parts of the complex speech mechanism. Acoustic recordings are valuable for some purposes however, and have been used with success by careful investigators. Both of the methods will be described in this chapter in so far as they have been employed in obtaining the data here presented.

Historically, experimental phonetics moved toward an exact science during the last quarter of the 19th century. The physiological methods used were adapted from those already in use in physiological laboratories. Rosapelly, working in Marey's laboratory, is credited with having first made recordings of speech processes by the kymographic method. He obtained and studied simultaneous records of a) speech breathing movements, b) vibrations of the larynx, c) movements of the lips in articulation, and d) air pressures from the mouth and nose during the processes of speaking (66, 71). Oakley-Coles developed the artificial palate which often gives important data as to bearings in mouth (49, 50, 58).

Rousselot gives credit to Rosapelly for his pioneering work. Rousselot developed the methods and became the leader in the field of experimental phonetics and may be considered the founder of the science of experimental phonetics. Rousselot's methods have been adopted with modifications by everyone working in the field since his time.

Early efforts to handle the problems of phonetics by acoustic methods were confined largely to the study of the vowel structure. Helmholtz, Hermann, Stumpf, and others employing methods then available, set the pattern for much of the work that followed. The development of the phonograph enabled investigators to make relatively accurate and permanent records of speech sounds which could be studied at leisure. Thus Marichelle studied phonographic grooves with a microscope and worked out a thoroughgoing analysis of the relationship of vowels and consonants within the train of syllables of speech. (50) The development of the telephone and the practical needs for further knowledge concerning the acoustic aspects of speech, especially as related to telephonic communication, has given further impetus to research in experimental phonetics. Advances in technology, especially in the application of electronics to the problems, have motivated research in this field.

THE RECORDING METHODS APPLIED TO THE PROCESSES OF SPEECH

Tracings (recordings) of the movements of the several parts involved are essential to an adequate analysis of the total speech process. Since the timing of the movements is of primary importance, the tracings must be simultaneous. For simplicity the speech mechanism may be divided into three divisions, although the mechanism functions as an integrated whole in the process of utterance:

1. the breathing mechanism which produces and regulates the air supply for utterance,
2. the larynx which produces the vocal tone, and
3. the articulatory mechanism which shapes the vocal cavities makes the strokes for the consonants and generally transforms the total effort of utterance into articulate speech.

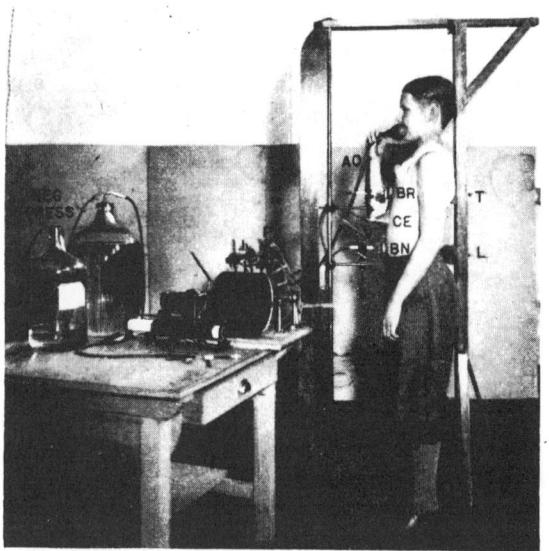

FIGURE 1. Stanchion

Frame for supporting apparatus for recording chest and abdominal movements. Accommodates subject standing or sitting. Two rigid blocks, T, thoracic, and L, lumbar, support the spine.

Vertical rod supports the bosses and applicator independent of the body wall.

AO—Mask for air outside lips, held by the subject. Leads by large tube to recording tambour of kymograph.

BR, BN—Bosses recording movements of body wall at rib-cage and at navel.

CE—Negative pressure applicator in epigastric region. Cf. Fig. 11, E. Neg. Press.

P—Recording tambours.

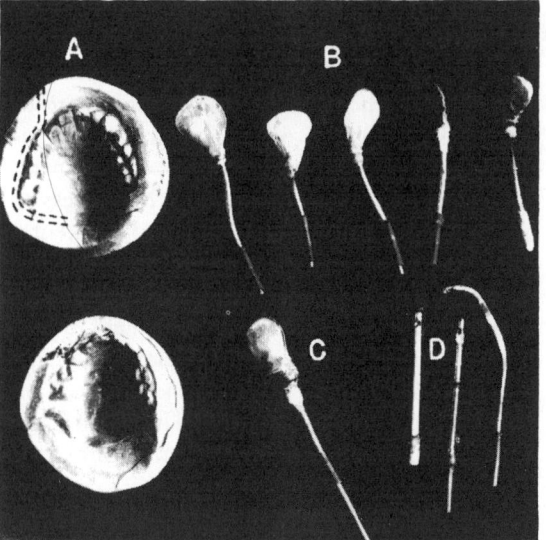

FIGURE 2. Tongue and Lip Markers

A—Casts of the palate of subject for fitting tongue markers. The dotted lines indicate the position of an air tube (D, curved form) outside jaw.

B—Various types of tongue markers with steel wire frames which support distended rubber coated with collodion.

C—Lip marker with steel wire frame.

D—Air tubes. The curved form passes outside jaw and taps mouth cavity behind molars.

These markers are connected by rubber tubes with the recording tambours of kymograph.

The apparatus and methods which have been used to obtain graphic records of the action of these several parts will be considered separately.

The Breathing Mechanism in Speech

Two aspects of the breathing mechanism have been recorded in parallel: movements of the chest muscles for the syllable pulse and movements of the abdominal muscles for the foot and breath group.

Movements of the Chest Muscles for the Syllable Pulse

The rapid pulses of the intercostal muscles for individual syllables have been generally overlooked by experimenters. The result is that the existence of the syllable as a physiological unit has often been denied or ignored. It is possible to obtain recordings showing the syllable pulse both in terms of the direct movements of the muscles themselves and indirectly in terms of the rapid fluctuations of air pressure within the chest. Four methods have been employed in studying this phenomenon. Three of these rely on pneumatic recording and involve (1) direct recordings of pressure changes within the chest from the tracheal tube of tracheotomized subjects, (2) pressure changes within the chest recorded by means of a rubber balloon in the stomach, (3) recordings of the pressure changes transmitted through the chest walls by means of a negative pressure applicator placed on the body wall, and (4) recording of action potentials from the intercostal muscles during speech. Each of these methods will be described next in some detail.

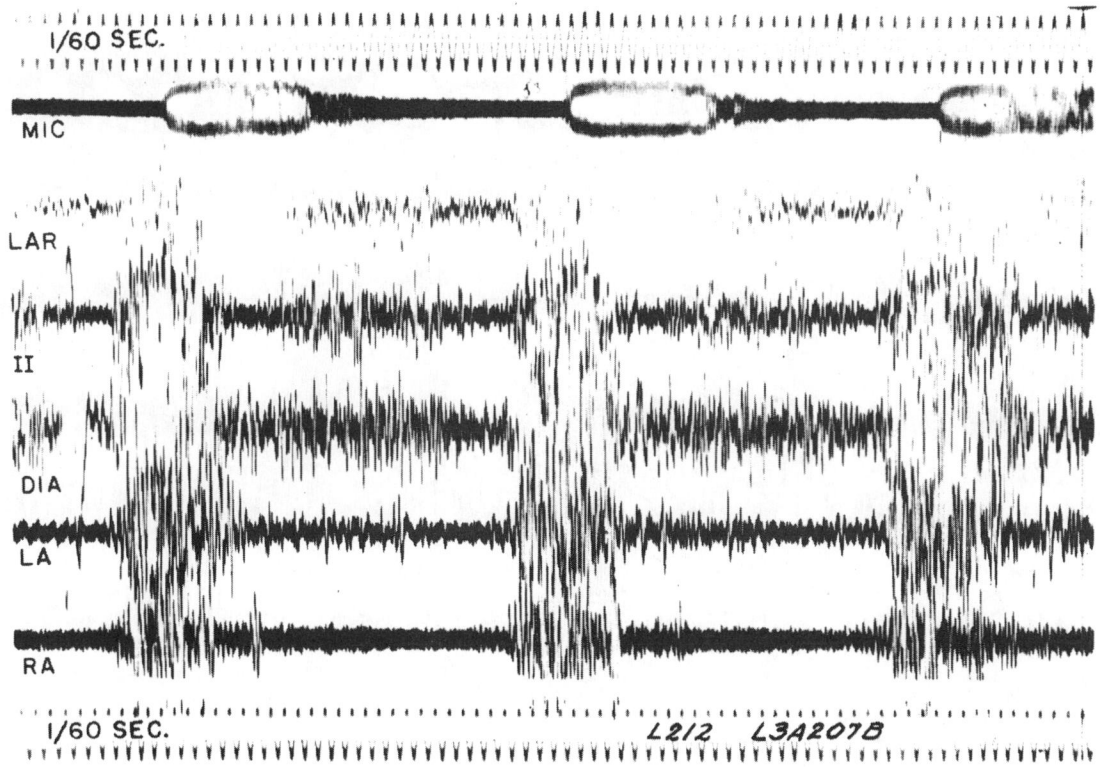

FIGURE 3. Action-Potential Recording of Essential Muscles of Speech

Syllables: *pup pup pup* at slow rate.

MIC—The opening of the vowel of each syllable is abrupt. The closure shows that the vibrations persist into the consonant.

LAT—Intrinsic muscles of larynx act well in advance of the vowel.

I I—Internal Intercostal muscles initiate the chest pulse for the syllable.

DIA—Diaphragm channel is affected by the I I and LA discharges. The actual diaphragm contractions occur (with the External Intercostals) at the close of the syllable and of the breath group.

LA

RA—The abdominal musculature is the first to act in an utterance, led by the contraction of the Rectus. The contraction of the Rectus leads off the breath group movement.

At this rate of utterance there is a breath group for each syllable.

---

1. Chest pulses recorded from the trachea. Disease of the larynx may make it necessary to provide an orifice for breathing below the larynx. Just above the sternum a tracheotomy tube is inserted into the trachea through which the subject breathes.

With such tracheotomized subjects who are able to speak normally, it was possible to get tracings directly of the sub-glottal variations of air pressure. A tight joint, easily separated for taking breath, led from the tracheal breathing tube to a taut tambour of ca. 5 cm. diameter. The membrane must resist pressures of 120-300 mm. water; the most satisfactory membranes were built of thin rubber layers cemented together. It is difficult to have such membranes as responsive at high as at low pressures; and yet it is important because the oscillations for the chest pulse may on occasion take place at a fairly high overall pressure of the abdominal breath pulse.

Tracings in great detail of sub-glottal pressures of this type were taken also from four laryngectomized subjects speaking with an artificial larynx.

An artificial larynx can be set up for the normal speaker, with a source of air pressure

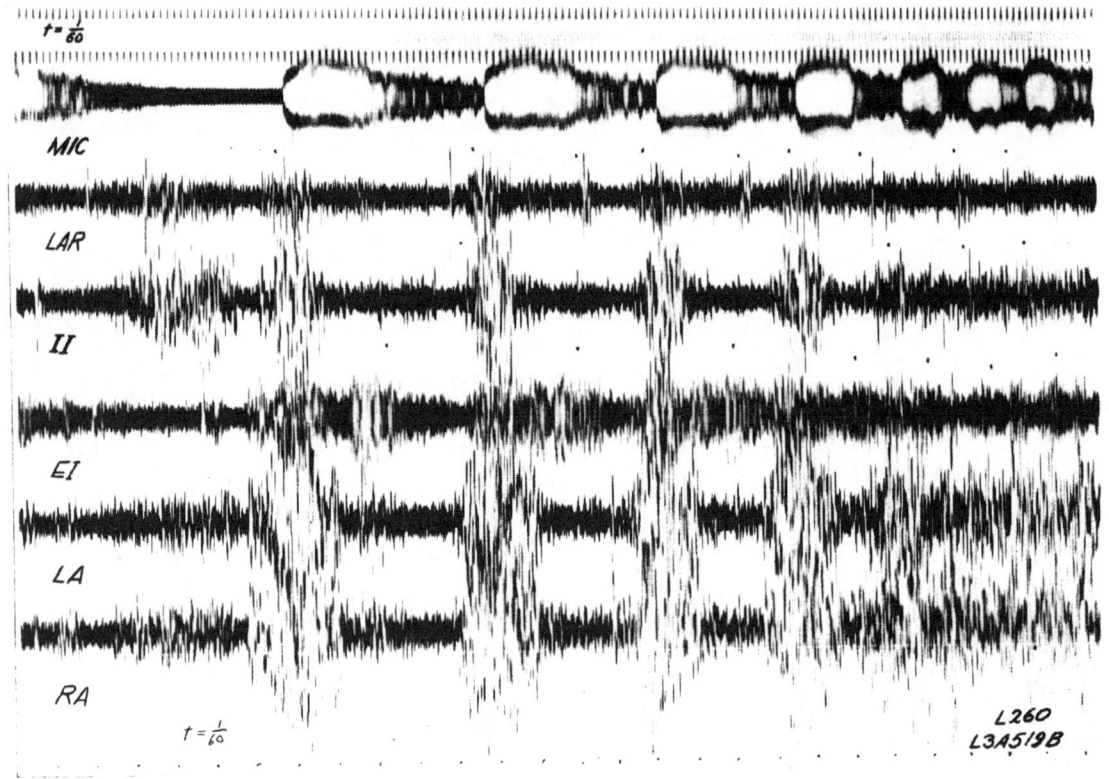

FIGURE 4. Action-Potential Recording of Muscles of Speech

Syllable *pup* spoken at increasing rate.
MIC—The vowel opens abruptly, but the vowel invades the arresting consonant, and when that drops, the releasing consonant also becomes voiced.
LAR—Clear pulses for the vowel begin well in advance of the vowel.
  I I—The pulses for the initiation of the individual syllables is very clear.
E I—The tracing is affected by potentials from the I I channel. The muscles from the External Intercostals contract between the artifacts from the I I channel.
LA
RA—The Lateral and Rectus abdominal pulses mark the distinct abdominal pulses for the breath group, up to the rate of 2.5 per sec. At that rate the abdominal muscles set for the long indeterminate type of breath group.

controlled by the hand, with the tube of the artificial larynx leading the tone and air pressure into the corner of the mouth. The subject "holds his breath", i.e. closes the glottis, while he articulates the syllables, the pulses of which he makes with the hand. As a source of air pressure a fire bellows is simple and convenient. If the bellows does not have a volume of 3–4 liters, a flask serving as an air chamber must be let into the line. The process requires an hour or so of practice but is not difficult. Tracings from such utterances with manual syllables correspond to tracings of the speech of laryngectomized subjects. Such a device is not expensive, and will settle once and for all the relations between the "chest pulse" and the "articulations".

Immediately after recovery from removal of the larynx a patient cannot utter the slightest sound by manipulating the articulatory apparatus; yet in a few hours he can learn to speak again with an artificial larynx. The air pulses from the trachea into the artificial larynx can easily be demonstrated by kymograms (Cf. Fig. 15, CT). When the tube from the artificial larynx leads the air flow and tone into the front of the mouth the movements of the articulations and the shaping of the mouth produce the consonants and vowels just as they did before the operation when the

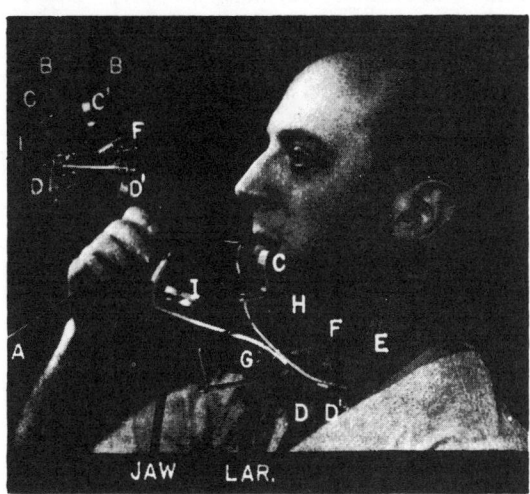 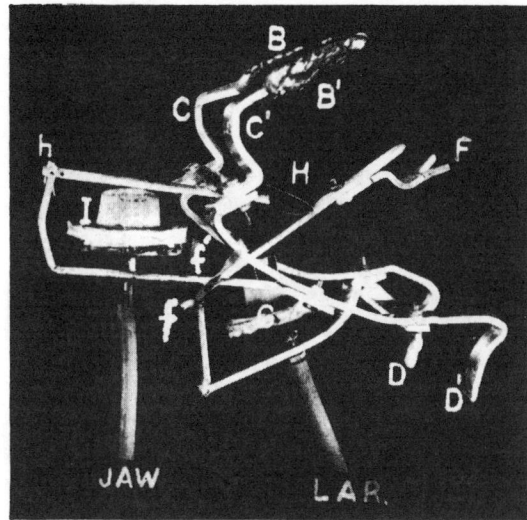

FIGURE 5. Jaw- and Larynx-Recorder

A —Tube for mouth pressure.
B, B'—Teeth grip for the upper anchorage of frame.
D, D'—Rests on the clavicles for lower support of frame.
C, C'—Frame supporting jaw- and larynx-levers.
E —Neck band.
F —Lever recording vertical movements of larynx.
F—Fulcrum for larynx lever.
G—Tambour for larynx movement connected with recording tambour of kymograph.
H—Lever recording movement of jaw.
I—Tambour for jaw movement connected with recording tambour of kymograph.

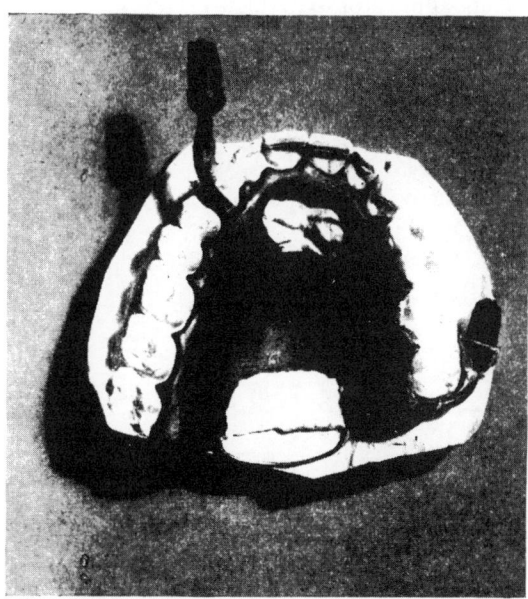

FIGURE 6. Artificial Palate with Windows for Recording Front and Rear Tongue Strokes on Kymograph

The two windows are shown when not covered with distended membrane. The front window opens directly onto palate. The rear window is extended by a wire loop.

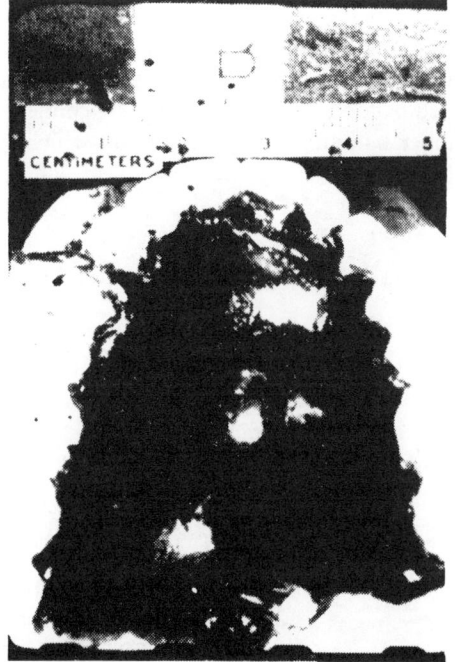

FIGURE 7. The entire surface of the artificial palate is covered with a rubber membrane coated with pigment

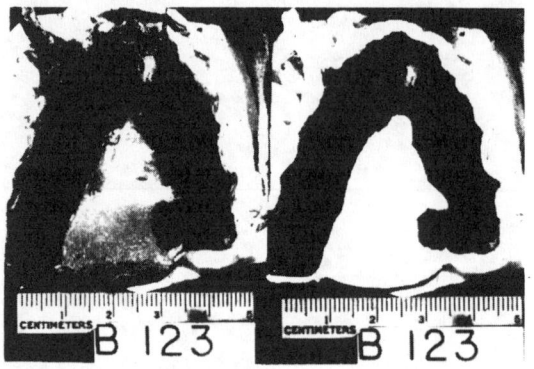

FIGURE 8. The surface on the artificial palate after the tongue stroke
The right hand figure has been cleared for better definition.

air flow and tone came into the mouth through the intact larynx. Although the reed of the artificial larynx is not subject to manipulation, the subject easily learns to control its vibration by adjusting the pressures above and below so as to start and stop the air flow through the reed.

2. Chest pulses recorded from a gastric balloon. The subjects swallowed a small rubber balloon which was then inflated and rose to contact with the diaphragm; a small rubber tube led to the recording tambour; the pressure of the inflated balloon was compensated by connecting a rubber balloon in a flask outside which was inflated to ca. 200 mm. water pressure; a septum was introduced into the tube leading to the recording tambour. The pneumatic tracings of the transmitted pulses parallel precisely the tracings taken directly of the air pressure pulses in the trachea (Cf. Fig. 16 GB).

3. Chest pulses recorded through the body wall. Indirect records of the changes of pressure within the chest can be obtained by means of an applicator placed on the chest- or abdominal wall and held in position by negative pressure. Tracings thus obtained parallel very closely those obtained by means of either the tracheal tube or the gastric balloon. The method has the advantage of not requiring specially selected subjects. Tracheotomized patients are relatively rare, and subjects have to be trained to swallow the gastric balloon.

The most responsive area for placement of the negative pressure applicator proved to be the epigastric region. Here the rectus abdominis musculature fans out leaving a relatively thin-walled area. Tracings have been obtained however from various areas over the entire trunk. A shallow aluminum cup with a narrow flange at the rim shaped to fit the contour of the body wall serves as an applicator (Cf. Fig. 1 CE, Fig. 11 E). Aluminum funnels are convenient material for the construction of such applicators. The applicator is held in place by a light negative pressure of 300 to 600 mm. of water provided by a siphon respirator (Cf. Fig. 11, A, C).

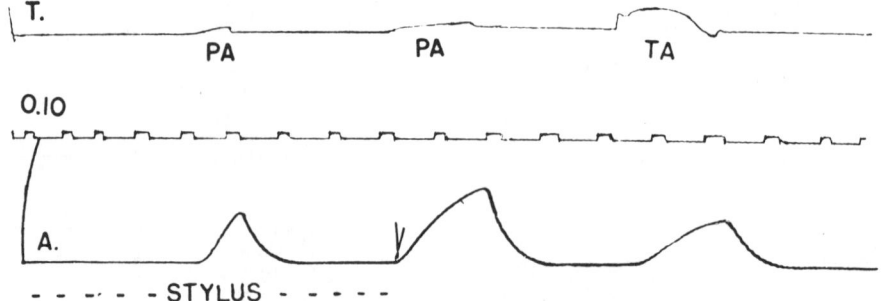

FIGURE 9. Artificial Palate Arranged for Recording Contacts on Kymograph
  T—Tongue marker slightly affected by the buccal pressure of the labials.
  Duration of the consonant of *ta* is clearly defined.
  A—Air pressure in mouth; stress is on *pa pa'* ta.
  The one record of the tongue contact for *ta* shows on the pigmented surface of artificial palate, Fig. 8.

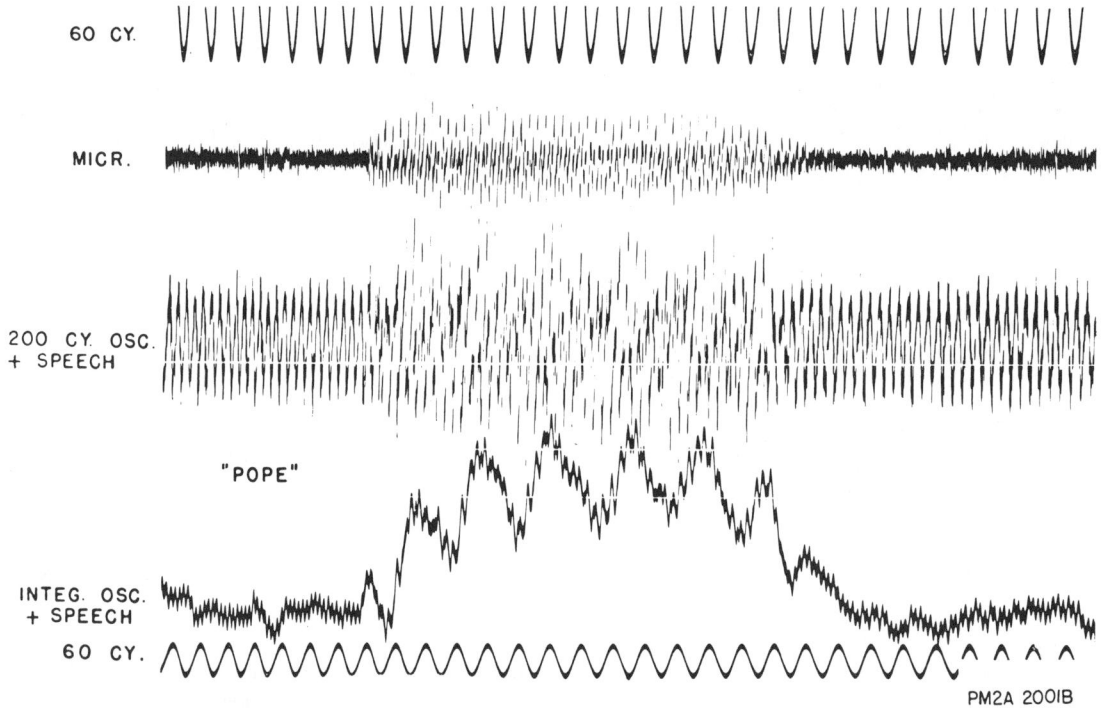

FIGURE 10. Interference Patterns of the Fundamental Cycles of Vowel
Syllable *pope* showing the interference patterns of the fundamental cycles of the vowel o. The integrated curve shows that the "cycles" are very irregular in duration.

Tubing with heavy walls connected the applicator with the aspirator, and the recording tambour. Between the applicator and the aspirator was a tiny check-valve made by grinding smooth the end of a bit of heavy-walled glass tubing and attaching a disk of very thin rubber over the lumen of the tube with a bit of rubber cement applied at one point. The valve was set to close when the pressure in the applicator fell below that of the aspirator. The check valve may be replaced by a capillary tube (Cf. Fig. 11, D).

In the transmission line between the applicator and the recording tambour a septum of thin rubber under tension was introduced into the tube to withstand the negative pressure; the distended, elastic septum balanced the negative pressure, so that the pressure was neutral in the section of the tube leading directly from the septum to the recording tambour. This makes a more sensitive recording system than is possible if the negative pressure is transmitted to the recording tambour. A convenient form of septum consisted of a rubber diaphragm stretched over the mouth of a thistle tube 3–6 cm. diameter; the thistle tube was inserted in a funnel and cemented in place with plastocene (Cf. Fig. 11, F). Hudgins has obtained good negative pressure tracings by connecting the applicator directly with a pneumodeik (34); the negative pressure in the line is balanced by a light coiled spring attached to the metallic diaphragm.

Any pulse transmitted through the tissues to the surface on which the applicator is placed affects the recording tambour. It is not the bulging of the surface under the applicator which gives the variation in volume. Instead the flattened edge of the applicator, slightly embedded in the yielding tissue, is thrown out by the pulse. The pulse causes an increase in the volume of the applicator and reduces the pressure further, and the change is recorded by the stylus. The sensitivity of the system can be tested by tapping on the chest wall; often the heart beat is recorded even when the applicator is applied to the lower rib cage or to the abdomen.

If a fairly large, triangular applicator is attached to the epigastrium, it is not affected by

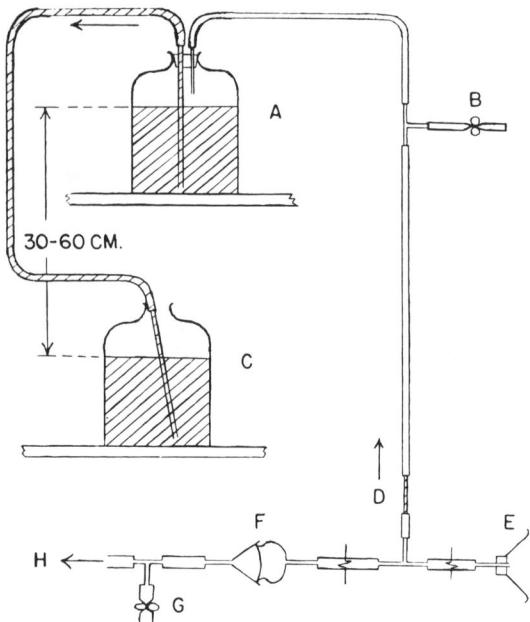

FIGURE 11. Simple Device for Negative Pressure
The slight vacuum is developed in the line E to F. F provides an elastic septum so that the line F to H, recording tambour, is maintained with neutral pressure.

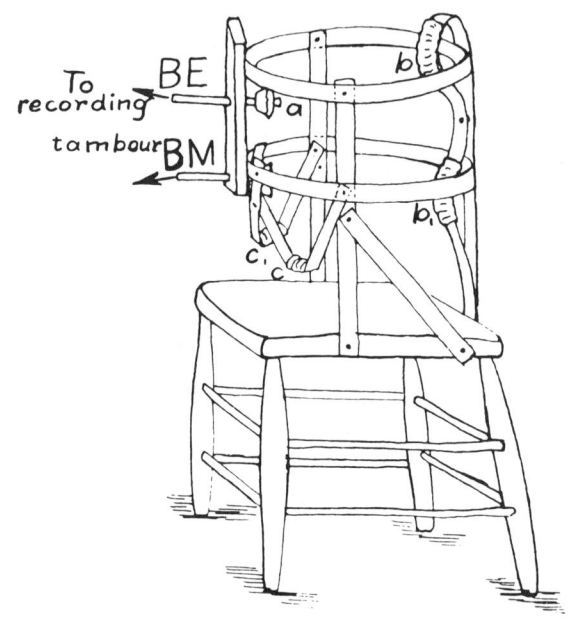

FIGURE 12. Chair for Recording Movements of Body Wall. Cf. Fig. 1
The spine is supported at b and b'.
The upper legs are anchored at c and c'.
BE, BM—The bosses are supported independent of the body wall.

the gross movements of the muscles and it is possible to get rather simple and clear tracings of the chest pulses; the fixation of the abdominal muscles is likely to interfere at rapid rates. At the navel level a large, oval applicator with the longer axis across the rectus abdominis will often give simple chest-pulse tracings, unaffected by the large abdominal contractions which move the applicator bodily without producing a record.

The detailed correspondence of tracings made from these negative pressure applicators to the tracings of the variations of air pressure within the chest is surprising; not only do the individual pulses appear but also the groupings of the pulses which are a marked feature of the air pressure tracings. Cf. tracings of the air pressure in chest with negative pressure tracings (87, p. 114-116, 206; 91, Figs. 17 and 21).

4. Oscillograph recording of action potentials. Action potentials from the muscles can be made to give direct records of the actual contractions of the intercostals which originate the syllable pulse. The placement of the electrodes for simultaneous recording of the muscles involved in speech is shown in Fig. 14.

With proper amplification it is possible to get simultaneous oscillographic tracings of the contractions of the various groups of muscles. For details of electrodes, amplification, and procedure, cf. 9, 79, 90.

The oscillograms show clearly the separate pulses of the intercostal muscles, and the grouped contractions, especially at rapid rates, of the abdominal muscles (breath groups). (85, p. 9, Fig. 3, p. 37, Fig. 4, 38)

There has been an exaggerated notion of the authority of an oscillogram. Any precision of the oscillogram must derive from a like precision of the contraction of the controlled muscles of the speech apparatus.

Movements of the Abdominal Muscles for the Foot and Breath Group

1. Tracings of the positive movement of the body wall in a given spot.

The apparatus (see Figs. 1 and 12) records the detail of the movements of the body wall in a

METHODS AND APPARATUS IN EXPERIMENTAL PHONETICS 43

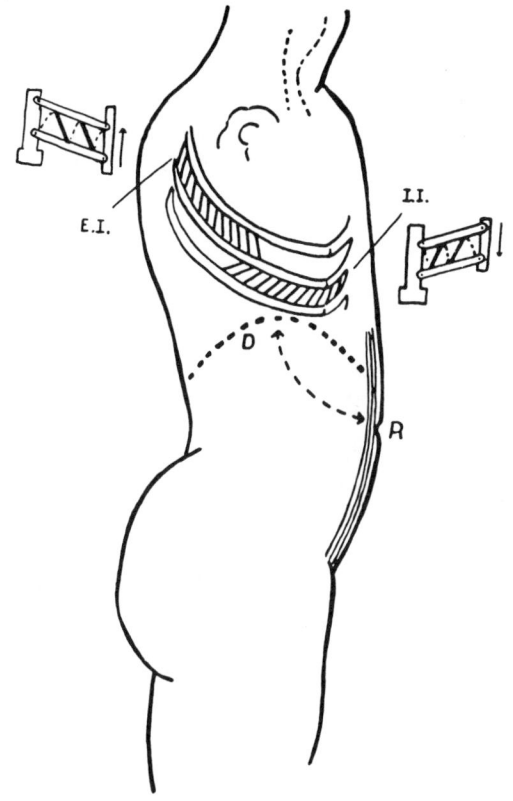

FIGURE 13. Diagram of the Two Musculatures of Speech
Chest pulse musculature:
E I—The External Intercostals which act to raise ribs in inspiration.
 I I—The Internal Intercostals which act to lower the ribs in expiration.
 These muscles act in opposition in the chest pulse.
Breath group musculature:
 R—The abdominal muscles led by the Rectus which exert pressure on the diaphragm through the liquid mass of viscera.
 D—Diaphragm which opposes abdominal muscles. Muscle of inspiration.
 These muscles act in opposition to produce the pulses of the foot and of the breath group.

given region. The tambour applied to the moving surface consisted of a thistle tube which was partly filled with parafin, leaving a cavity of ca. 1 cm. in diameter and 1.5 cm. in depth; the thistle tube was covered with a tense, thin rubber membrane. A boss of cork 2 cm. long and 8 mm. in diameter was attached to the center of the membrane, and rested directly against the chest-

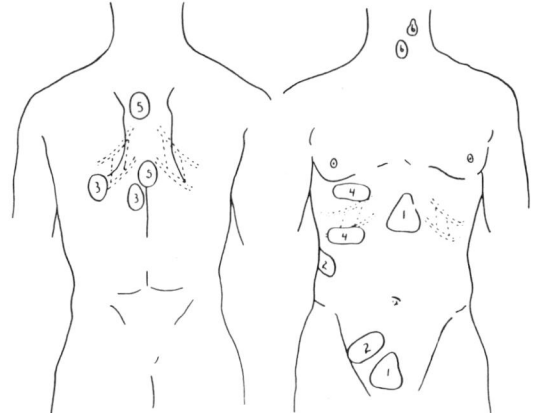

FIGURE 14. Placement of Electrodes for Recording Action Currents of the Muscles of Speech
1—1 Rectus abdominis.
2—2 Lateral muscles of abdomen.
3—3 Diaphragm.
4—4 Internal Intercostals.
5—5 External Intercostals.
6—6 Internal muscles of larynx.

or abdominal wall. The free end of the boss was pressed against the body wall until the other end forced the membrane back into the cavity. The tension of the membrane kept the boss in contact with body wall as it receded in the process of expiration during speech. A T-tube with a clamp introduced into the line leading to the recording tambour permitted the equalization of pressure within the system after the boss had been adjusted in position. Tests show that such tambours will respond to 25-30 movements per sec.

Such tambours must be supported independent of the body wall on a rigid frame not attached to the subject. Various types have been used: chair (Fig. 12) with heavy metal strap to which supports could be bolted; and several forms of "stanchion" are figured in cuts. The stanchion (Fig. 1) provided two adjustable points of support for the spine, and a vertical rod to which the applicators and the tubes for chest and abdomen could be attached. Such a frame accommodates the subject standing or sitting.

The contraction of the musculature of the body wall will cause an *outward* movement, although the resulting compression produces an expiratory pulse. During the larger breathing movement of the phrase, however, the abdominal walls and the rib cage show a gradual recession, followed by the inflation due to the inspiration for the next phrase.

2. Negative pressure tracings of the pulses of the feet and breath groups. (The method is described, p. 40, 41.)

When properly placed on the abdomen a negative pressure applicator records the pulses of the feet and the breath groups which originate in the abdominal musculature. It is possible, with care, to place one applicator on the abdominal wall so that it records primarily the foot and breath-group pulses. A simultaneous tracing of the chest pulses of the syllables is necessary to show the timing of the syllables in the foot and breath group movement, so that the coordination of the constituent syllables in the foot and breath group can be studied.

3. Oscillograms of the action potentials from the abdominal musculature. (The method is described, p. 42.)

Electrodes were placed on the abdominal muscles, the intercostals, and in the proper area for the diaphragm, so that contractions of the intercostals for the chest pulses and the contractions of abdominal muscles for the foot and breath-group pulses could be recorded simultaneously. As the action-potential method is the one way to get the detail of the intercostal contractions for the chest pulses of the syllable, the simultaneous recording of the abdominal contractions is of primary importance for the study of the detail of the coordination of larger units with the constituent syllables.

Action of the Larynx

The methods of recording laryngeal vibrations directly from the walls of the larynx have been described by Rousselot p. 97. It is important for some purposes to have a direct recording showing the incidence and duration of the laryngeal tone. Electric applicators can be used to pick up the tone. The same purpose can be served, however, by tracings of the air pressures both inside and outside of the mouth. (33)

Vertical movements of the larynx have proved to be significant factors in the articulation of surd and sonant *stops*. To record these movements the recording lever must be rigidly supported independent of other moving parts. Hudgins and Stetson (35), using a modified version of the apparatus described by Rosapelly (70, p. 98) and Zwaardemaker (107, p. 357), succeeded in anchoring the supporting device firmly to the clavicles below and the upper jaw above. Sen, using the same device in Hudgins' Laboratory (77) at the Clarke School, studied the vertical movements of the larynx as a factor in differentiating between aspirated and non-aspirated *stops* in Bengali dialects.

Articulatory Processes. Contacts of Articulatory Members to Opposing Surfaces

Movements of the articulatory organs may be recorded in terms of their contacts with the opposing surfaces. Such records give important clues to the action and timing of the articulatory member, both with relation to the syllable pulse from the chest and with relation to other articulatory members. Contacts of the lips, lips and teeth, and tongue with the alveolar ridge and with the hard palate were recorded by means of lip- and tongue-markers.

Lip- and tongue-markers were constructed to record the strokes of lip and tongue in the production of the consonants. The markers were made with a thin wedge-shaped cross-section. It is essential that they be very sensitive but that they do not collapse, whatever the pressure. Lip markers were constructed of thin mica bound at the thin edge of the wedge with thin "fish-skin" (animal membrane) fastened with rubber cement, and with sides of "fish-skin". Another satisfactory form which became routine was made by stretching very thin rubber tightly over a flat steel wire loop of the proper shape, the ends of which were thrust into a flattened cork which constituted the thick end of the wedge. The cork received the small tube leading to the kymograph. The thin wedge of taut rubber was coated repeatedly with ricinated collodion. The collodion dried to a wall more rigid than the rubber which was merely a temporary support for the collodion wall.

The tongue-markers also were constructed with a collodion wall laid on over taut rubber. The frame of flattened steel wire was shaped to a plaster cast of the subject's palate, and thin rubber was stretched over the wire frame mounted so as to make a thin wedge. The wall next to the palate was repeatedly coated with collodion until quite rigid; the surface receiving the stroke of the tongue was given one or two coatings to make a firm but resilient wall. The tube from the tongue-marker was led out through a convenient gap in the teeth. The tongue- and lip-markers stand use better if the edges at the wire are bound with narrow strips of "fish-skin" laid into the first moist coat of collodion (Cf. Fig. 2).

It did not prove possible to get satisfactory tracings with lenticular rubber bulbs, or with capsules of thin, taut rubber such as Rousselot used; they do not respond to the rapid variations of pressure, and the tracing of the double or of the abutting consonants does not show the two maxima. Lip- and tongue-markers must respond to fluctuations of 25 per sec. The tongue-tip trill is a convenient signal for testing recording apparatus up to 30-40 per sec.

The wedge-shaped markers with resilient walls were thin enough so that they did not introduce a thickness of more than a millimeter between the lips or between the tongue and the palate. These markers and their fittings had, of course, to be kept air-tight; a leak betrays itself very quickly in the tracing. The tongue-marker must fit the palate; a layer of dental wax may be necessary so that air does not pass to falsify a tracing of outside air made concurrent with a tracing of the tongue strokes. The lip- and tongue-markers, the mouth pressure tubes, and the mask for outside air were held in position by the subject. (Fig. 2.)

The tracing of the consonant can be called a record of the consonant movement only in so far as the movement of the consonant results in contact of lip or tongue with the opposing surface. In general, the tracing is a record of consonant contacts, with the variations of pressure. The tracings of the consonant contacts for abutting consonants (including doubles) delineate the back stroke of the arresting doublet and the beat stroke of the releasing doublet which occur in contact and at rapid rate. It was in this case that Rousselot's apparatus failed to respond.

Contacts of the tongue for the lingual consonants have also been recorded by a method that employs the familiar artificial palate. The original purpose of this device was the combination of the palatographic and the kymographic methods of recording (92). The modified artificial palate, however, may be readily employed to replace the tongue markers described above for recording lingual contacts both in the anterior and posterior areas of the mouth. Artificial palates molded to fit the palates of the individual subjects were made of vulcanite following the dentist's technique. Two "windows" were cut in the finished mold, one in the region of the alveolar ridge, the other at the posterior edge of the hard palate. Thin walled phosphor bronze tubes, 1.5 mm. diam. were shaped to fit the contour of the palate and embedded in the vulcanite during the process of vulcanizing. The tubes provided outlets for the "windows" within the palate with their outer ends leading to rubber tubes connected to recording tambours. (Figs. 2 A, 6, 7.)

The windows were covered on the upper surface in contact with the hard palate, with a layer of animal membrane reinforced with a heavy layer of collodion to give them a rigid backing. The "windows" were covered on the lower side with which the tongue comes in contact by a membrane of condom rubber. A thin coating of collodion adds resiliency to the membrane of these windows which become capsules formed in the wall of the artificial palate. The rapid strokes of the tongue for the front linguals "t, d, n, s", and "l" and the posterior linguals "k, g, and ng", strike the flexible membranes of the capsules and the contacts are recorded. (Fig. 1, Stetson, Hudgins & Moses, Pal. changes, 1940.) (92, Fig. 1.) Figs. 6 and 7 show the artificial palate lying in a cast of the subject's upper jaw. The dotted lines of Fig. 2 A indicate the position of a metal tube which may be used to record the air pressure behind the consonant constriction along with the contact. Figures 8 and 9 (Stetson, Hudgins & Moses) show a palatogram-kymogram combination obtained simultaneously by this method.

Recording Air-Pressures

The pressure changes in the chest are direct functions of the action of the breathing muscles. The chest pressure is only slightly affected by the articulatory processes which occur above the larynx. Records of chest pressure changes during speech obtained by methods described above show only minor differences in amplitude for syllables having consonants and vowels, as compared with syllables having vowels alone. (Fig. 18, 19, 20, 21.)

Pressures above the larynx, on the other hand, although due to the chest pulse for the most part, are radically modified by the articulatory processes. Hence tracings that show the pressure changes above the larynx taken simultaneously with pressure changes below the larynx provide important clues to articulatory processes.

Kymograph recording of the pressure just outside the mouth has been a standard procedure since Rosapelly and Rousselot. The technique of Rousselot was modified in that the volume of the mouthpiece was increased and an escape for air provided. A firm rubber mouthpiece was fitted about the mouth, with an elastic border which did not interfere with the movements of jaw and lips. The border was made elastic by slicing the edge into a comb; the border was made air-tight by cementing the wrist section of a rubber glove inside the mouth-piece and turning the cuff out over the sliced edge. The mouthpiece had a volume of ca. 200 cc., and ventilation was always provided in the mouthpiece and sometimes near the recording tambour to be rid of reverberation and to prevent the air pressure from backing up while speaking. The tube leading to the recording tambour was large (1 to 1.5 cm.). The recording tambour was of very thin, taut rubber, diam. of 5 cm. The mouthpiece was pierced to provide for lip- and tongue-markers and for the mouth-pressure tube at the corner of the mouth. The range of oscillation provided was larger than that of Rousselot's tracings of outside pressure. Rousselot's rather rigid membrane was intended to show sound waves. These tracings were intended to show variations of pressure rather than sound vibration. However, the sound vibrations were usually present in one of the three tracings: 1) of the consonant, 2) the mouth pressure, or 3) the outside pressure. The tracings of pressure just outside the mouth are not comparable to tracings of pressure in the chest; the constriction of the larynx and the variations of mouth volume make the series unlike.

Tracings of air pressure from the nose, which indicate the action of the velum, were recorded by the familiar nasal olives. This is a standard practice in experimental phonetics. Usually a single olive, a small blown glass bulb open at both ends which fits snugly into the nostril, gives an adequate record of the pressure changes in the nose. The single olive does not completely obstruct the air flow from the nasal cavity, and thus interferes less with the normal speech process, than do olives in both nostrils.

Tracings of air pressure changes inside the mouth provide records of another important aspect of the process of articulation. Pressures build up behind the constrictions of both the releasing and the arresting consonants. The rate of rise of this pressure, its maximum amplitude, and the terminal shape of the pressure curves provide significant information. A record of the inside air pressure (A in the records) is readily obtained by inserting a small metal tube into the mouth so that it taps the oral cavity behind the consonant constriction. The tube is placed so that it does not interfere with the consonant constriction. It may enter the mouth at the corner for a recording of the labial and front lingual consonants. In order to tap the pressures behind the posterior sounds "k and g", however, the tube must reach well back into the mouth. For this purpose a tube is laid along outside the lower molars and curved sharply at the end to enter the oral cavity posterior to the last molar. The dotted line, Fig. 2 A, illustrates the position of the tube. Indeed, the pressures for all of the consonants can be recorded with the tube in this position and there is practically no interference with the articulatory processes.

Recording the Movements of the Jaw

The movement of the lower jaw plays an important role in both the shaping of the vowel cavities and in the articulation of consonants. In ordinary speech a rapid opening of the jaw occurs with each vowel (syllable). For the syllables with vowels having a narrow front orifice the jaw movement is of small amplitude but none the less present, while for the syllables with open vowels the movement of the jaw is relatively large. There is evidence also that the jaw is a factor in the articulation of labial consonants. Studies of the maximum rate of movement of articulatory organs have shown that the jaw is capable of a higher rate than the rate of the lips with the jaw fixated. The implication is that at rapid rates of syllable utterance the jaws carry the lips in the articulation of labial consonants. (36)

Records of jaw movements are readily obtained by several methods. The simplest device supports the active recording element on a rigid pair of plastic spectacle frames. The recording element is similar in structure to the rubber-covered coiled-spring pneumograph commonly used in recording respiration in physiological laboratories; but it is much smaller and more delicate. A coiled spring 10 cm. in length and 1.5 cm. in diameter was covered with thin-walled rubber tubing made of either condom rubber or of surgical drainage tubes. Cork stoppers, into which the ends of the spring were inserted, serve both for the attachment of the tubing and for the introduction of a glass tube outlet to the connecting rubber tube of the recording tambour. The ends of the recorder are attached to the eyeglass frame and to a tape looped under the chin with a slight tension when the mouth is closed. Movements of the lower jaw distend the "pneumograph" longitudinally, inducing pressure changes which are communicated to the recording tambour.

Methods of Recording Vowels

There has been some instrumental observation of jaw movements, and of the position of the tongue with simple apparatus; but the bulk of the recording of vowels and of vocalization has been done with acoustic apparatus.

Physiological

The artificial palate has been used to delineate the position of the tongue where it is in contact with the hard palate; this gives a slight indication of the differences in position for the vowel.

Direct measurements with disks have been used to show the fundamental tongue positions. (20)

Extensive X-ray studies have been made of the longitudinal section of the vocal canal during the utterance of a vowel. The median line of the tongue is indicated by a metal cord or chain, and a barium paste outlines the surfaces. (73, 74)

The reciprocal relations of the front and back orifices in the utterances of the vowels were demonstrated by Marichelle, in an unpublished study, in which the front orifice was defined by wedges between the teeth, and the back orifice was gauged by use of the artificial palate.

Acoustic

The acoustic analysis in the main has been concerned with the modulation of partials by the varying cavities. The vowel has been treated as an acoustic quality, though it is usually recognized that the basic explanation must be in terms of cavities and movements.

Much of the work by Helmholtz, Stumpf, D. C. Miller, Crandall, Gemelli has been done with prolonged vowels; the vowel has reached an approximately steady state, and the analysis by Fourier's or Vercelli's method has seemed adequate. A system of one and two "formants" has been worked out and has general vogue.

But it is apparent that the usual vowel of actual speech does not come to a steady state; and the fact that the vocal folds constitute a "relaxation oscillator", in which there is a damping or accelerating factor in each cycle, makes the application of a mathematical method out of the question.

There is nevertheless an acoustic modification of the sound complex which issues from the larynx. It may be that interference and absorption play a part along with resonance.

It is possible to segment the vowel, and show that the vowel quality inheres in the beginning, the middle and the end of the acoustic pattern. Playing back the same vowel of two identical variable-density films on two photoelectric playbacks, in varying phases, reversing one of the films so that the end of the one film of the vowel is heard along with the beginning of the other film of the vowel, or mixing the segments of the vowel, do not affect the vowel quality.

Potter and his colleagues at the Bell Telephone Laboratories have shown that the sound spectrum which consists largely of "white noise" is radically modulated by cavities and movements. They have noted empirically the regions in the spectrum most subject to this modulation. It is especially noteworthy that their recordings show the changes of the beginning and end of the vowel due to the opening and closing of the orifices made by consonant constrictions. The "kinks" in the 'bars' representing the zones of modulation are due to the position of the opening or closing consonant constriction, and define the consonant as front (lip), median (front tongue), or posterior (back tongue). (42, 43, 64, 82)

ANALYSIS AND INTERPRETATION OF THE RECORDS FROM THE PROCESS OF THE SPEECH MECHANISM

Pneumatic Recording Systems

The various systems which employ pneumatic kymograph recording must include a recording member. For much of the work the recording tambours were of rubber. For the lip- and tongue-markers, and for the negative pressure tracings, they were small, 1-1.5 cm., flexible but not elastic. Perished rubber, or rubber in which a permanent dimple had been made by deforming the sheet rubber over a boss of the size of the diaphragm, was used. The rubber was derived from condoms, and the "animal membrane" used was from "fish-skin" condoms. The recording diaphragms for the air pressure tubes and for the other applicators were taut rubber of 5-8 cm. diameter. The recording parts of the commercial Marey tambours were rebuilt. The recording stylus and the post vertical to the membrane were made of light bamboo. The writing stylus was short, ca. 6 cm., pivoted on an axle made of the tip of a small cambric needle and tipped with a glass or thin celluloid film; mass was reduced to a minimum and vibration and overthrow were eliminated by damping.

Reference marks were made at the beginning of each series to show the exact vertical relation of the stylus tips: these marks were used in determining simultaneous points. All tracings were taken with a time line from either a small 50-per-sec. fork, or a Jacquet time marker giving fifths of a second. In measuring the tracings these fifths were divided into tenths and the hundredths estimated. The measurements were made with a protractor in reference to the nearest fifth indicated by the time line. Thus the unit of measurement was 0.02 sec., with fractions estimated. This is sufficiently minute for the purpose and as close as the limits of error of the method warrant.

It is important to note that in making such records the pneumatic transmission at such rates consists of a low-pitched sound wave, a travelling condensation-rarefaction, not an air flow. There is no measurable lag in such apparatus, the volume of air is not important, but tubing with rigid wall and smooth bore and with few or no sharp angles is important; rarely reverberations may give difficulty. These can be filtered out by inserting lengths of capillary tube in the transmission lines (8).

Many of the later recordings were made with a substitute for the Marey tambour, the pneumodeik, which was developed in the course of the work in phonetic recording. The pneumodeik, with its metal diaphragm, is durable, needs little attention, and is sensitive enough for practically all recording. It is not quite as sensitive as a small, loose rubber diaphragm in skilled hands. But since it is quite stable, and can be calibrated, it has been used extensively in the laboratories of both Stetson and Hudgins (34).

Processing of Kymographic Tracings

The figures in the text are photographic reproductions of the kymograph tracings. It is now convenient, with reversible film negatives, to make photographic prints from smoked paper with black lines on white ground. These prints were produced by using the smoked paper itself as the negative. The ground was cleared in some cases. Often both negatives and positives were made of a very "hard" thin printing paper, clearing by managing exposure and development. In a few cases the time line has been retouched, but all other tracings have not been retouched.

A number of subjects were always used, and a large number of measurements were made of each type of record. The kymograph sheets used for cuts were not mutilated, and the entire series of records taken is filed for convenient reference, and has proved valuable. The detail of procedure, and of the apparatus used, was written on the smoked sheets, usually before they were fixed; and, if necessary, notes were added during the measuring process.

If records are made and preserved in large quantities, the method of handling becomes important. A type of thin "label" paper has been used, selected by testing so that it would not curl when dipped in alcohol. The records are attached about the drum with as little starch paste as possible; the later bath in alcohol granulates the paste and it gives no trouble; mucilages are to be avoided.

The kymograms were fixed by passing them face down across the surface of the fixative, without wetting the back of the sheet. The fixative consisted of a solution of bleached shellac in alcohol, with a cc. or so of glycerin or sorbitol, and a little castor-oil, per litre. The solution is kept as dilute as possible. It is tested occasionally, as it evaporates, with fresh smoked paper. There should be barely enough shellac to fix the smoke so that it will not rub off. Such a record is thin and flexible and convenient for filing. It will dry in a minute or so and is ready for immediate study. The reference lines for measurement, and any further comments, are scratched in the fixed smoke with small chisels ground out of No. 5 needles. Care is taken that these etched lines do not cross any tracing of the record. The records are labeled, each one in full, and adequate titles written in large at the top of the record. They are filed vertically in modified filing cases, with labeled manila dividers, so that they can be easily consulted. Many questions can be answered by an inspection of a series of records side by side.

For some of the later recording, "Teledeltos" paper has been used in a polygraph. It is excellent for photographing; annotations can be made in pencil or in ink. The paper is furnished by the Western Union Telegraph Company and can be used with any form of kymograph or polygraph.

Syllables, both open and closed, when in series, have been measured from the détente of the releasing consonant to the détente of the initial consonant of the next syllable. Isolated syllables, if closed, have been measured from the détente of the releasing consonant to the détente of the arresting consonant; if open, from the détente of the releasing consonant to the end of the vowel. This method of measuring syllables accords best with other studies, and has the advantage of giving an accurate rate per sec., and of eliminating the erratic length of contact of the initial consonant of a group or series.

In the tracings the letters and combinations have their usual English values. The vowels are the English short vowels unless otherwise indicated. Occasionally digraphs are used for a single vowel: "*ee*" or "*ea* = *long* "*e*" (tea); "*ay*" = long "*a*" (pay).

Reading the Tracings of Motor Phonetics

It is essential to read the evidence for an experimental phonetics in the actual data presented; only a little can be put in the form of phonetic characters, and statistics. The actual events and their concurrence can only be presented in the form of annotated simultaneous tracings. Great pains have been taken to label the tracings in full and to supply them with legends.

The kymograph tracings represent both 1) movements and contracts, and 2) changing air pressures, by means of the rise and fall of line tracings.

1. A positive stroke to contact, the increase in pressure of the lips or tongue, the opening of the jaw, the bulge of a muscle, the rise and expansion of the chest are all marked by the rise of the curve; the reverse, of the stroke leaving contact, the diminishing pressure, the closing of the jaw, the recession of chest or abdominal wall, are all marked by the fall of the curve.

2. In the chest (C), the mouth (A), and outside the mouth (AO), rising air pressure is indicated by a rising curve and falling air pressure by a falling curve. If the pressure becomes negative, as in the intake of air, the air pressure curve falls below the base line.

The oscillograph and microphone tracings indicate intensity by variations in amplitudes; in some cases a volume meter has been used. It is important to note that the level of ground noise due to minor disturbances is well below threshold.

In action-current recordings there is usually some leakage of the stronger muscle pulses into the tracings of neighboring muscles. This is noted in the legends of the figures.

Constant reference to the time line is important. Any change which occurs within an interval of 0.05 sec. must be discontinuous and figure as a stroke, not a changing shape. Simple movements at a maximum of 10/sec. consist of beat- and back-strokes of 0.05 secs. each. 2.5-3 per sec. is the upper limit for a series of syllables with abutting or doubling consonants ("*put-put-put-, pup-pup-pup-*"). (Cf. Appendix X: Demarcation of Syllables.)

SUGGESTED READINGS

This is a selective list of references to observational techniques used in speech production research. The classification scheme should not be taken too seriously, as many of the measurement devices (e.g., strain gauges) may be used in multiple applications.

Cineradiography/Cinefluorography

Houde, R. A. (1968). A study of tongue body motion during selected speech sounds. *SCRL Monograph 2*, Speech Communications Research Laboratory, Santa Barbara, CA.

Kent, R. D., Carney, P. J., & Severeid, L. R. (1974). Velar movement and timing: Evaluation of a model for binary control. *Journal of Speech and Hearing Research, 17*, 470-488.

Moll, K. L. (1960). Cinefluorographic techniques in speech research. *Journal of Speech and Hearing Research, 3*, 227-241.

Perkell, J. S. (1969). *Physiology of speech production: Results and implications of a quantitative cineradiographic study.* Cambridge, MA: MIT Press.

Electroglottography

Childers, D., & Krishnamurthy, A. K. (1985). A critical review of electroglottography. *CRC Critical Reviews in Biomedical Engineering, 12*, 131-161.

Fant, G., Ondrackova, J., Lindqvist, J., & Sonesson, B. (1966). Electrical glottography. *Quarterly Status and Progress Report (Speech Transmission Laboratory, Royal Institute of Technology, Stockholm), 4*, 15-21.

Fourcin, A. (1974). Laryngographic examination of vocal fold vibration. In B. Wyke (Ed.), *Ventilatory and phonatory control systems.* London: Oxford University Press.

Electromagnetic Devices

Hixon, T. J. (1971). An electromagnetic method for transducing jaw movement during speech. *Journal of the Acoustical Society of America, 49*, 603-606.

Perkell, J. S., & Cohen, M. H. (1986). An alternating magnetic field system for tracking multiple speech articulatory movements in the midsagittal plane. *Technical Report, 512, Research Laboratory of Electronics*, MIT, Cambridge, MA.

Schonle, P. W., Wenig, P., Schrader, J., Grabe, K., Brockmann, E., & Conrad, B. (1983). Ein elektromagnetisches verfahren zur simultanen registrierung von bewegungen im bereich des lippen- unterkeifer- und zungensystems. *Biomed. Technik, 28*, 263-267.

Electromyography

Basmajian, J. V., & Deluca, C. J. (1985). *Muscles Alive* (5th ed.). Baltimore: Williams & Wilkins.

Bouisset, S., & Morton, D. (1973). Comparison between surface and intermuscular EMG during voluntary movement. In J. E. Desmedt (Ed.), *New developments in electromyography and clinical neurophysiology. Vol. 1.* Basel: S. Karger.

Harris, K. S. (1981). Electromyography as a technique for laryngeal investigation. In C. L. Ludlow & M. D. Hart (Eds.), *Proceedings of the conference on the assessment of vocal pathology.* ASHA Reports 11, 116-124.

Hirose, H., Gay, T., & Strome, M. (1971). Electrode insertion techniques for laryngeal electromyography. *Journal of the Acoustical Society of America, 50*, 1449-1450.

Loeb, G. E., & Gans, C. (1986). *Electromyography for experimentalists.* Chicago: University of Chicago Press.

Fiberoptic Viewing

Fujimura, O., Baer, T. & Niimi, S. (1979). A stereofiberscope with a magnetic interlens bridge for laryngeal observation. *Journal of the Acoustical Society of America, 65*, 478-480.

Sawashima, M. & Hirose, H. (1968). A new laryngoscopic technique by use of fiberoptics. *Journal of the Acoustical Society of America, 43*, 168-169.

General Instrumentation References

Abbs, J. H. & Watkins, K. L. (1976). Instrumentation for the study of speech physiology. In N. J. Lass (Ed.), *Contemporary issues in experimental phonetics* (pp. 41-78). New York: Academic Press.

Borden, G. & Harris, K. S. (1984). *Speech science primer*, (2nd ed.). Baltimore: Williams & Wilkins.

Magnetic Resonance Imaging

Baer, T., Gore, J. C., Boyce, S., & Nye, P. W. (1987). Application of MRI to the analysis of speech production. *Magnetic Resonance Imaging 5, 1*, 1-7.

Palatography

Fletcher, S. G., McCutcheon, M. J., & Wolf, M. B. (1975). Dynamic palatometry. *Journal of Speech and Hearing Research, 18*, 812-819.

Photoelectric Methods for Glottis, Larynx, or Velar Port (Transillumination)

Ewan, W., & Krones, R. (1974). Measuring larynx movement using the thyroumbrometer. *Journal of Phonetics, 2*, 327–335.

Frøkjaer-Jensen, B. (1967). A photo-electric glottograph. *Annual Report of the Institute of Phonetics of the University of Copenhagen, 2*, 5–19.

Lisker, L., Abramson, A. S., Cooper, F. S., & Schvey, M. H. (1969). Transillumination of the larynx in running speech. *Journal of the Acoustical Society of America, 45*, 1544–1546.

Photoelectric Methods for Lips or Jaw

Kelso, J. A. S., Bateson, E., Saltzman, E. L., & Kay, B. (1985). A qualitative dynamic analysis of reiterant speech production: Phase portraits, kinematics, and dynamic modeling. *Journal of the Acoustical Society of America, 77*, 266–280.

Tuller, B., & Kelso, J. A. S. (1984). The timing of articulatory gestures: Evidence for relational invariants. *Journal of the Acoustical Society of America, 76*, 1030–1036.

Respiration–Chest Wall Movements

Baken, R. J., & Matz, B. J. (1973). A portable impedance pneumograph. *Human Communication*, Autumn, 28–35.

Gelfer, C., Harris, K. S., Collier, R., & Baer, T. (1986). Is declination actively controlled? In I. Titze & R. C. Scherer (Eds.), *Vocal fold physiology: Biomechanics, acoustics, and phonatory control*. Denver: Denver Center for the Performing Arts.

Hixon, T., Mead, J., & Goldman, M. (1976). Dynamics of the chest wall during speech production: Function of the thorax, rib cage, diaphragm, and abdomen. *Journal of Speech and Hearing Research, 19*, 297–356.

Strain Gauges

Abbs, J. H., & Gilbert, B. W. (1973). A strain gauge transducer system for lip and jaw motion in two dimensions. *Journal of Speech and Hearing Research, 16*, 248–256.

Hixon, T., Mead, J., & Goldman, M. (1976). Dynamics of the chest wall during speech production: Function of the thorax, rib cage, diaphragm, and abdomen. *Journal of Speech and Hearing Research, 19*, 297–356.

Muller, E. M., & Abbs, J. H. (1979). Strain gauge transduction of lip and jaw motion in the midsagittal plane: Refinement of a prototype system. *Journal of the Acoustical Society of America, 65*, 481–486.

Ultrasound

Keller, E., & Ostry, D. J. (1983). Computerized measurement of tongue dorsum movement with pulsed-echo ultrasound. *Journal of the Acoustical Society of America, 73*, 1309–1315.

Sonies, B. C., Shawker, T. H., Hall, T. E., Gerber, L. H., & Leighton, S. B. (1981). Ultrasonic visualization of tongue motion during speech. *Journal of the Acoustical Society of America, 70*, 683–686.

Watkin, K. L., & Zagzebski, J. A. (1973). On-line ultrasonic technique for monitoring tongue displacements. *Journal of the Acoustical Society of America, 54*, 544–547.

Velar Monitoring (Mechanical)

Horiguchi, S., & Bell-Berti, F. (in press). The velotrace: A device for monitoring velar position. *Cleft Palate Journal*.

X-Ray Microbeam

Fujimura, O., Kiritani, S., & Ishida, H. (1973). Computer controlled radiography for observation of movements of articulatory and other human organs. *Comput. Biol. Med., 3*, 371–384.

Nadler, R., Abbs, J. H., & Thompson, M. (1985). The new nationally shared X-ray microbeam facility: Status report. *Journal of the Acoustical Society of America, 78* (Suppl. 1), S38 (A).

Chapter III

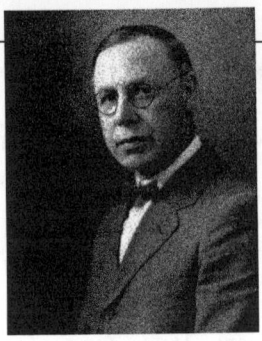

COORDINATION OF THE MOVEMENTS OF SPEECH

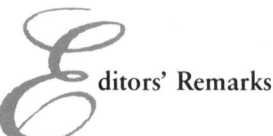ditors' Remarks

Chapter 3 is an important chapter in the monograph. The number of topics covered and concepts introduced are manifold; however, a single theme predominates. This is best seen in Stetson's own words: "The syllable then is constituted by a ballistic movement of the intercostal muscles. Its delimitation is not due to a 'point of minimum sonority' but to *the conditions which define a movement as one movement* [our emphasis]. In the individuality of the syllable the sound is secondary: syllables are possible without sound. *Speech is rather a set of movements made audible than a set of sounds produced by movements* [our emphasis]." It is the primacy of the syllable and the movement definition of the syllable that is the major force in *Motor Phonetics* and in this chapter.

Stetson begins the chapter by reviewing his well-known work on the fundamental types of movement. The syllable is defined with reference to this general view of action, and consonants and vowels are portrayed as movements that shape the ballistic chest pulse. Vowels emit the pulse; consonants delimit the syllable pulse. He goes on to describe how different kinds of movements alter the style and identity of different utterances. In particular, he introduces for the first time in the monograph, evidence of sudden transitions in syllable structure when speaking rate is increased (e.g., Figure 26). "It is certain that such changes and reversions are not matters of the relations of acoustic patterns, but are matters of the relations of movements." Both the use of rate manipulations and the suggestion that the structure of phonetics derives from articulatory organization are remarkable. From these insights Stetson creates his motor phonetics. A few other points are worth noting. One is Stetson's characterization of the vocal folds as a relaxation oscillator, that is, as a *nonlinear* system in which dissipative losses over a cycle are taken fully into account and compensated for. Such nonlinear models of vocal fold action are just now being treated seriously. A second point is that Stetson provides us through the monograph with many *trajectories* from different articulators, but makes no quantitative analysis of the trajectories themselves or the coordination among articulators. Progress in this realm is sorely needed.

THE MOVEMENT OF THE SYLLABLE AS THE FUNDAMENTAL UNIT OF EXPERIMENTAL PHONETIC ANALYSIS

Since the syllable is the simplest possible utterance in a monosyllabic breath group, it is convenient to consider first the syllable pulse. The syllable pulse is the simplest basic movement and is essential to the consonants and vowels which constitute the phonemic units so often assumed. If movements are the essentials in speech, why not consider the movement of the "sound" as the fundamental unit, as Rousselot actually did in his tension-tenue-détente analysis?

The answer is that the "sounds" and their movements cannot be discussed without involving their function in the syllable. The nature of the "sound" depends on what it does in the syllable. The distinction between the vowel and the consonant, or between a "syllable-forming sonant" and a true consonant must depend on the part the "sound" plays in the syllable. In this, Saussure was nearer right than Rousselot. The distinction between consonants, implosive and explosive ("appuyante et appuyée"), and their different fate in the course of phonetic changes, can be explained only by reference to their function in the syllable. The movements of the "sounds" often overlap and often fuse; they are not always separate. But by common consent a syllable is always a separate event in the speech series. And while investigators may not find it easy to determine the principle of syllable division, no one has assumed that two syllables could in any sense overlap or coincide.

When teachers and demonstrators give what they think are "separate sounds", they are actually uttering syllables; the vowels and, on occasion, the liquids and nasals constitute separate syllables, as in "*oh, a, I, rr...., ll....*"; long drawn out fricatives, "*sss....*" etc., become vowel substitutes, the other consonants are given either with a brief vowel which the consonant releases as in "*buh, puh*", or which the consonant arrests as in "*eff, ess*". The syllable is the smallest unit which can be uttered.

The fundamental unit for phonetic analysis is the movement of the syllable, a single breath pulse which is sometimes released by a consonant movement and sometimes arrested by a consonant movement. The syllable pulse may be released or arrested by the chest muscles alone ("*Oh, a, I, tea, eat*"). The division of the syllables is the division of these chest pulses one from another. The delimiting consonants are integral parts of this chest-pulse movement; they either release or arrest the chest pulse; the vowel on the other hand is due to the shaping of the vocal canal by an articulatory movement to emit the chest pulse. These articulatory movements are auxiliary movements to the chest pulse. When abutting consonants appear between syllables, the constriction is maintained throughout the pair; the first consonant of the pair arrests the chest pulse of the first syllable and the second consonant releases the chest pulse of the second syllable. A "double consonant" is a case in which the arresting consonant of the first chest pulse and the releasing consonant of the next chest pulse are the same consonant repeated. It is possible to demonstrate these movements experimentally, and to determine their coordinations.

THE THREE TYPES OF SKILLED MOVEMENT AND APPLICATION TO THE MOVEMENT OF THE SYLLABLE

In discussing any system of skilled movements, there are three fundamental types of movement to consider:

1. The movement of fixation: opposing groups of muscles hold the member in position. When a person is about to speak, the chest is partly inflated and is often held in that position for a short time before any syllable is uttered. In such a case the chest is fixated, poised in readiness, before speech begins.

2. The "controlled" or tense movement: in this type at least two opposing groups of muscles work together in producing the movement. Both the antagonistic muscle-groups are contracted throughout the movement. The direction of the movement can be changed after it is under way; such a movement is relatively slow, and "controlled" throughout its course.

Any slow adjustment is of this type; when one traces a curve slowly the "controlled" movement is employed. Writing is a series of rapid strokes. A forgery by tracing can always be detected by the minute changes of direction in a "controlled" movement, changes which are visible under the microscope. The slow expiration of air in a prolonged vowel constitutes a "controlled" movement. The large breathing movement of the entire phrase is a slow, "controlled" movement during which the rapid pulses of the syllables occur, like ripples on a wave.

3. The ballistic movement: the entire movement consists of a single pulse. It is impossible to change the movement during its course. The member is indeed thrown from one limit to the other like a projectile, as the name implies.

A study of the action of the muscles in such ballistic movements shows that the movement is started by a sudden contraction of the positive muscle-group which immediately relaxes. During at least half of the course of the movement neither of the antagonistic muscle-groups is contracted, so that the moving member flies free. At the end of its course the movement is usually arrested by the contraction of the negative muscle-group. The movement is a movement by momentum.

When a tennis stroke is made, a sudden contraction of the extensors of the arm starts the stroke; the extensors immediately relax, during the first quarter of the excursion, and the arm and racket are carried through the stroke by their momentum; at the close of the stroke the flexors of the arm may come into play and arrest the arm. All rapid movements are of this type. In speech, the rapid movements of articulation and the syllable pulse are ballistic. If one is unfamiliar with a language, one is always impressed by the high speed of its movements (86, p. 18 f; 90).

ANALYSIS OF THE BALLISTIC AND TENSE MOVEMENTS WITH SPECIAL REFERENCE TO THE SYLLABLE

In the simplest possible case, the ballistic movement is stopped by the muscles themselves, as is the movement of the conductor's baton, of the violinist's bow, or of the writer's pen. The antagonist muscles involved divide into two groups: the positive group which starts the movement, and the negative group which arrests the movement; in case the movement is repeated, this negative group returns the member to the starting point.

When the arrest is almost instantaneous, the member is returned at once to the starting point, as in the case of a rapid, repeated movement, the action of the positive muscle group results in a beat stroke, and the action of the negative muscle-group results in a back stroke which returns the member to the original position.

The movement of the conductor's baton or of the violinist's bow is arrested by the antagonist muscles. So the syllable movement of "*oh*" or "*a*" is arrested by the chest muscles. The movement of the hand in clapping is arrested by the movement of the opposite hand; the stroke of the cymbal in the right hand is arrested by the movement of the cymbal in the left hand. So the movement of the syllable pulse in "it" or "up" is arrested by the articulatory movement of the tongue or of the lip, which closes the vocal canal and compresses the air column and so acts on the moving chest walls. If the member when arrested is held in position at the lower limit of the movement, the interval required to take up the momentum and relax the arresting negative muscle group is as long as the interval required for a back stroke to return the member to its original position for the next beat stroke. Such a movement is to be seen in beating three-four time so that the baton follows a triangular path. This interval during which the negative muscle-group contracts, arrests the movement and then relaxes, may be called "the relaxation phase". It is an interval equivalent to the duration of the back stroke, and is sometimes called a "condensed back stroke" or a "back stroke in contact with an obstacle". This back stroke or relaxation phase includes the preparation for the next beat stroke.

The beat stroke is always ballistic; it occurs very rapidly and can hardly be longer than 40-100 millisec. On the other hand, the interval involved in the back stroke varies greatly. In the slow beating of time, beats may occur at the rate of two in three seconds, i.e. with a period of 1.5 sec. per movement. Assuming that the interval of the beat stroke is 0.050 sec., the back stroke, or relaxation phase, would be at this maximum, 1.45 sec in duration. At maximum speed, a movement can be repeated ca. 10 per sec. At such high speed the back stroke as well as the beat stroke is ballistic, and the back stroke has a duration of 0.050 sec. The back stroke, or relaxation phase (including preparation for the coming beat stroke) may vary, then, from 1.45 sec. to 0.050 sec.

The significant points in the application of this movement analysis to the movements of speech are:

1. The nature of the movement constituting the pulse for the syllable, including the vowel and the consonant (p. 56); the chest pulse and the auxiliary movements.

2. The nature of the movement constituting the stress group of the foot and the breath group (p. 58); the abdominal supporting and grouping movements.

SPEECH AS THE ACTIVITY OF A MOVING MEMBER

The vocal apparatus constitutes a tubular member inside the trunk which acts like the arm and hand in the quick raps of the coppersmith or the rapid strokes of the penman.

The apparatus for a skilled movement, like the taps of the hammer or the strokes of the pen, is not of course the musculature of the moving hand and fore-arm merely; there must be supporting movements of the upper arm, and a shoulder girdle posture. The strokes are delivered with shifts of these posture muscles of the shoulder and upper arm which support and direct and furnish pivots at the shoulder and elbow for the obvious ballistic movements of the hands.

The connections of the moving member of arm and hand for posture and support consist of bony levers, pivot joints, and tendons. Some of the connections of the tubular member of the speech apparatus are more unusual. The pivots of the ribs at the spine, and of the jaw are obvious, but the rapid and nicely adjusted movements of the tongue are peculiar. The abdominal muscles and the diaphragm are connected by the liquid mass of the viscera; and the chest is connected with the articulatory organs by a column of air under varying pressure (Cf. Fig. 13).

The apparatus of the skilled movement of the syllable is not of course the musculature of articulation merely; there must be a posture fixation of the rib cage and abdomen for the beginning of utterance, and a slow movement for the descent of the rib cage and the recession of the abdomen as the phrase progresses. The syllable pulse is supported and integrated by the movements of the abdominal muscles for the foot and the breath group.

The functions of the speech apparatus, however, the time constants, the relation of posture (fixations), the slow tense supporting movements, and the ballistic pulses are all characteristic of a single moving member. The maximum rate is ca. 8-12 per sec. (not 16-18 per sec. as would be the case if two or more ballistic members were alternating as in piano- or in flute-playing).

The unit movement of speech is the pulse which produces the syllable, a pulse of air through the glottis made audible by the vocal folds in speaking aloud and stopped and started by the chest muscles or by the auxiliary movements of the consonants. The larynx itself does not initiate the syllable nor control the process of articulation; this is quite apparent in the case of speech with an artificial larynx. The larynx makes possible the vocalization of speech. In just one thing is the larynx a prime mover; it determines the pitch of the tone. The initiation of the tone is due to the pressure differential above and below the larynx. The principal problems of the process of speech lie above and below the larynx.

A familiar way of treating speech divides the physiological apparatus into resonators, reed, and bellows. But the bellows is not like that of an organ, furnishing air under pressure to the glottis. Negus' statement that the larynx is a valve is easily misunderstood; only in the case of the glottal stop (which does not occur in English) does the larynx figure as a valve in speech. The chest-abdomen musculature is like a bellows for blowing the fire; when the bellows is inflated there is an increase of volume but there is no increase of pressure within.

In speech there are two fundamental groups of muscles:

1. The abdominal muscles working against the diaphragm (+ chest) which maintain the posture and the slowly changing adjustment of the phrase in speech and produce the movements of the foot and breath group (Fig. 13). The larger muscles of the rib-cage fixate the attachment of the diaphragm. The pressures from the abdominal muscles are transmitted through the viscera to the diaphragm. Thus the chest is maintained in position for the pulses of the intercostals.

2. The internal intercostals working against the external intercostals make the syllable by a

momentary pressure pulse (Fig. 13, I.I.-E.I.). The internal intercostals draw the ribs down, deflating the chest; they are the muscles of expiration which produce the pulse. The external intercostals draw the ribs up, opposing the internal intercostals, and arresting the pulse.

While the intercostals make a rapid series of syllable pulses, the abdominal muscles make a single movement against the opposing diaphragm for the group of syllables. This constitutes the breath group of one or more feet. The main stress of the group is produced by the culmination of this abdominal movement.

Thus the intercostals make a rapid series of syllable pulses at rates as rapid as 8–10 per sec., and the larger movements of the abdominal-thoracic musculature group and stress the syllables. These breath groups (of a single foot) may follow each other at the rate of 3–4 per sec. There is kymographic and action-potential evidence of these two musculatures (Figs. 3 and 4, DIA, RA, II, and EI). The pulses produced by the intercostals and the abdominal muscles have been recorded in various ways (Cf. p. 36 Figs. 15, 16, 17, 20, 28 etc.).

The breath group is an abdominal movement; the driving rectus and parietal muscles of the abdomen reciprocate with the diaphragm and thoracic muscles. This movement groups the syllable pulses and adjusts the chest-abdomen to the slight reduction in volume due to the emission of the chest pulses.

The breath group movement gives the overall form of the foot and of the breath-group series of syllables, which shows in the stresses of the feet, and in the elimination and restoration of syllables. It is evident that the syllables are parts of the breath group, and variations in the rate or the stress of the breath group may modify the component syllables radically. Since the syllables are parts of the breath-group pattern, the pattern conserves the individual syllables; they may be reduced, or even eliminated but the proper modification of the rate and stress of the breath group will restore them.

The breath group may consist of one or more feet; the feet may consist of one or more syllables. Thus it is possible to have a breath group composed of a single syllable, or of 10-15 syllables.

In speech, the rapid movements of the consonant and the movement of the syllable pulse are ballistic. The moving member in the case of the syllable consists of the driving and arresting muscles of the chest wall and the air column on which they act; the air column connects the chest muscles to the articulatory muscles of the consonant.

If the syllable consists of a vowel only, OVO,

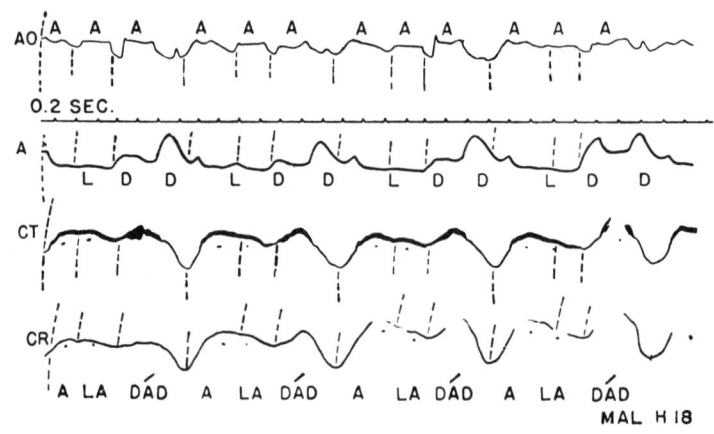

FIGURE 15. Pulses directly from Trachea

Syllables: *a la dad'*.
AO—Air outside: vowels and consonants.
  A—Air pressure in mouth; marks rise of pressure for consonants.
CT—Air pressure from trachea: chest pulses and breath groups.
CR—Air pressure tracing from negative pressure applicator which repeats the tracing of the tracheal pressure (CT) in remarkable fashion.

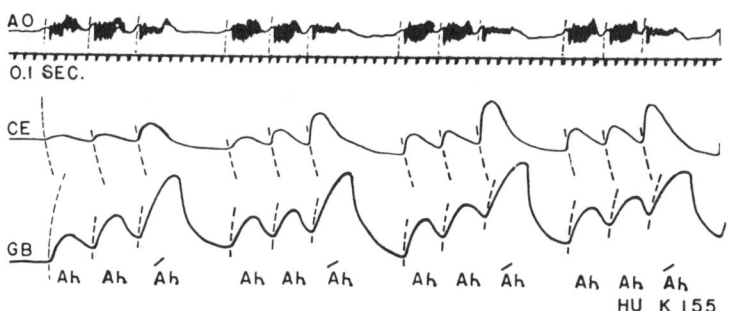

FIGURE 16. Pulses from Gastric Balloon

Syllables: *ah ah ah'*.
AO—The vowels and their vocalization.
CE—Negative pressure tracing of chest pulses from epigastrium.

GB—Tracing of pressures from gastric balloon which parallels the tracing of the epigastric pulses (CE).

the positive chest muscles (Inter. intercostals) start the wave of compression in the air column and the negative chest muscles (Exter. intercostals) stop the compression and take up the momentum of the chest wall. (The compression backs up slightly against the resistance of the glottis, if it is phonating, and of the tortuous vocal canal.)

If the syllable consists of a vowel and a consonant, OVC, the positive chest muscles start the wave of compression in the air column, the consonant stroke stops the compression wave, and the compressed air column helps to take up the momentum of the chest wall.

If the syllable consists of a consonant and a vowel, CVO, the positive chest muscles start the wave of compression in the air column, which is momentarily blocked and then released by the consonant stroke, and the negative chest muscles stop the compression and take up the momentum of the chest wall.

If the syllable consists of consonant, vowel, consonant CVC, the positive chest muscles start the wave of compression in the air column, which

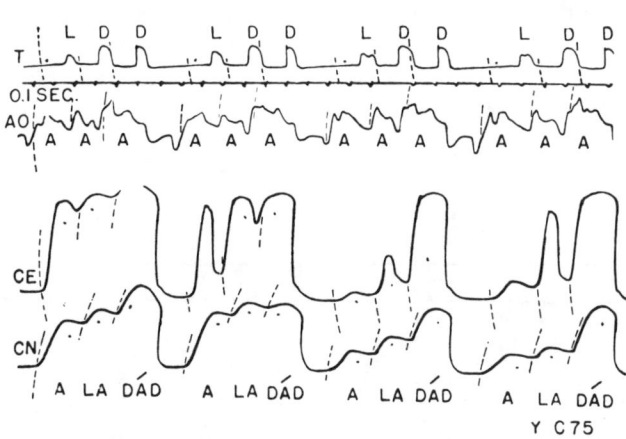

FIGURE 17. Pulses from Epigastric and from Navel Levels

Syllables: *a la dad'*.
CE—Negative pressure pulses from epigastric level; sometimes from chest pulses, sometimes from abdominal pulse for breath group.

CN—Negative pressure pulses, at the navel level, delineating the breath groups.

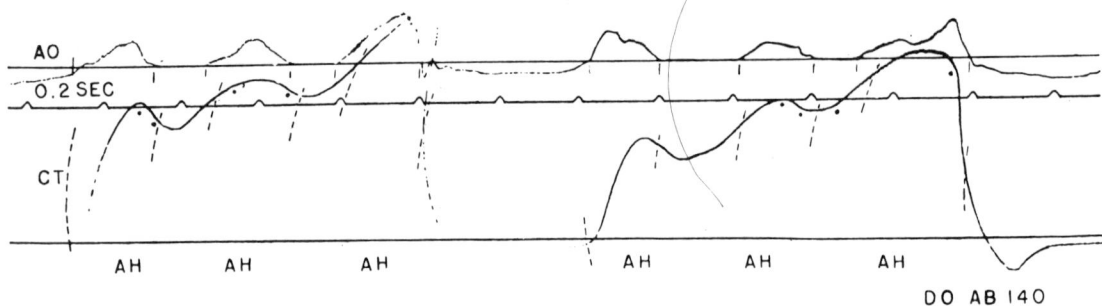

FIGURE 18. Chest Pulses directly from Trachea
Syllables: *ah ah ah'*.
AO—Syllable pulses outside mouth.
CT—Pulses from trachea showing syllable pulses and breath groups of abdominal muscles.

is momentarily blocked and then released by the consonant stroke, and the arresting consonant stroke stops the compression wave and the compressed air column helps to take up the momentum of the chest wall.

CHARACTERISTICS OF THE SYLLABLE AS A MOVEMENT

The syllable, then, is constituted by a ballistic movement of the intercostal muscles. Its delimitation is not due to a "point of minimum sonority" but to the conditions which define a movement as one movement. In the individuality of the syllable the sound is secondary; syllables are possible without sound. Speech is rather a set of movements made audible than a set of sounds produced by movements.

The consonants are not mere noises floating in the stream of sound. They are auxiliary movements, connected by the compressed air column with the chest muscles, and they have a function in releasing and arresting the chest pulse which constitutes the main movement of the syllable.

The syllable may consist of an expiratory movement or chest pulse released and arrested by the intercostal muscles. This is the case with the single syllable consisting of a single vowel, OVO: "*a, I, Oh*" in English, "*a, y, ou, eu, an, in, un, on*" in French. The articulatory shaping for the vowel may be set beforehand and the syllable occur when the rapid release and arrest of the chest pulse take place.

Fig. 23 gives tracings of a syllable composed of a repeated vowel in comparison with a similar

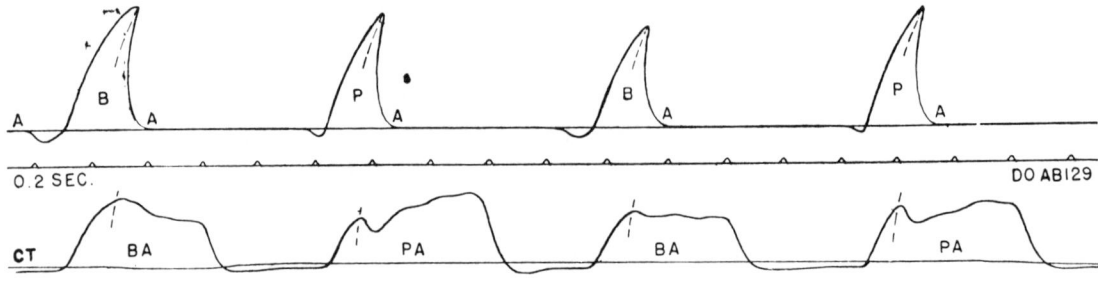

FIGURE 19. Chest Pulses directly from Trachea
Syllables: *ba pa*.
A—Air pressure in mouth for consonants *b* and *p*.
CT—Chest pulses from trachea with distinctive forms.

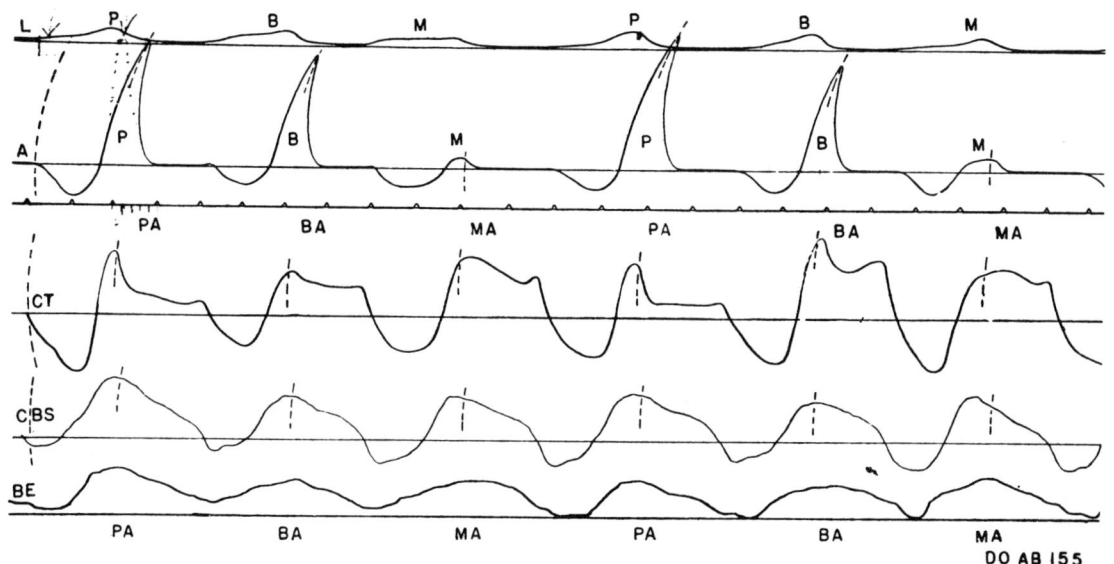

FIGURE 20. Pulses directly from Trachea

Syllables: *pa ba ma*.
  L—Lip marker.
  A—Air pressure in mouth. Typical low pressure for *m*; nasal outlet.
  CT—Pressure from trachea.
  CBS—Boss on lower sternum. The breath groups of the overall rib-cage-abdomen movement.
  BE—Boss on epigastrium. Parallels movements in abdominal musculature for breath groups of CBS.

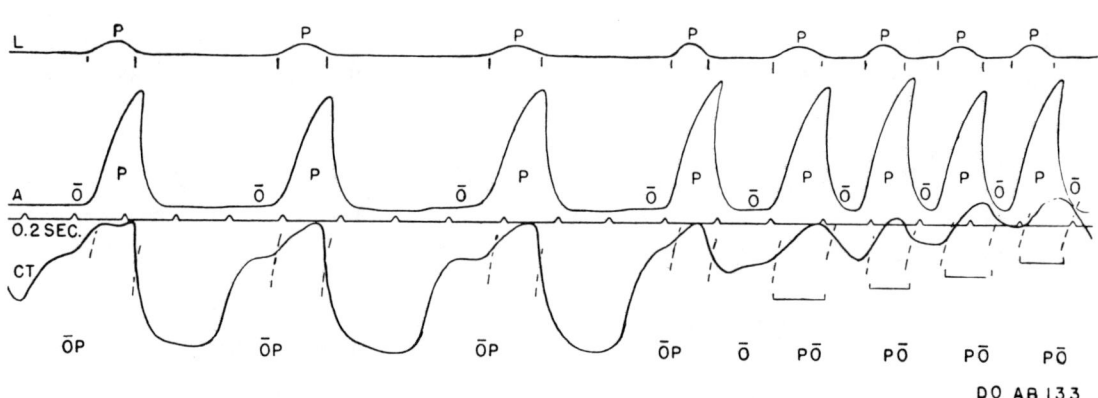

FIGURE 21. Pulses directly from Trachea

Syllables: *ope, ope* at increasing rate.
  A—Air pressure in mouth.
  CT—Air pulses from trachea. Characteristic of arrested and released syllables. First three syllables in separate breath groups. At syllable 4 a single indeterminate breath group begins.

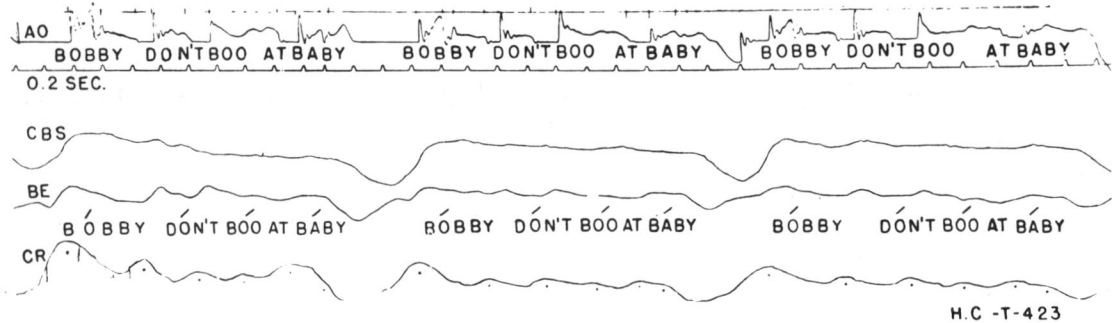

FIGURE 22. Chest Pulses

Syllables: *Bobby don't boo at Baby.*
AC—Air outside defining consonants and vowels.
CBS—Boss on sternum indicating the breath group of four feet.
BE—Boss on epigastrium indicating breath group and feet.
CR—Chest pulses indicated by negative pressure from the Rectus abdominis.

syllable with a releasing consonant. The variations in the chest pressure show the separate syllables when with and when without the consonant.

The articulatory conformation may not be that of a vowel; any continuant will do; "*f, s, v, z, r, l, n, m*" will all form syllables provided there is a chest pulse. If the articulatory conformation is maintained, as many syllables are formed as there are new ballistic chest pulses. Thus the series of "*n*"'s discussed by Sievers in "*berittenen*" (75 p. 94).

The "*n*" can be developed into an indefinite series; one has only to fixate the vocal apparatus in position for "*n*", and give a series of chest pulses, and a series of syllables is the result. In Fig. 111 "*runnin' an' neighin'*" and Figs. 88 and 89, "*Lil' 'll lie low*", the tracing of the chest pressure shows that the pressure does not rise because of the consonant closure; on the contrary, the minimum pressure occurs during the releasing consonant and the pulse is only partly under way when the releasing consonant opens. The maximum chest pressure occurs between the consonants of the syllable. In forms like "*runnin' 'n' neighin'*" it seldom happens, as Sievers assumes, that the "*n*" position is retained; this does occasionally take place, but as a rule the

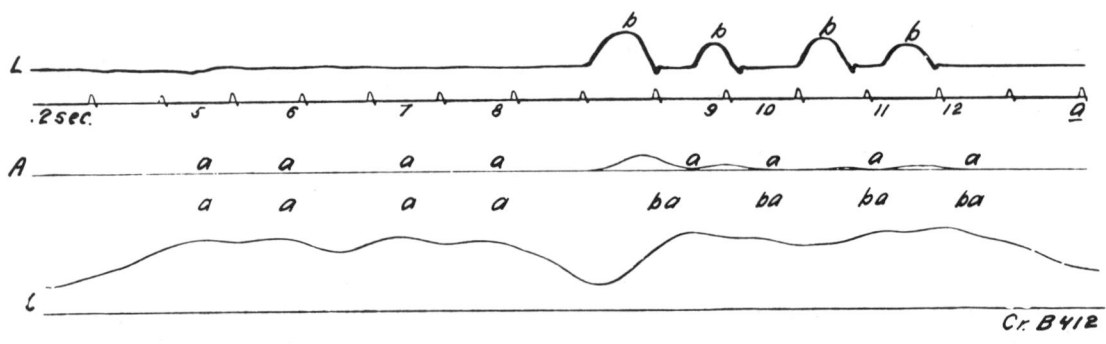

FIGURE 23. Chest Pulses directly from Trachea, glottis vibrating freely

Syllables: *a a a a ba ba ba ba.*
L—Lip marker.
A—Air in mouth; tracing defective.
C—Syllable pulse from trachea; distinct pulse for each syllable.

tongue makes a definite stroke for each syllable. The same observations hold for the series of "*l*"'s in "*lil' 'll lie low*".

Klestadt gives pneumographic tracings of speech in which each syllable is clearly indicated by a chest pulse (41).

Bloomer and Shohara published a preliminary study of respiratory movements in which the syllables are evident (7).

These syllables, OVO, are ballistic movements with chest release and chest arrest. If the movement were not chest-arrested it would trail off in a sigh or a moan. If a consonant is incorporated, we may have the chest pulse released by the consonant, or the chest pulse arrested by the consonant. All phoneticians are agreed that the releasing and arresting consonants are unlike. Compare Fig. 27 where "*eat....*" becomes "*tea....*"

The rate of the syllable movement is rapid; it is possible to repeat a single vowel like "*a, a....* at the rate of 5–7 per sec. The highest speed is obtained when the syllable has an occlusive releasing consonant; "*ta, ta....*" can be repeated at the rate of 7–12 per sec.; the rate depends slightly on the rhythmic grouping and is equivalent to the maximum repetition time ("tapping time") of the subject.

It is interesting that the chest muscles are capable of producing 8–12 pulses per sec. This is the highest speed of small and well-coordinated muscles like those of the hand. Tracings such as those shown in Fig. 24 prove that the muscles involved in the syllable movement cannot be the larger muscles of diaphragm and abdomen; the intercostal muscles of the chest must function.

"Long" vowels are distinctly slower, if the characteristic quality is preserved. "*Tea, too, tay*" can be repeated at the rate of 4.8–5.2 syllables per sec.

Rousselot's reading of a selection from the Chanson de Roland shows an average rate of 4.9 per sec. for 110 syllables; a reading of the same selection some five years later gives an average of 4.5 syllables per sec. (70, p. 1055; 72, p. 96)

The duration of the syllable depends somewhat on the force with which it is uttered. Increased force of utterance involves a greater contraction of the positive muscles of expiration, and this requires a longer time for the process of arresting the movement. Sometimes this increase in length shows in the vowel, when the negative chest muscles which arrest the movement come into play during the latter part of the vowel. This is unusual in the Romance languages, but quite common in English in which most of the "long" vowels have a "vanish" during which the arrest of the syllable movement begins.

It is possible to prolong a syllable at will, if the syllable is "open" or if the syllable ends with a voiced continuant like "*m, n, l, r,* etc.". In beating time, so that the baton describes a "figure-eight", this movement may be prolonged after the pulse of the beat; in the same way the beat stroke of the syllable may be arrested by a back-stroke process which continues the course of the movement in a slow, "controlled" form. Movements of this sort, which begin with a ballistic pulse and are continued as a "controlled" movement, are very common in all fields. In unusual cases, a vocal movement of the "controlled" type begins, perhaps in the utterance of a fricative, and is finally merged into a ballistic pulse; in such cases, the preceding movement is counted part of the syllable generated by the ballistic pulse. It is after this fashion that the preliminary slow movement of the orchestral conductor merges into the entering beat stroke of the selection.

FUNCTION OF THE VOWEL IN THE MOVEMENT OF THE SYLLABLE

The characterized factors of the syllable, the vowel and the consonant, constitute the familiar phonemes which the phonemic systems are concerned.

The fundamental classification of such phonemes has already been indicated:

Vowels which emit the syllable pulse.
Consonants which delimit the syllable pulse.

Consonants have two fundamental functions:

Releasing the syllable pulse.
Arresting the syllable pulse.

The compound consonants which function as a single syllable factor, and the abutting consonants at the syllable frontier will be handled in the discussion of the movements and functions of the consonants.

It will be convenient to postpone the detailed classification of the vowels and consonants until the processes involved have been studied in detail.

In popular phonetics the vowel is counted the core of the syllable and is often identified with the syllable. Such a "sound" often constitutes the bulk of the syllable in point of duration and is quite prominent as a matter of quality. So much so that Marage (48) and Devaux-Charbonnel (16), reasoning from the prominence of the vowel in acoustic records, have counted the vowel the important item. The importance of the vowel in the syllable is reflected in the common term "syllabic". The very term "consonant" stresses the importance of the vowel. A. G. Bell (2) was surprised to find, however, in dealing with the speech of the congenital deaf, that the specific vowel is less important than the consonants. But he showed that the function of the vowel is important even if the quality is negligible. He demonstrated that a reading is quite comprehensible if a single indeterminate vowel is substituted for all the vowels of the passage. The Semitic writing systems seem to treat the vowel as secondary by putting the consonants on the line and marking the vowels, ad libitum, as mere "points".

For audibility, however, the vowels are essential. In singing, the vowel becomes primarily important, and the consonants often lose their function and are neglected.

Sievers and others have stressed the fact that a syllable may be composed of a consonant like "*m n, l, r*" counted in some sense as a vowel. One can go further. The action of the vocal folds is not essential to the syllable. A syllable may be composed of "*sh......*" or of "*pst*". In whistling through the teeth we have a series of syllables composed of nothing but a long drawn "*s*".

The syllable, however, involves a chest pulse and the vowel is a more or less open conformation of the vocal canal for emitting this pulse. The chest pulse and the delimitation of the pulse by consonants are made audible by the action of the vocal folds.

The function of the vowel in the ballistic pulse of the breathing apparatus which produces the syllable is entirely different from the function of the consonants. The consonant has a function in the movement of the syllable, it constricts the vocal canal to delimit the chest pulse; the vowel on the other hand is a shaping movement to emit the chest pulse. The articulatory movement which produces the vowel conformation usually involves a movement of the jaw as well as of the lips and tongue. The coordination is simple; just as in violin playing the fingering changes the pitch of the tone produced by the bow, so the vowel shaping determines the timbre of the tone produced by the chest pulse. When the syllable disappears the vowel perforce goes with it; but the consonant as a distinct auxiliary movement may transfer to a neighboring syllable.

Rousselot has shown that the vowel is heard not only when the position has been reached, but also while the organs are quitting position and moving to a new vocalic formation (Cf. Potter, Kopp and Green). Visible Speech (64). In speech at the ordinary rate of 4–7 syllables per sec. it is impossible to hold the vowel position; there must be constant change of the shaping movement and the vowel cannot be acoustically a steady-state tone. It is apparent that the diphthong is a compound vowel in which the changing movement is vocalized during the syllable pulse. Many of the English vowels are really diphthongs, not only such recognized forms as "the long *i*" and "*oi*" but also the "long" vowel with "vanish", which is characteristic of the English pronunciation. The apparent simplicity of the vowel sounds of a language when produced and when heard is due to the simple, definite articulatory movement which produces the vowel. At the rate of 12–18 per sec. successive events fuse to qualitative aspects of the mass of sound. The rate of succession of the syllable factors is well within that range. Every emitting vowel shape, however complex it may seem on analysis, is physiologically a simple movement, capable of a rapid rate of utterance, of 7–10 syllables per sec. Only a movement of that type can be handled in speech. In all languages the stress and rate however light and approximately uniform, modify the duration of the syllable and vary the vowel quality. But the syllable is recognized as the same syllable with the same emitting vowel, in spite of variations. The inevitable changes which occur constantly in producing syllables, and the conditioning when the language is learned, lead the user to recognize the vowel as the same in spite of extensive change.

The Functions of the Vocal Folds

For various reasons, the action of the vocal folds has never been counted to be like that of the other organs of articulation. It is true that the glottis closes or opens the vocal canal, just as do the other organs of articulation. But in the main this closure is not absolute and there is a tendency to treat the action of the vocal folds as if they merely added a quality to the outgoing breath pulse. The breath pulse is said to be 'voiced" or "unvoiced".

There are very real reasons for this usage. It is only rarely, as in the "glottal stop" (coup de glotte), that the larynx acts a a true consonantal organ. In the production of the vowels and of the voiced consonants, the action of the folds is not consonantal. The vocal folds have no part in the delimitation of the syllabic movement, as has the movement of a consonant. In fact, the larynx does not initiate any syllabic or consonantal or vocalic movement. It is an open question whether the larynx can be said to initiate a tone. While the pitch is due to the action of the larynx, the inception of the tone is due to the pulse of the breathing apparatus for which the vocal folds may be adjusted in the various types of vocal attack. At first sight it would seem that the difference between a voiced occlusive ("*b, d, g*") and an unvoiced occlusive ("*p, t, k*") must be due to the action of the larynx alone. And yet both A. Graham Bell and Rousselot report cases in which speech with an artificial larynx presented satisfactory voiced and unvoiced occlusives, when in these cases the difference between the voiced and unvoiced occlusives must have been due to the management of the pressures above and below the artificial larynx, and not to the larynx itself, the reed of which is not under control but is ready to sound at any and all times. There can be no question as to the accuracy of these two observers—though oddly enough the importance of the case for the theory of the voiced occlusives occurred to neither of them. Bell (2) might have found important evidence against his theory of continuous breath-pressure during speech. Rousselot (69) was concerned solely with the question of the vowels.

The notion of the vowel as a "position" has more in its favor than the notion of the consonant as a position; the vowel prolonged does become a position. The classification of the vowels based on systematic observation by A. Melville Bell and Henry Sweet was in terms of tongue position supplemented by the position of the lips and larynx mass.

The development of methods of acoustic recording led to the theories of the vowel quality in acoustic terms by Helmholtz (29), C. Stumpf (93), D. C. Miller (53), Crandall (12), Gemelli (19), et al.

Working with prolonged vowels and applying harmonic analysis, they came to fair agreement as to the "formants" of the vowel. The prolonged vowel is characterized by the prominence of one or two zones in the frequency spectrum which are definite for each vowel, and which are independent of the pitch of the "larynx tone" produced by the glottis. Gemelli's analysis was based on the disposition of the characteristic regions of the frequency spectrum in relation to each other, and does not assume the formant bands (using the analysis of Vercelli, which includes anharmonics).

The assumption in all these cases was that the band of frequencies, reinforced for the formant, was composed of (changing) partials of the periodic larynx tone. There was some obvious evidence which controverted this view. Whispering is a common form of speech with intelligible vowels, obviously without a larynx tone. In the artificial larynx a free-swinging reed with well-defined period and partials does not give satisfactory vowels. A weighted reed resting against a seat which gives many close-spaced frequencies and indeterminate noise within a limited range, and which speaks and stops abruptly with variations of pressure, produces fair vowels. Even in the slow, careful speech studied by Gemelli (19), Curry (13), et al., it was difficult at times to locate in the oscillogram the few "typical cycles" (cicli tipici) which the theory demanded for the specific vowel quality; the effect of the releasing consonant often extends well into the vowel, and the effect of the arresting consonant appears so early in the vowel that little remains of a "pure vowel" unaffected by either consonant.

The notion that the vowel quality depends on the partials of definite cycles is barred by testing the phase relations. If two films printed from an original vowel, and therefore identical, are played back simultaneously in various phase relations, the vowel quality is not affected by any phase relation between the two series of vowel oscillations. One of the identical films may be played back in reverse concurrent with the other film, without disturbing the vowel quality.

The shape or movement heard in the vowel is not due to an overall pattern involving the entire vowel, but to cues which appear in any part of the vowel duration. Perhaps this might have been expected in view of the fact that the vowel starts from a variety of preceding cavity shapes and consonant constrictions, and the rate of movement of the different members involved in the incipient vowel is different; the jaw, the lips, the back and the front of the tongue do not move at the same rate (36). After having approximated the normal shape, the vowel pattern shifts to prepare for a variety of consonant constrictions and cavity shapes which may follow a spoken vowel. Therefore a single overall pattern is not possible and the vowel must be recognized, though modified, by various interpenetrating movements.

The presence of two formants in many prolonged vowels, and the earlier formulations of vowel positions, provoked the study of the cavities of pharynx and mouth. Grandgent (20) in 1890 had undertaken actual measurements showing a two-cavity system for the vowels.

Paget developed plastocene models of coupled resonators to represent the cavities of (steady-state) vowels. X-ray photographs were used by G. O. Russell and others to determine the positions of the organs in the vowel series. The cavities are formed in the front and back regions of the mouth and pharynx, modified as to volume by the tongue and jaw movements, and modified as to orifices by the lips and by the tongue approaching the palate in the median range.

Meantime, the evidence from whispering and from the artificial larynx was reinforced by observations which showed that the vocal folds constitute a relaxation oscillator of irregular cycle to which an analysis of the Fourier or Vercelli type does not apply; and specific experiments show that vowels can be produced from noises unrelated to the human voice. The essential is a range of frequencies 250-3500 Hz within which most of the frequencies are represented; the acoustic material for the vowel may be a white noise rather than a complex tone. See Fig. 10 showing five cycles of a vowel, mixed and integrated.

The brief duration of the vowels in ordinary rapid speech makes it impossible for resonances to develop from varying partials of a specific larynx tone of changing frequency. Moreover, the glottal output is not a series of regular cycles but a series of irregular cycles of damped oscillations and often without pitch.

The term "modulation" used by the Bell engineers is better than the term "resonance" as applied to the process whereby the energy distributed through this range of the sound spectrum is concentrated in certain zones. The changing shape of the cavities plays the principal part in intensifying the bands of frequency which the Bell engineers call "bars". The work has been empirical, searching out the ranges of frequency which seem characteristic and which show changes most obviously. There is as yet no precise indication of the changing shapes of mouth and pharynx, or of the interaction of the cavities responsible for the modulation. And there is no question that the shapes change.

Relations of Vowel and Consonant

Most striking are the changes of the modulatory bars by the influence of the releasing and arresting consonants. (3, 64) Where a consonant opens from its constriction, it changes the modulating cavity by producing a rapidly enlarging orifice. This change of the modulating cavity changes the vowel "bars"; the most indicative bars are said to be "kinked" at the beginning by the consonant. When a consonant arrests the syllable, the consonant produces a rapidly diminishing orifice, changing the modulating cavity and "kinking" the vowel bars in the opposite direction. In forms like "gag" or "bob" the reversal of the warp is very apparent, and at no point in the vowel are the bars free from the warping of one consonant or the other.

The function of the vowel shape is not only to emit the syllable with a specific quality—often variable in many languages—but also to make audible the releasing and arresting factors of the syllable. The earlier analyses of acoustic records (e.g., Marichelle (50), Gemelli (19)) show the

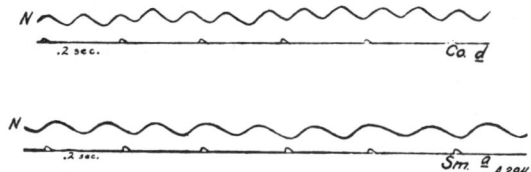

FIGURE 24. Chest Pulses Registered from Nostril. Glottis open. Maximum rate
N Co d—About 11 per second.
N Sm a—About 8 per second.
Rate of chest-pulse movement is as high as that of any articulatory movement.

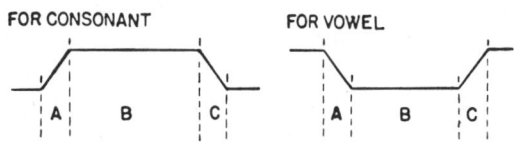

FIGURE 25. Rousselot's Diagram of Movement of a "Sound"
A—Tension-arrivée (Followers of Rousselot change "tension" to "arrivée").
B—Tenue.
C—Détente.

influence of the consonant on the vowel, but the visible-speech patterns make apparent the place of consonant constriction from which the vowel shape opens or the place of consonant constriction to which the vowel shape closes. And for the first time in acoustic recording, the syllable unit is usually apparent. The treatment by Potter, Kopp, and Green confuses consonants, which are vowel-like in appearance, with the vowels, and does not take note of the rapid rate-of-change which must be heard as a discontinuity, and which requires a ballistic movement to produce. But when allowance is made for those two ambiguities, the patterns of visible speech are significant confirmation of kymograph and action-current recordings of the syllable unit with the syllable factors.

The vowel makes the releasing factor and the arresting factor of the syllable audible. The consonant constriction may involve airflow and sudden contacts which produce noises to be heard at close range; but such noises are mainly inaudible across the ordinary room, and the place of the consonant constrictions is indicated in the changes of the vowel bars of the visible-speech pattern (Fig. 36). Although the kymograph, oscillograph, and visible-speech recordings all show the chest-release and the chest-arrest of syllable forms OVO, CVO, OVC, the usual phoneme writing as V, CV, VC obscures the syllable factors. The syllable pulse, in the chest-released forms, is released by the chest muscles (the internal intercostals) into the vocal canal which is shaped for the vowel. Meanwhile the air pressures in the mouth and just outside the mouth are equal, and the vibration of the glottis starts as the oscillograph oscillations, and the 'bars' of visible speech assume the vowel pattern at once. The syllable pulse, in the chest-arrested forms, terminates with the opposing contraction of the antagonist chest muscles (the external intercostals) with an abrupt fall of the air pressures, and with a vowel pattern which diminishes in intensity, but shows little change in form. In a

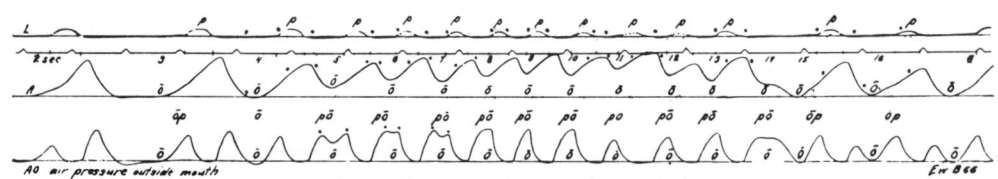

FIGURE 26. Changes at Syllable Frontier with Changing Rate
Syllables: *ope ope* . . at increasing and decreasing rate.
L—Lip marker *p*. Dots show limits of laryngeal vibration. Pressure rises with rate.
A—Air in mouth indicates shifting from arresting to releasing consonant.
AO—Air outside. Indicates shift from arrested to released syllable.
At syl. 5 *ope* becomes *poe*.
At syl. 15 *poe* reverts to *ope*.

language with heavy stress, like English, the stressed vowels in slow, careful type of utterance tend to diphthongize in the familiar "vanish"; the quality of the end of the vowel is modified toward schwa. The chest release and the chest arrest may or may not be phonemic.

In all these cases in which the vowel functions as an indicator of the type of release and of arrest of the syllable, it is most important to note that the consonant and the vowel are fused in a basic unit movement in the syllable. Sequences like CVO CVO CVO (ordinarily written CV CV CV) *pay, pay. . . . , tea, tea. . . .* , however rapid, never show any interaction of the vowel with the following consonant, although at rapid rates the vowel phonation of the preceding syllable may invade a surd releasing consonant which gradually becomes sonant (Cf. Fig. 26).

Sequences like OVC OVC OVC (VC VC VC) "*ape, ape. . . . , eat, eat, . . .*" show the arrest by the consonant and introduce an intersyllabic pause, if the syllables "*ape*", and "*eat*" are maintained; if the rate per sec. is increased beyond 3.5 per sec., the syllables become "*pay, pay. . . .* and *tea, tea. . . .*" (Fig. 27) which are now chest arrested, while the arresting consonant has shifted to the releasing function in the next syllable. The consonant is fused with the vowel in the form OVC, "*ape, eat*"; but the consonant does not affect the following vowel unless the syllable is re-organized as "pay, tea", with the consonant functioning in the releasing position. Thus the vowel in its interaction with the consonant helps in indicating the structure of the syllable.

Confusion of Vowel and Consonant

Although the function of the vowel (the emitting shape) as a factor in the syllable is quite distinct from that of the releasing and arresting consonants, phonemic schemes often confuse the vowels and consonants. This is made easy by the properties of two groups of consonants:
1. the semi-vowels;
2. the liquids and nasals.

The semi-vowels are related to the vowels in this fashion: If the vowel shaping of /i/ is made a stroke to the limit of the constriction, and suddenly released, the consonant *y* (j) results. "*E, E*",—OVO, and "*ye, ye*"—CVO gives the contrast. If the vowel shaping of /u/ is made a stroke to the limit and suddenly released, the consonant "*w*" results. "*Ou, ou*"—OVO, and "*woo, woo*"—CVO gives the contrast.

In a series of syllables in which the conditions of rate and stress force an elimination of syllables, the /i/ and /u/ are often reduced to the related consonant strokes, e.g., "petunia, Rouen".

The liquids and nasals, "*l, r, m, n, -ng*", are continuants with slight constriction, and therefore may function as vowels, i.e. as "syllabic consonants", e.g., Hrdlička, sympto*m*. Though any continuant may be given the function: "*whew*" (aspirated whistle), "*shhh*", "*pst*".

If the functions of the factors in the syllable are kept in mind, the difference between the vowels and consonants is always clear, and the reasons for a change of function can always be traced.

The apparent interchange of function of consonant and vowel has helped to confuse the distinction between consonant and vowel for those who look on the phoneme as the independent, basic unit, and do not realize the basic function in the syllable which is the distinguishing trait of consonant and vowel. If an articulation emits the syllable pulse, whether it is characterized by consonant timbre, or even by an extraneous white noise, it is a vowel. If an articulation, whatever its timbre, releases or

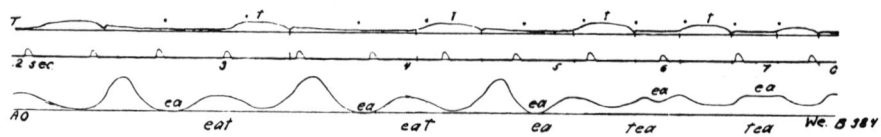

FIGURE 27. Changes at Syllable Frontier with Changing Rate
Syllables: *eat eat . . tea tea*.
T—Tongue marker. Dots indicate limits of laryngeal vibration.
AO—Air outside.
At syl. 4-5 *eat* becomes *tea*.

COORDINATION OF THE MOVEMENTS OF SPEECH

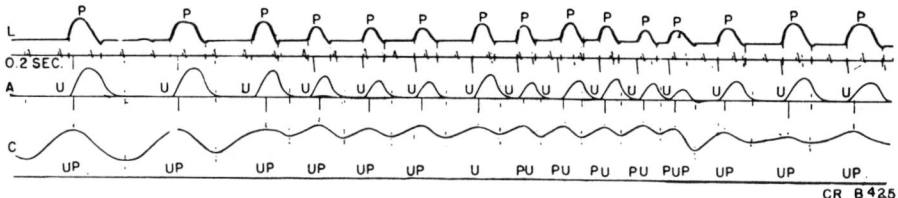

FIGURE 28. Pulses Recorded directly from Trachea
Syllables: *up up*.
L—Lip marker.
A—Air in mouth.
C—Air pulses from trachea. Typical forms for arresting and releasing consonants.
At syl. 8-9 *up* becomes *pu*.
At syl. 13-14 *pu* reverts to *up*.

arrests the syllable pulse, it is marked by an auxiliary stroke and is a consonant.

Tense and Lax Vowels

The contrast noted by Passy (61, p. 96) between the "tense" vowel of the French "site" and the "lax" vowel of the English "sit" is due to the fact that the French site is arrested partly by the chest muscles, so that the "*te*" may tend to become a separate syllable in emphatic speech. The English "sit", on the contrary, is arrested by the consonant movement alone. The complete "relaxation" of the English vowel is of the arresting chest muscles (external intercostals). In the French "site", on the contrary, there is a contraction of the arresting chest muscles (external intercostals) along with the consonant movement at the close of the chest pulse.

Duration of Vowels

It has long been customary to speak of the "length" of the vowel. The study of oscillograms shows that the vowel cannot be separated from the consonant of the syllable. Gemelli's records give the gradual transition of the acoustic pattern of the consonant to the acoustic pattern of the vowel; the change is continuous; and the vowel flows gradually into a following consonant. In reality, the "long" and "short" apply to the syllable not to the vowel.

The ancient doctrine of vowels (syllables), which are long by position, implies that an arresting consonant which belongs to the syllable in question lengthens the vowel (syllable); and the studies of syllables in the laboratory confirms this lengthening. If the consonant (or compound consonant, "cluster") belongs to the following syllable it does not lengthen that syllable. Experimental studies show that such releasing consonants overlap the vowel process and do not add to the duration of the syllable.

Languages with a heavy word stress have syllables of varying duration, and the quality of the vowel is affected. In the stressed syllables the vowels tend to lengthen, and even to diphthongize (Brechung); in the unstressed syllables, which are uttered at rapid rate, the vowels are reduced and

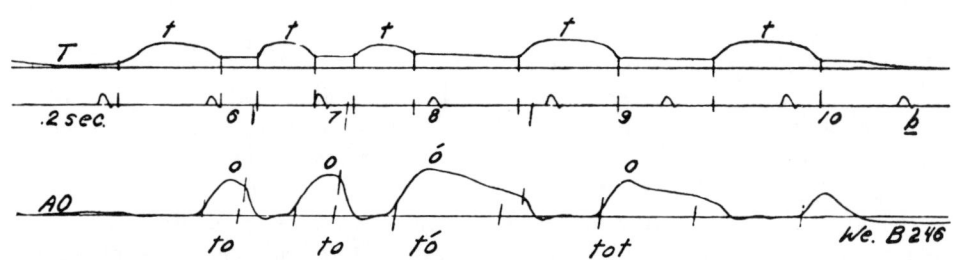

FIGURE 29. Whispered Syllables
Syllables: *to to to' tot*.
T—Tongue marker.
AO—Air outside. Slow descent in pressure in each syllable without mid-sag. Stress on third syllable.

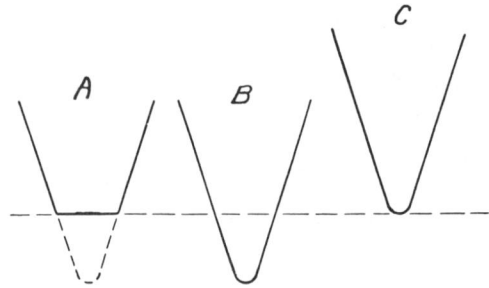

FIGURE 30. Diagram of Stroke to Obstacle
A—Stroke interrupted remains in contact during part of back stroke.
B—Stroke with obstacle withdrawn and self-arrested.
C—Stroke which barely touches obstacle.

may even disappear with the syllable.

It is a familiar fact that the English "long" vowel may be shortened and reduced but that the English "short" vowel cannot be prolonged; the quality of the "short" vowel depends on the rapid utterance of the vowel. If the short syllable is heavily stressed, an arresting continuant will be prolonged; or the intersyllabic interval will be prolonged. The time is necessary for neutralizing the momentum of the heavy stress. The "*e* mute" of the French and the "dark *e*" of the English are cases of a vowel reduced to its lowest terms; there is as little as possible vocalic movement from the neutral or "resting" position of the vocal apparatus, and the vowel is as brief as possible. Since the "short" English vowels, cf. "*pat, pet, pit, put*", are also very brief, they seem to approach the "dark *e*" in quality; and they also cannot be prolonged. The difficulty of singing words like "mother" and "heaven" is a familiar illustration of the change in vowel which must occur if the vowel is prolonged.

The French vowels are all rather brief and there is little apparent change during the vowel. In the utterance of the "long" English vowel, on the other hand, the vocalic apparatus is shifted to the next sound, while the vowel is still sounding, and a secondary quality is always heard at the close. This is very marked in vowels having the heavy word stress common to the Teutonic languages.

The movement of the jaw is often part of the characteristic of certain vowels, and this involves a variation in the duration of the syllable (21, 27, 28, 52, 59).

In a language like French, where the word stress is very light and variable, it is possible for an observer like Verrier to assume "isochrony", i.e. that the syllables tend to be of equal duration.

In some languages the vowel duration is phonemic; e.g. Finnish. The contrast between long and short is observed. Often the conditioning from generation to generation preserves such a contrast, although the qualities have changed radically. Thus in English the traditional "long *i*" (as in "pine") contrasts with the "short *i*" (retained as in "pin") and the traditional "long *e*" (as in "he") contrasts with the "short *e*" (as in "hem"). This illustrates the effect of conditioning in determining the habitual associations of the articulations.

The Vowel System

It is customary to speak of the "vowel system" of a language, of which such traditional contrasts are a part. The extreme vowel positions may be thought of as /i/, /a/, and /u/; and the specific series of vowel positions can be indicated between them, and there may be combinations in which a position of one series is fused with a position of the other series. Each language has its "cardinal vowels" which usually include the extreme positions. Although the classification of the vowels is physiological, not acoustic, the vowel positions chosen in a given language are less obvious than the bearings of the consonants. Within this range of recognized vowels, various changes due to rate and stress appear, which are notated in terms of the system, though the gradations may actually be continuous. Between the stressed form "the" and a completely unstressed "the" there is an indefinite series, unrecognized in any phonetic notation.

Physiological Traits of the Vowels

There is still very little exact knowledge of the movement complexes of the vowel. Although palatograms show some of the bearings, kymograph tracings show the movement of jaw and velum, moving pictures show lip positions (early, Marey-Marichelle), kymograph tracings show details of air flow and air pressure in the chest and vocal canal, X-ray profiles, both 'stills' and movie films (too few frames per sec.) show something of the changing shapes of the vowels, and the visible-speech patterns show changes produced by the opening and closing of the consonants, the data are not adequate; the changes are rapid and often millimeters are significant.

For the systematic indication of the vowels the older physiological descriptions are revised, or standard works are cited. Some have suggested that the visible-speech patterns developed in the Bell Telephone Laboratories might well become standard indication of the stable vowels. They do not, at present, indicate the significant detail of the vowel range of the various languages; but it is possible that the method can be made more delicate especially for particular purposes.

However objective a frequency spectrum indication of the vowels may be, or however clearly differentiated, such a record might define standard vowels in given conditions but it would do nothing toward explaining the movements which underlie the vowels and which determine the relations and the changes of the vowels in every language. It is not a matter of "diachronous change" but of the synchronous changes which figure from sentence to sentence in everyday speech. The same vowel may appear in a single English sentence as 1) prolonged with 'vanish', 2) as approaching shwa, and 3) as a null form; changes of rate and stress in that same sentence will give a new series for that same vowel. It is certain that such changes and reversions are not matters of the relations of acoustic patterns, but are matters of the relations of movements.

THE FUNCTION OF THE MOVEMENTS OF THE JAW

The jaw figures in the movement of the lips for the labials, and may be primary at maximum rates, because the jaw movement is more rapid than that of the lips. And the jaw has a secondary part to play in some linguals since it shifts the general position of the tongue.

But the primary function of the jaw is in opening the vocal canal for the emission of the syllable.

The releasing consonant stroke closes the vocal canal so that the action of the chest muscles compresses the air; then the rapid back stroke of the lip or tongue, with the opening of the jaw, releases the air. The beat stroke, and often the back stroke, occur during the beat stroke of the chest. At rapid rates the back stroke of the consonant, the opening of the jaw, and the back stroke of the chest, tend to coincide, as well as the beat strokes. The opening and closing of the jaw marks the series of syllables.

In a series of syllables with arresting consonants like "*up, up*...." the syllable pulse is started by the chest muscles; it is "chest-released". The jaw parts as the mouth is opened for the syllable emission, although the vowel movement is at minimum. But the syllable pulse is stopped, arrested, by the consonant stroke; the jaw movement is essential to the arresting "*p*", and the opening and closing of the jaw indicates the syllable movement.

The shaping movement of the vocal canal, which gives rise to the vowel quality, is often accompanied by the opening of the jaw.

As the syllable closes, the jaw often closes because of the adjustment for the new vowel and for the arresting and releasing consonant movements at the syllable frontier.

The neutral vowel, shwa, and the reduced vowels which approach shwa, have the least vowel movement and such syllables may be produced without any jaw action whatever.

"Long" vowels and diphthongs involve a more pronounced opening of the jaw. The common tendency in English to diphthongize all stressed "long" vowels makes the jaw movement prominent.

THE MOVEMENT OF THE CONSONANT

Although the same "sound" has sometimes been counted both a vowel and a consonant, in one form or another, a distinction has always been drawn between the vowels and the consonants. It is the custom to recognize a vowel "*i*" and a consonant "*i*" (the consonant "*i*" in English is often spelled "*y*" as in "yes"; in French it is often unchanged, as in "rien, dieu"); a vowel "*ou*" and a consonant "*ou*" (written "*w*" in English but unchanged in the French as in "oui"). The difficulty of making distinctions has given rise, as we have seen, to the term "semi-vowel" which is sometimes applied to the liquids "*l*" and "*r*" and to the nasal "*m*" and "*n*". Sievers has been at pains to point out that the same "sound" may function in rapid alternation as a consonant and as a vowel; "berittenen" has already been cited. But aside from the practice of dividing "sounds" into the "syllabic", which is supposed to be the core of the syllable, and the "consonant", which is supposed to be added to the vowel, there has been little attempt to define the function of the consonants. Often the consonant has been considered quite secondary to the vowel. Marage defined the consonant as a supralaryngeal noise preceding or following the aero-laryngeal vibration of the vowel; he felt that the consonant occupies but a small place in the syllable, and therefore should be subordinated to the vowel (16, 48).

Rousselot applies his general analysis of the tension-tenue-détente to the consonant; this describes the position of the organs and can be made to explain the important difference between the implosive (arresting) and the explosive (releasing) functions of the consonant (Fig. 25). The study of historic phonetics has shown that there is an important distinction between the consonant which closes a syllable and the consonant which opens a syllable. The implosive consonant which closes the sylable is called appuyante when it abuts the explosive consonant of the next syllable which is called appuyée. The different fate of these consonants in the evolution of the Romance languages led to this distinction. The terms imply that the explosive consonant of the abutting pair is somehow supported and so buttressed against change, while the implosive is supporting and may disappear. Rousselot defines the explosive consonant as consisting primarily of taking-position and holding-position, while the implosive consists primarily of holding-position and quitting-position. F. de Saussure counts the implosive-explosive junction important for the division of the syllables. But these analyses do not touch the fundamental question of the relation of the movement of the consonant to the movement of the syllable.

The consonants are to be divided into releasing consonants which start the syllable movement and arresting consonants which stop the syllable movement. "Explosive" and "appuyée" are other names for the releasing consonant; "implosive" and "appuyante" are other names for the arresting consonant.

The Arresting Consonant

In a series of syllables like "*up, up....*" the syllable pulse is started by the chest muscles; it is "chest released". But the syllable pulse is stopped, arrested, by the consonant stroke. The consonant closes the vocal canal, and the rise of air pressure in the pharynx and chest takes up the momentum of the chest wall and brings the movement to a stop. Figs. 26, 27 and 28 show that the highest chest pressure of the pulse occurs when the consonant stroke closes the vocal canal. The lowest chest pressure between the syllable pulses occurs well after the consonant. The next syllable pulse does not begin until after the back stroke of the arresting consonant. There is a hiatus in the sound, for vocalization of the vowel of the next syllable does not occur until the delayed rise in chest pressure.

The pressure in the mouth has the typical arresting form; the closure of the lips brings the rise in mouth pressure which accompanies an arresting consonant. The curve has the rounded form due to the gradual subsidence of pressure; the chest pressure sinks as the chest muscles prepare the next pulse.

When the pressure just outside the mouth is recorded with a modified form of Rousselot's apparatus, the tracing shows something of the variations in the chest pressure, interrupted, of course, during the closure of the consonants. The pressure just outside the mouth varies with the mouth pressure which derives from the chest pressure, but is radically modified by the valve of the glottis and the changing volume of the pharynx-mouth cavities. The mid-sag in the pressure outside is not due, however, to any change in the chest pressure, but to the enlargement of the mouth cavity as the mouth opens, which affects the pressure in the mask before the mouth. There is a corresponding rise in pressure in the mask when the mouth cavity is rapidly diminished as the mouth closes. The point of minimum chest pressure is well marked in the tracing of pressure outside and the rapid rise for the next vowel is clearly indicated; the vocalization usually appears in this tracing if the membrane is sensitive. Tracings of whispered syllables do not often show the mid-sag; the glottis is open enough to sustain the mouth pressure in spite of changes in volume and the curve of pressure outside merely shows a steady decrease in pressure during the syllable. Fig. 26 may be compared with Fig. 29.

Passy notes that the English can differentiate "an aim" and "a name", i.e. an arresting consonant may persist in English where it would shift to the releasing position and transfer to the next syllable in French. (61) This is true, but only at a moderate rate. If "*an aim*" is said faster and faster it soon becomes "*a name*". The "*n*" has shifted from the arresting function in "*an*" to the releasing function in "*name*". The arresting consonant adds to the duration of the syllable and, as the rate increases, tends to shift to the releasing position in the next syllable where it does not require extra time. Binet and Henri (4) found that at maximum speed the syllables of the digits with consonant arrest required more time than those with open syllables. This change can easily be studied in experimental series. Fig. 26 shows "*ope, ope. . . .*" becoming "*poe, poe. . . .*" and as the rate slows reverting to "*ope, ope.*" Fig. 27 shows "*eat, eat. . . .*" becoming "*tea, tea.*" Fig 28 shows "*up, up. . . .*" becoming "*pu, pu. . . . .*" and reverting to "*up, up. . . .*" The reversion to the original form, and the increase in chest pressure and decrease in the consonant stroke at rapid rate will be considered later.

The Releasing Consonant

This consonant releases the syllable pulse. The stroke of the expiratory chest muscles and the beat stroke of the consonant occur at the same time. The consonant stroke closes the vocal canal so that the action of the chest muscles compresses the air, then the rapid back stroke of the consonant releases the air. The beat stroke and often the back stroke of the consonant occur during the beat stroke of the chest. At a rapid rate the back strokes of the consonant and chest muscles, as well as the beat strokes, tend to coincide. The releasing consonant never adds to the length of the syllable and it actually accelerates the syllable movement. The coordination is much faster than that of the arrested syllable. The rate may be as high as 9—12 per sec., which is the maximum rate of a skilled movement.

Tracings show that the pressure in the chest continues to fall during the arrested syllable when the consonant closure occurs, while the pressure in the mouth rises. Although the consonant muscles and the chest muscles contract at the same time as the releasing consonant, the chest pressure does not begin to rise until the middle of the consonant contact. For the actual relations cf. Fig. 48, syl. 10–12, Fig. 50, syl. 4–5, pp. 91, 92. This lag of .03–.05 sec. is due to the size of the cavities involved. In speech the consonant muscles quickly close a cavity of 200 c.c. at most, while the chest muscles act on a limited area of the walls of a cavity of 2500 c.c. at least. The pressure conditions in a rapid series of open syllables permit vocalization to begin immediately after the releasing consonant and to continue up to the releasing consonant of the next syllable. This has led some to assume that the median releasing consonant belongs to both syllables. (103, p. 357) But the consonant belongs to the syllable in which it functions.

The Releasing and Arresting Consonant as Two Functions of One Movement

The consonant stroke seems now to open and now to close the vocal canal; how can it be counted the same thing in these different cases? When the tongue moves from the neutral position and makes a quick stroke to the palate as in "*a-la*" or "*hut*" there seems little question that the stroke is made to the palate. In the word "*hut*" the stroke must occur in that fashion; but in the case of "*la*" or "*to*" the tongue may be in contact with the palate *before* the essential stroke occurs. While the same spot is involved, there seems at first sight a radical difference between the essential stroke of the releasing consonant in "*ta*" and "*la*", which seems to be *from* the hard palate, and the essential stroke of the arresting consonant in "*at*" and "*al*", which is *to* the palate. Apparently the arresting and releasing strokes are in opposite directions, although they move over precisely the same path. But the movement shifts from arresting to releasing and back again, and at a fairly rapid rate; therefore it is improbable that the entire coordination of the movement changes with this change of function.

The consonant movement involves an obstacle, an opposing surface to which and from which the stroke of the consonant plays. The detail of such movements to an opposing surface will help in understanding the arresting and releasing functions of the consonants. It is sometimes said that a rapid movement is likely to be followed by a "rebound"; in reality, the return movement, the back stroke, is not due to elasticity, but to the accurately timed contraction of the negative muscle-group which arrests the member and returns it to the starting point. It is this rapid back stroke which is sometimes called the "rebound". In case the movement is arrested by an obstacle, the opposing surface, precisely the same sequence may occur. The momentum of the movement is taken up by the obstacle, and the negative muscle-group acts at the proper time and returns the moving member. The time consumed proves to be precisely the same as if the opposing surface had not intervened. Plotted against time, the movement would have presented a u-shaped or v-shaped path at the end of the stroke. The opposing surface truncates this u-shaped or v-shaped curve and gives a flattened form (Fig. 30), but the time relations are the same as if the movement had been completed with self-arrest and normal return (Fig. 30). When the movement barely reaches the obstacle, barely flicks the opposing surface, the curve of the complete movement is practically normal, and the truncation is eliminated; the member does not remain in contact with the surface (Fig. 30). This means that although the movement is to a surface, the holding in position is eliminated. Many of Rousselot's records show such forms (70, p. 597, Fig. 387, p. 390, 949, Fig. 631, p. 952, Fig. 635, 636; 86, p. 29).

This normal movement may be modified by eliminating either the excursion to the opposing surface, or the excursion from the opposing surface. A blow can be delivered to an opposing surface when the member is in actual contact with that surface. The essence of the blow, of the beat stroke, is the sudden contraction of the positive muscle-group which exerts pressure on the opposing surface. Such blows delivered to a surface with which the member is in contact are very common. In piano-playing and in typing the finger is often in contact with the key struck; precisely the same movement can be executed with the finger resting on the surface of a table. In the case of the stroke to the piano- or typewriter-key, the back stroke may be of large amplitude, and may be the most obvious thing in the movement; this is true of "staccato" playing.

Translated into terms of phonetics this would mean in the case of the explosive "*t*" that the tip of the tongue may be in actual contact with the palate when the blow is delivered *to* the palate. The beat stroke actually occurs, although the tongue tip is in contact with the opposing surface at the time of the sudden contraction of the positive muscle-group. The methods of recording employed to date have not been very satisfactory for showing this sudden pressure against the opposing surface, nevertheless it does appear in some records published (72, p. 77, Fig. 68). In the word "*pap-pa*" the lips are still in contact when the "*p*" of the second syllable occurs, but the sudden pressure which is the beat stroke of the releasing "*p*" shows clearly. The beat stroke is not eliminated although the excursion of the lips does not return the member to the original position; contraction of the positive muscle-group, and a pressure is a stroke.

The "condensation of the back stroke", the elimination of the excursion from the opposing surface, is as often observed. When the blow is struck to the opposing surface there may be no "rebound"; the momentum may be taken up by the obstacle and the negative muscle-group does not return the member to the original position. The relaxation of the positive muscles and the preparation of the next movement may occur while the member remains in contact with the surface to which the blow is struck. In the pronunciation of the word "*hut*" the tongue may deliver the stroke of the "*t*" to the palate and remain in contact during the relaxation process. This is the "condensation of the back stroke". The tongue may or may not leave the palate at once; in any case the excursion from the palate has nothing to do with the consonant arrest.

This analysis of the consonant stroke makes the arresting consonant and the releasing consonant modifications of the one movement. The essential thing is a stroke to the opposing surface, which may be given in contact, and which may or may not be followed by a back stroke from the surface. When the beat stroke occurs in contact the only apparent movement may be *from* the palate in the releasing consonant. When the back stroke occurs in contact the only apparent movement may be *to* the palate in the arresting consonant.

The study of the tracings proves that all consonants, whether continuants or occlusives, have essentially the same function of releasing or arresting the syllable movement (Cf. later material on the double consonant and on other abutting pairs).

The time relations of the consonants show that they are all essentially the same process. Rousselot says that "attributing to each consonant the interval necessary for its production, the consonants are all of about the same length; there are but slight differences:

Strong continuants require c. .180 sec.
Weak   "   "   " .150–.160 sec.
Strong occlusives   "   " .140 sec.
Weak   "   "   " .120 sec. (70, 72)".

E. W. Scripture quotes similar values from Grégoire (21, p. 161, 263, 418; 76).

These values compare very well with the intervals of rapid movements in other fields. The interval .180 sec. is equivalent to a rate of 6.6 per sec.; .120 sec. is equivalent to a rate of 8.3 per sec.; 6.6–8 per sec. is well within the limits of the "tapping time", or "repetition time" as measured for rapid movements of the hand. Such repeated movements involve, of course, the beat stroke and the back stroke. The ordinary method of taking "tapping time" involves a stroke to an opposing surface. The records, however, are like those taken of a free movement with self-arrest. The ballistic stroke (contraction phase) of most of the consonants can be executed with great rapidity, in .020–.040 sec., a fact which has important bearings on the functions of the consonant in the syllable movement.

Detail of Consonant Movement

The lingual occlusives "*t/d*" and "*k/g*" show the stroke and the opposing surface very clearly but these are not so apparent in the case of the other linguals.

The lingual continuants "*s/z, sh/j* (French *ch/j*), *ch/ch* (French *tch*), German *ch*, etc." all constrict the vocal canal but may not close it. The organs however spring into position with a ballistic stroke and quit the position with precisely the same type of back stroke as occurs in the case of the occlusives. The fundamental distinction lies in the fact that they may not completely close the canal; in other respects their action and their time relations are much the same. The fact that the breath is escaping gives them a continuous sound during the movement while the corresponding closure of the occlusive is silent; but this does not affect the function of the continuants in the least (Cf. Fig. 45). Figs. 31 and 32 show forms in which the pressure in mouth rises for the continuants just as for the occlusives, and there is often little difference in the consonant contact. It is the difference between a tight and a leaky closure.

The labials include the occlusives "*p/b*" and the continuants "*f/v*". The movements of the lips are fairly obvious; in reality, the lower lip is primarily the moving member.

The tongue may be substituted for the lower lip. With a little practice, all the labials can be

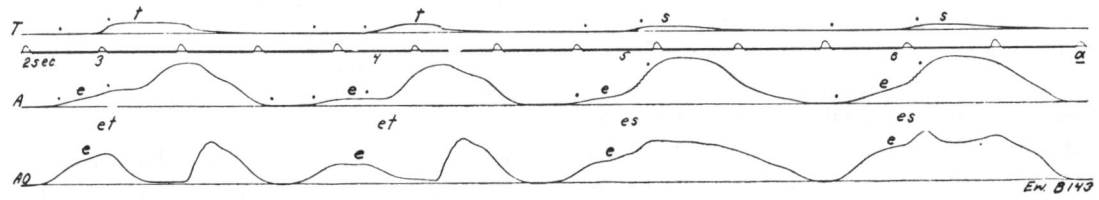

FIGURE 31. Comparison of Occlusive and Continuant (Excellent test for the Tongue Marker)
Syllables: *et et es es*.
  T—Tongue marker. Contacts of the *t* are slightly stronger than those of *s*.
  A—Air pressure in mouth. Both unvoiced stop and unvoiced continuant, have high pressure.
  AO—Air pressure outside mouth. The stop *t* shows zero air pressure outside, but the continuant shows high pressure.
  Dots show the limits of laryngeal vibration.

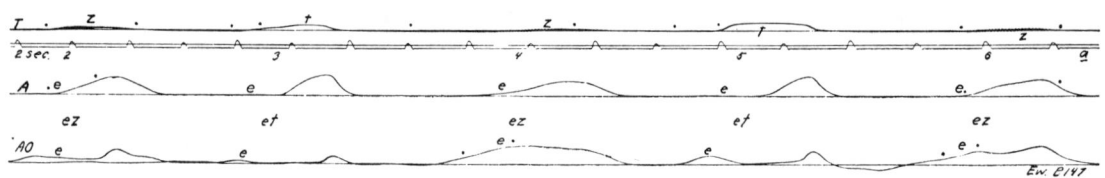

FIGURE 32. Comparison of Voiceless Stop with Voiced Continuant
Syllables: *ez et ez et.*
T—Tongue marker. *z* shows vibration only. *t* has definite stroke.
A—Air in mouth. Rise of air pressure for stop is more abrupt.
AO—Air outside mouth. The pronounced flow of air for the continuant contrasts with the small flow of the stop.

made successfully with the tongue striking the upper lip (or the lip and teeth).

The base of the tongue plays against the palate and the velum in producing the gutturals "*k/g*", German "*ch*" (hard), Greek gamma, and French "*r grassyée*". The tongue is primarily the moving member.

The glottis figures in two sounds. The aspirate "*h*", common in English and occurring on occasion in French (60), is, strictly speaking, not a consonant. Statements like Clédat's (10, p. 73) are merely traditional. It is really a modification of the vowel and cannot occur in the arresting position. The rarer glottal stop (coup de glotte) figures as a consonant.

In addition to the consonants considered there are two other classes. The first class contains the vowels which narrow the canal to such an extent that when they take the extreme position and open abruptly they may function as consonants; "*ou*" = consonant "w", and "*i*" = consonant "y". These have no peculiarities save that they are often associated with the vowels and may arise in vowel combinations. Although these vowel-related consonants are sometimes called "semi-vowels", a second class has a better claim on the term because they leave the vocal canal so open that they may easily figure as vowels: the liquids "*l*" and "*r*" and the nasals "*m, n, -ng*". Since these "sounds" are all vocalized and allow the breath to escape freely they may figure as vowels. On the other hand, they constrict the vocal canal sufficiently to function in the arrest and release of the syllable movement.

Voicing of Consonants

As a whole, the consonants are divided into two parallel series, the "voiced" and "unvoiced" (sonant and surd). It is evident that the quality is due to the action of the vocal folds which are often supposed to act independently, like the other organs of articulation. But the vocal folds do not come into play as a separate factor. Instead, they are activated by the pulse of air from the chest. And there are reasons for thinking that the difference between the voiced and unvoiced consonants is not due to the direct action of the vocal folds, but rather to the coordination of the articulatory apparatus and the chest. When the pressure in the buccal cavity is practically that of the chest, there is no flow of air to activate the vocal folds. When the pressure in the buccal cavity is reduced by the consonantal release of air, or when the expiratory muscles increase the chest pressure, the vocal folds are activated. The experience of the subjects with an artificial larynx has already been cited.

A study of the mouth pressure for surds and sonants in rapid speech shows that the difference in pressure, expressed by the terms "fortis and lenis", is more fundamental than the voicing of the consonants, and persists after the voicing distinction is lost, i.e., after both surd (fortis) and sonant (lenis) are voiced. Musehold's statement that the velum is momentarily lowered for "*b, d, g*" is quite mistaken. The airflow necessary for the occlusives "*b, d, g*" is provided by the descent of the larynx mass. The velum is closed for all consonants except the "nasals" "*n, m, -ng*". The relation of these accessory movements which change the quality of the consonants is somewhat the relation of the movements of the vowel to the syllable movement. The movements occur together but they do not condition each other, though they cooperate in producing the given consonant (35; 56, p. 75).

TYPES OF SYLLABLES AS DETERMINED BY THE CONSONANTS

In dealing with the function of the auxiliary consonant stroke in the syllable movement there are four types to consider:

1. A syllable movement arrested by its own negative muscle-group (the inspiratory muscles) may be called the syllable movement with chest-arrest. This is the case in uttering "*a, a* . . . ." or "*ta, ta* . . . ."; OVO or CVO.

2. The syllable movement is arrested by the consonant stroke; this is the syllable with consonant arrest, thus, "*at, at*", "*tat, tat*". (Cf. Fig. 37, "up" and "*pup*"; OVC, CVC).

Many movements are arrested by an obstacle. When the finger of the typist hits the key, the momentum of the movement is taken up by the obstacle, not by the counter action of the negative muscle-group. This very common form may be called ballistic movement with arrest by obstacle. Sometimes the obstacle is another member, the movement of which puts it in the path of the ballistic movement. Thus one claps one's hands; an orator arrests the blow of the right hand in the palm of the left. This is the movement with auxiliary arrest; it is the type of syllable movement with consonant arrest. The consonant stroke is the obstacle arresting the chest pulse.

3. The beginning of the ballistic movement may be initiated in different ways. Often the chest muscles start the syllable movement themselves; this is the movement with chest-release, thus "*a, a* . . . ." and "*at, at* . . . ." (Cf. Fig. 37, "*up*"; OVO, OVC).

4. An auxiliary consonant stroke may release the chest pulse, thus, "*ta, ta*", "*tat, tat*". In snapping the fingers the movement of one finger releases the movement of the other. When one puffs out a candle, the closed lips suddenly release the air compressed by the muscles of expiration. This is the chest pulse with consonant release (Cf. Fig. 37, "*pup*"; CVC).

Elaborate combinations of movements are frequent in complex habits. In the playing of wind instruments, auxiliary movements sometimes release the chest pulse as in the case of "triple-tonguing"; the movement is very seldom arrested by an auxiliary movement. A whistled note is sometimes brought to a close by a consonant stroke resembling the "*t*" stroke.

In flicking a coin or shooting a marble, the finger holds the thumb (or the thumb holds the finger) during a growing tension which is finally released by the auxiliary movement. In coughing, the pressure of the chest compression is finally released in the throat.

The movement of shaking down the mercury in a clinical thermometer involves an arrest produced by the movement of the other hand which intercepts the beat stroke of the hand holding the thermometer; the movement of the left hand is actually substituted for a self-arrest by the muscles of the right hand. It is possible to produce somewhat the same shaking movement with the right hand alone, with self-arrest. A refractory fountain pen is often subjected to the same treatment. In movements of plucking and picking, the thumb and fingers arrest each other's movements in closing on the object.

In the ordinary forms of syllable movement with chest-arrest, the muscles of the breathing apparatus are connected with each other by an intervening system of bones, cartilages and joints. This is the rule with antagonistic muscle-groups. At first sight it seems difficult to think of the muscles of the tongue or of the lips functioning as the negative muscle-group for the breathing apparatus; the muscles of the tongue and lips are not attached to the chest. How can the lips and tongue act as antagonists to the chest muscles? An examination of the entire speech mechanism shows that the column of compressed air in the chest and vocal canal becomes the intermediary between the expiratory muscles of the chest acting as the positive group and the muscles of the consonant apparatus acting as the negative group. At the end of the syllable, the sudden closure (or constriction) of the vocal canal by the consonant movement stops the escape of air, raises the air-pressure, and thereby arrests the beat stroke and takes up the momentum of the movement. The movement of the consonant apparatus is harnessed to the movement of the breathing apparatus as effectively as the organist's finger is connected with the valve at the pipe in an organ with pneumatic action. When the syllable pulse is chest-arrested, the muscles of the rib-cage act directly on the moving mass of the chest walls to take up the momentum and arrest the syllable movement. But when the syllable pulse is consonant-arrested the muscles of lips, tongue, velum, do not act directly on the mass of the chest walls. Instead, they close the vocal canal, and cause compression of the air column, which reacts on the moving mass of the chest walls. This consonant-arrest therefore takes more time since the air pressure must rise before force is exerted. The compressed air must be released, usually by the détente, and the process adds to the duration of the syllable. Often the syllable arrest is a combined consonant- and chest-action. But as the rate of the syllable utterance increases, there is no time for the delaying process of consonant-arrest and the arrest must become a chest-arrest. This is the determining factor in the shift of the arresting consonant to the releasing position in the next syllable, or in the dropping of the arresting consonant if the shift is not possible.

Fig. 33, A, B, represents schematically the possibilities of coordination of the articulatory apparatus with the chest movement.

The slow, continuous movement of expiration, punctuated by the consonantal movement, does not occur in normal speech. There is no experimental evidence of such a correlation, and the series of syllables in "*lil' 'll lie low*", and "*runnin' 'n' neighin'*" (Figs. 88, 89) do not show any tendency to maintain continuous chest pressure while the syllable is initiated by the "n" or the "l". The early efforts of the deaf to speak may approximate this form; but it cannot give intelligible speech.

In some cases the articulatory apparatus is fixated as in A II, and the syllable is due entirely to the breathing apparatus. This is the case with a series of vowels (Cf. Fig. 23).

But in most cases, the chest pulse is released or arrested, or both, by the movement of the consonant. The scheme B I, II represents a series like "*tat, tat; tat. . . .*". For details of such movements (Cf. Fig. 36).

The events of a series of syllables as represented by various investigators are presented in Fig. 36. The observations of F. de Saussure of the implosion-explosion division of syllables and of the explosion-syllable-point-implosion structure of the syllable itself, are not based on experimental work; but the concepts are essentially physiological, as he notes in the text (75, pp. 79–80). The diagrams of Fig. 36 are drawn from experimental studies.

Saussure conceives of a series of syllables such as "*ab ba* and *vak*" as being separated by the implosion-explosion junction, at "*ab: ba*" and indirectly "*ba: vak*". In the opening "*ab*" the explosion occurs at the beginning of the vowel "*a*" and increases to the syllable point; the implosion process begins in the vowel, but concludes in the implosion of the consonant "*b*". The syllable "*ba*" leads off with the explosion of the "*b*"; the implosion continues to the syllable point in the vowel, when the implosion begins and runs to the end of the syllable in the vowel. The syllable "*vak*" opens with the explosion of the consonant "*v*", culminates at the syllable point in the

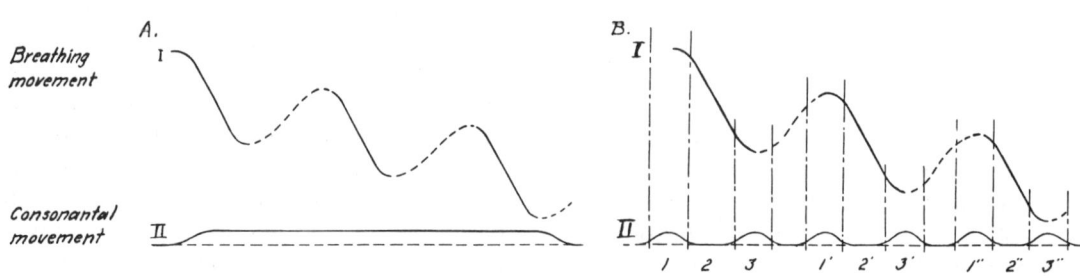

FIGURE 33. Coordinations of the Articulatory Apparatus with the Chest Movement

AI—Breathing movement shows pulses for each syllable.

II—Consonantal movement is a fixation, as for "*n, n, n,*" or "*a, a, a*". Syllable is due entirely to the breathing apparatus.

BI—Breathing movement shows pulses for each syllable.

II—Consonantal movement releases and arrests each chest pulse; "*tat, tat, tat*".

This is the more common form, but any syllable may be chest released or chest arrested, e.g. "*at*" or "*ta*".

COORDINATION OF THE MOVEMENTS OF SPEECH

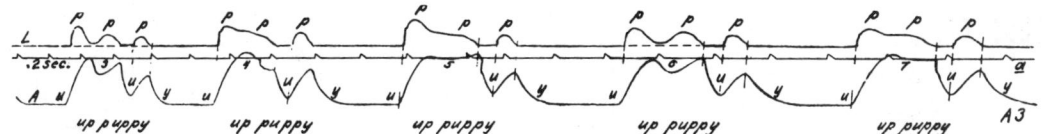

FIGURE 34. Comparison of Double and Single Consonants (Kymograph is increasing speed)

Syllables: *up puppy*.

L—Lip marker. The arresting *p* is given with more force than the releasing *p* of the first syllable of puppy. The consonant curves show degrees of fusion.

A—Air pressure in mouth. The two maxima are distinct in all the doubles of the excerpt. As indicated elsewhere, it is mathematically possible that such curves result from separate chest pulses.

Difference in the duration of the double and of the single consonant is very apparent; there is every indication of the two movements of the lips in the double.

---

vowel, when the implosion continues through the vowel into the closing consonant "*k*".

Marichelle bases his diagram (not shown) on his analysis of wax phonograph grooves. He makes the consonants integral parts of the syllable, and counts the transition from the constriction of the consonant to the more open vowel and the reverse process the significant articulations. He does not attempt to indicate this movement of articulation on his diagram; but he does stress the effect of the consonant constriction on the cycles of the vowel, both in the explosive and implosive articulations (50, pp. 80–83). Marichelle is aware that the consonant is perceived in the totality of the syllable, and not as a separate unit: he gives detailed experimental confirmation of this view (50, p. 83, Pl. 10).

Rousselot's scheme is derived from Saussure's

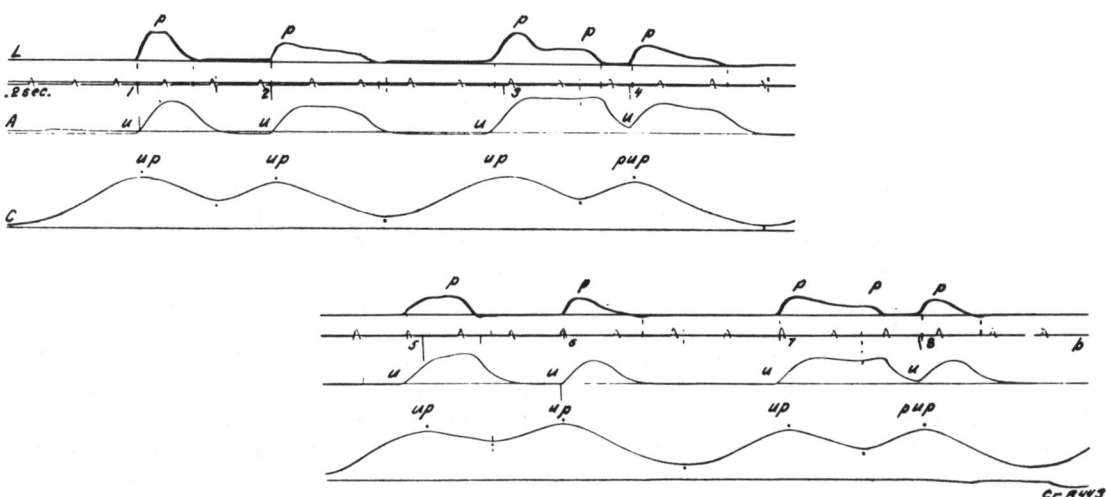

FIGURE 35. Relation of the Consonant Contacts to the Chest Pulses in Double and Single Consonants; Chest Pressure directly from the Trachea

Syllables: *up up, up pup*.

L—Lip marker; Syl. 1, 2, 4, 5, 6, 8 show single, arresting forms of the *p*. There is a slight tendency to double the final syl. 2, 4. Syl. 3-4, 7-8 have typical doubling forms with the stress on the arresting consonant.

A—Air pressure in mouth. Syl. 1, 5, 6, 8 are typical arresting forms. Syl. 2, 4 are finals which tend to double. The doubles, syl. 3-4, 7-8 are typical with the rounded rise of the arresting phase and the sharp drop at the détente of the releasing phase.

C—Chest pressure. In the case of the single arresting consonants the minimum occurs after the détente of the *p*. In the case of the double, 3-4, 7-8, the minimum occurs during the releasing doublet and not in the middle of the double.

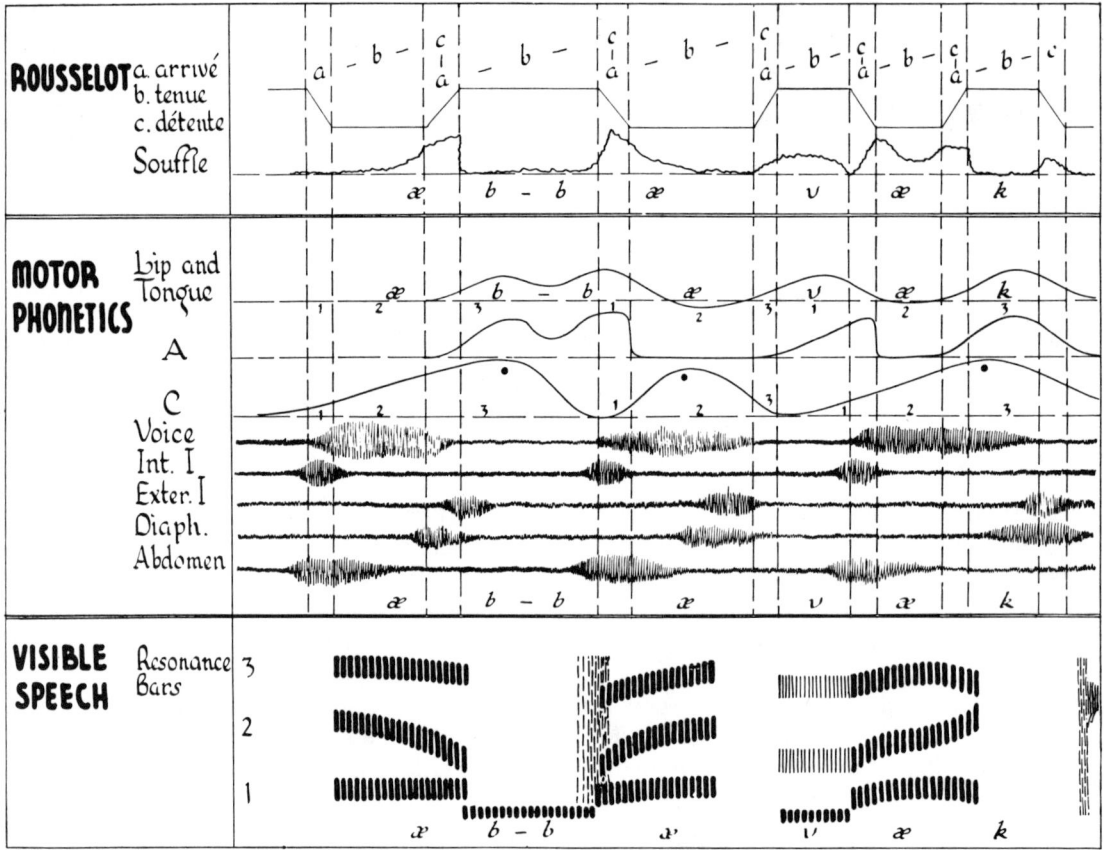

FIGURE 36. Comparison of the Representation of Syllables by Rousselot, Motor Phonetics and Visible Speech
Syllables: *ab-ba vak*.

Rousselot: *Arrivée*. Since the arrivée of a vowel must also be the détente of a consonant, the zones c and a of the syllables coincide.

Souffle. Corresponds to the tracing of the air pressure outside when the mouth mask is used in motor phonetics tracings.

Motor Phonetics: Lip and Tongue tracing indicates the consonant contacts of the syllables. The contact is continuous through the double of *b-b*.

A—Air inside the mouth. The pressure rises for the consonants; the forms of the releasing and arresting are characteristic.

C—Chest pressure, registered by different methods, shows the relation of the chest pulses to the releasing and arresting consonants in the syllable.

Voice Microphone line marks the vibration of the vowels.

Int. I. Contraction of the internal intercostals which initiate the chest pulse.

Exter. I. Contraction of the external intercostals which arrests the chest pulse.

Diaph. Contraction which terminates the breath group movement.

Abdomen Contraction which initiates the breath group movement.

Visible Speech: Resonance Bars. The 'kinking' (warping) of the bars toward the upper, or the middle, or base line indicates the place of the consonant constriction. For *b* and *v* the bars are warped toward the base line. For *k* the bars are warped toward the upper level of the syllable pattern. The term "hub" (visible or invisible) is a method of explaining the warping of the vowel bars by the consonants. *b-b* and *v* show the baseline resonance of voiced sounds; *b* shows "fill" with voicing. The détente of the *k* shows a "spike" with "fill".
Cf. Figure 114, App. XIII.

explosion-implosion conception of the syllable, but applied by Rousselot to the basic articulation which he conceives to be the "sound" (70, p. 334-5, Figs. 116, 117; 72, p. 25, Fig. 12).

In the first curve of Rousselot, Fig. 36, it will be noted that the "détente" phase of one articulation is identical with the "tension" phase of the next (c_1 and a_2; c_2 and a_3 etc.). If the syllables "ab-ba" had been represented as separated there would have been a complete cycle for the articulation of each "b", and the series would have been a_1 b_1 c_1, and a_2 b_2 c_2. If, however, the syllables had been "at-la", the overlapping of phases would have been more extensive than in the preceding figure, for the "tenue" of the "t" would be identical with that of the "l", the "tension" of the "t" would serve for the "l", and the "détente" of the "l" would serve for the "t".

In the second curve of Rousselot, Fig. 36, "Souffle", there is shown diagramatically the air pressure just outside the mouth; it falls to zero, of course, during an occlusion, and rises the moment the vocal canal is opened. The curve is nearly the reverse of the curve of the air pressure in the mouth, given in A below. It is to be noted that any variations of pressure during an occlusion cannot of course appear in the "Souffle" curve (Cf. Fig. 112).

Fig. 36, "Motor Phonetics", gives a group of curves representing the events of the syllable in terms of movements. Only the outline of the coordination (of movements, contacts and air pressures) is given here; the system of movements will be treated more fully later.

In the first syllable "ab" there is no releasing consonant; the chest pulse, curve C, is chest-released. The descending stroke, 1—3, represents the rapid movement of the pulse; in 1 the sudden contraction of the chest muscles occurs, compressing the chest. During phase 2 the momentum of the chest continues the compression and a stream of air flows freely through the vocal canal. In phase 3 the movement of the consonant closes the canal and blocks the flow of air; the rapid rise in air pressure arrests the chest movement. In this case the consonant movement replaces the contraction of the negative muscle-group of the chest. The actual connection between the chest and the accessory movement of the consonant is effected through the column of compressed air in the vocal canal.

Between the syllables "ab" and "ba" (between 3 and 1) the chest muscles readjust for a new compression. The lips remain in contact but the muscles of the lips relax in preparation for the releasing stroke of the "b" in "ba" (1 of the next syllable). In this second syllable "ba" the rapid contraction of the chest muscles recurs in 1, the pressure suddenly rises because of the consonant closure, but is suddenly released by the back stroke of the lower lip from the upper, and the air flows freely through the canal in phase 2 as before. In phase 3 the inspiratory muscles of the chest itself contract to stop the momentum of the chest, forming an open syllable "ba". The syllable movement is chest-arrested and the air pressure remains at zero (3) because there is no consonant closure.

Between the syllables "ba" and "vak" (between phases 3 and 1) the chest muscles readjust for the new compression.

In the third syllable "vak" the consonant and the syllable movements are coordinated in phase 1. Phase 2 shows the free flow of air with zero pressure in mouth. The coordination in phase 3 is precisely that of the arresting consonant in "ab".

The maxima of the air pressure are of rounded form when the arresting movement closes the canal, and the fall in pressure is abrupt when the releasing consonant opens the canal (Cf. Fig. 37, syl. 4). An actual tracing which will give something of these relations will be found in Fig. 35.

The project of the Bell Telephone Laboratories, which is concerned with "Visible Speech", is like that of Marichelle (50), some fifty years earlier, in that a visual representation of the acoustic patterns of speech is the purpose of an experimental study. Steinberg and French (82, p. 4), Kopp and Green (43, p. 74), confirm Marichelle's finding that the syllable is perceived as a unit in which the consonants are apparent primarily in their effect on the vowel. Although the acoustic recordings in wax which Marichelle studied gave small indication of the syllable division, possibly Marichelle's first-hand experience in the instruction of the deaf led him to stress the syllable and the syllable division.

The acoustic patterns are presented in "Visible Speech" as 'spectrograms' in which the changing sound components at different frequency levels are translated into concurrent bars, each of

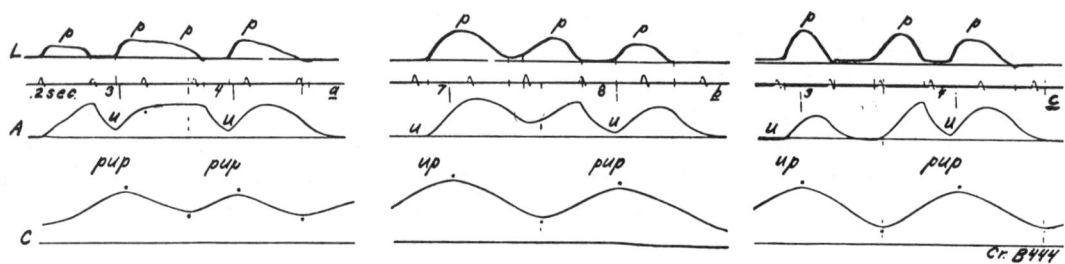

FIGURE 37. Stages of a Double Becoming Single. Reverse of the Development of the Double. Chest Pressure is recorded directly from the Trachea

Syllables: *pup pup, up pup, up pup.*

L—Lip marker. At *a*, syl. 3-4, the form is double; there is no very distinct indication of the two *p* lip strokes. At *b*, syl. 7-8, there are two distinct contacts but they are still adjoining, and there is slight contact throughout. At *b*, syl. 3-4, the two *p*'s are quite distinct; a definite intersyllabic interval appears.

A—Air pressure in mouth. The form *a*, syllable 3-4, is a double, but not marked.

At *b*, syl. 7-8, the double form is pronounced; the two doublets are very distinct.

At *c*, syl. 3-4, the two components are separated and have become characteristic arresting and releasing forms.

C—Chest pressure: The minimum pressure occurs during the releasing doublet. The minimum becomes more and more pronounced until the actual separation occurs.

which concentrates on one of a series of bands of frequency. The bands of frequency were chosen to bring out the prominent and most obviously modulated spectrum zones which represent the influence of the changing cavity-orifice of the vocal organs.

The method brings out strikingly two important traits of the syllable:

1. The fairly well-defined "resonance bars" mark the pattern of modulation of the vowel which is usually the core of the syllable. Up to a rate of ca. 3 per sec., the vowels of the English syllables are easily recognizable.

2. With Marichelle, the consonants are to be read in large part by the influence of the consonant constrictions on the vowel. In consequence, the syllable must be perceived as a whole, not as a series of consonant, vowel, consonant..

While the vowels and the influence of the consonants on the vowels are well portrayed, the actual movements, contacts, and air pressures of the speech process must be inferred. In the attempt to make the main acoustic features prominent, variations of intensity are omitted in the present form of the apparatus, and it is therefore impossible to catch the pulse of the syllable which

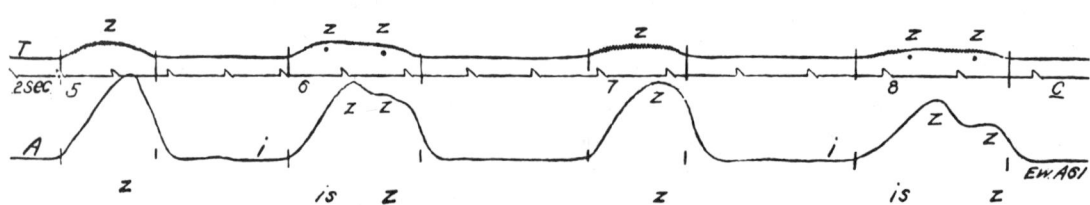

FIGURE 38. Double and Single Continuant

Syllables: *Z is Z.*

T—Tongue marker. The two maxima are apparent though not as clearly defined as in the case of stops. The vibration of the voiced consonant is clearly seen in the original. A continuant consonant is harder to record; the consonant contact is never complete, of course.

A—Air pressure in mouth. Forms are rather rounded in contrast with the releasing curves of stops. In syls. 6 and 8 the arresting consonant is stronger than the releasing—true throughout the series.

is so important for recognizing the individual syllable and the groups of syllables.

The findings can be collated with the movement process of a motor phonetics, as Fig. 36 shows (See also Fig. 114, App. XIII).

The opening of the vowel of "*ab*" is marked by the appearance of the "resonance bars" for the "*ae*"; the second bar is 'kinked' down at the arrested end because the arresting "*b*" prescribes a closure at the lips, and the modulation of the vowel shows the change of the volume-orifice, as the lips produce the closure. The authors speak of the 'hiddenhub' of the labials which is down toward the base line; but it is rather the visible effect on the vowel of the change of cavity-orifice as the lips come together for the stop.

The constriction for the "*b*" brings a sudden discontinuity because acoustic conditions are abruptly changed, but there is no "spike", i.e. there is no disturbance at all in the frequency levels, because the *closure* is not marked by a sudden emission of air under pressure. The "stop gap" means the interval of consonant closure. Since the "*b*" is a sonant, it will have a "voice bar", showing that the vocal folds are vibrating. There will be no 'spike' since there is no release of air between the doublets. When the arresting member of the double appears there is no release of air between the doublets. But when the releasing "*b*" opens in "*ba*", the 'spike' portrays the sudden release of air under pressure, and the slight stop-gap fill indicates the aspiration as the air escapes in the English syllable before the vowel sounds. Just as the "resonance bars" of "*ab*" were kinked, so the resonance bars of "*ba*" will be kinked down as they sound after the vowel. But as the mouth opens and the "*ae*" prescribes the normal cavity-orifice, the resonance bars become horizontal at the usual levels.

Assuming that the rate of the syllables is 4—5 per sec., discontinuities will appear between consonant and vowel, and between vowel and vowel. They indicate the very brief intervals during which the ballistic movement of the consonant closure, or of the vowel shaping, is so rapid that the modulation cannot follow the cavity-orifice change. This indication of a ballistic movement contributes to the perception of the total syllable movement. Both sounds and silence, continuous and discontinuous change, figure in the motor patterns of speech.

The third syllable "*vak*" shows the voiced interval of a sonant labial (without the spike and aspiration of the opening English stop), with the downward kink of the "resonance bars" indicating the labial opening. The "resonance bars" kink upward as the syllable is arrested by the "*k*" because, this time, the constriction is in the back of the mouth, the reverse of the lip closure.

The Microphone line gives the envelopes of the syllables. The consonants show slightly, with the exception of the "*k*" in "*vak*", which is a surd. The vowels constitute the principal acoustic events.

The internal intercostals contract to release the pulse of each syllable; the fact that the contraction is a momentary impulse is apparent.

The external intercostals contract to arrest the pulse of each syllable.

The Rectus abdominis contracts in anticipation of the breath group involved; the syllables are assumed to occur no faster than three per sec., and an abdominal stroke (breath group) for each syllable is possible. If the syllable rate exceeds three per sec. the abdominal muscles fixate or make a slow, 'tense', phrasing movement.

The action-current tracings give the muscle action for the syllables and for the foot- and breath-group-units. Acoustic and pneumatic recordings can give only indirect evidence of the movements of the foot and the breath group.

In order to make the diagram, any reference to the foot or breath group has been omitted. The syllables "*ab-ba vak*" must be considered as feet in a breath group (Cf. Figs. 35 and 37).

The feet are produced by the abdominal muscles which make the stress of the foot and group the syllables.

The breath group is the movement of expiration involving the abdomen-chest adjustment which groups the feet in the breath group.

CERTAIN DIFFERENCES IN THE SYLLABLE AS MODIFIED BY THE AUXILIARY MOVEMENTS OF RELEASE AND ARREST

When the syllable has a consonant release, the length of the syllable movement is not affected; the consonant movement fuses with the syllable movement. The syllable may be very short, a rapid ballistic movement, with chest-arrest, or it may be indefinitely prolonged, changing into a controlled movement. The consonant release does not limit the duration of the syllable.

On the other hand, when the syllable movement has a consonant arrest, the length of the syllable is conditioned. The ballistic stroke of the syllable is arrested by the consonant movement and the syllable movement cannot be indefinitely prolonged into a controlled movement. Its maximum length, therefore, is that of a ballistic movement, .13 sec. at the most. In a group of 40 cases studied (3 subjects), the maximum is .13 and the minimum .05 sec. The arresting consonant may be prolonged, or a pause may occur after the syllable, but the syllable beat stroke is, of necessity, brief. This means that the vowel of the syllable, with arresting consonant, will always be a relatively brief vowel.

Thus, the records of "closed" syllables (syllables with arresting consonants) show a short duration of the vowel: *patte*, .16 sec. (including the "*p*"); *patelin*, .10 sec. ("*pa²*") (72, p. 86). *Beat*, .14; *bid*, .14; *bin*, .10; *bit*, .06 sec. (37). These may be compared with *pa*, .24; *pate*, .28 (*pa-*); *bee*, .50; *bonjour*, .68 sec. (*bon-*); in all of which the syllable is "open". E. W. Scripture quotes Gregoire's observation that for some reason in *pâté sucrée* the "*t-s*" shortens the vowel and lengthens the occlusion (76). The "*t*" has become an arresting consonant, and the syllable "*pat*" is now closed, therefore the vowel shortens. The position of the tongue against the palate is maintained from "*t*" to "*s*", and the back stroke phase of the first syllable occurs during that interval, therefore the occlusion is lengthened.

In English (and in German as well) the prevailing form of the syllable is actually both released and arrested by a consonant; it is consonant delimited, CVC. This is true of the simplest possible vocabulary of 300 words suggested for deaf children (22). It is true of the first 500 words, and of the first 1000 and 2000 word lists of the most frequently used words (96).

The common syllable is not the consonant-vowel, CVO, which many think of. At least 80 per cent of the syllables are arrested by a consonant (OVC, CVC); at least 70 per cent are both released and arrested by a consonant (CVC). This means that arresting consonants and abutting consonants are very common; a heavy stress on such syllables will produce the changes in the stressed and unstressed syllables to be discussed later.

The number of different syllables runs very high; at least 5000 are in use in English and German, and more than half that number of syllables occur frequently in French. It is not possible to handle the individual syllables in a European language. Therefore, the syllables are made into classes according to the characterized syllable factors. There are the syllables which are released by a given consonant or by chest action, the syllables which have a given vowel shape, and the syllables which are arrested by a given consonant, or by chest action. Each syllable belongs to two or three of these classes. The aspects which characterize these three syllable factors (releasing, vowel shaping, and arresting) prove to be limited; there may be 5—20 vowels, and 10—50 consonants; these constitute the alphabet of the language; they are the familiar "sounds" or "phonemes".

The compound consonants are very common. They are composed of two or more simple consonant strokes together which characterize releasing and arresting syllable factors. The 300-word vocabulary cited above includes some 37 compound consonants; common words in English are as likely to contain compound consonants as simple consonants.

As can be inferred from Sievers' discussion, not all syllables which end in a consonant are actually closed syllables. If the vowel is long in duration, the arrest of the syllable movement, and possibly the change to a controlled movement, will be well under way before the consonant is uttered. In such cases the consonant occurs with the latter part of the syllable movement but is not an integral part of it. Such consonants are often noticeable in singing where the prolongation of the vowel leaves the consonant dangling. Often the consonant is given as an explosive and really constitutes an inconspicuous, added syllable (88, Cf. Fig. 75, syl. 2).

The tradition in English orthography, which makes a spelling like "*mate*" and "*hate*" indicate a "long *a*", while "*mat*" and *hat*" indicate a short *a*", harks back to the days when the "*e*" was the sign of a second syllable, and the first syllable was therefore open: *ma-te, ha-te* while "*mat*" and "*hat*" were closed syllables (Appendix X: The Demarcation of the Syllable).

Chapter IV

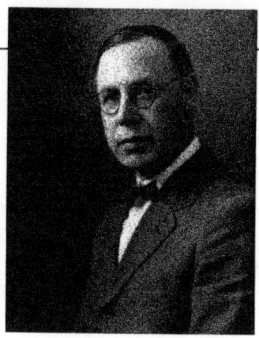

INFLUENCE OF THE PHONETIC UNITS ON EACH OTHER

Editors' Remarks

The highlight of Chapter 4 is Stetson's emphasis on the modification of articulation as a major focus of study in experimental phonetics, which is still true today. According to Stetson, "The two great causes of phonetic modification are changes of rate and stress" (p. 89). By gradually increasing speaking rate, he sought to establish the main factors that modify syllabic structure. A number of beautiful examples are provided that seem worthy of more detailed investigation using modern techniques. Stetson emphasizes that speaking rate forces movements to coalesce or drop out because rate determines duration. In a certain sense this is true, but he also recognizes that definite changes in coordination among articulators occur, even though no attempt is made to quantify or even express qualitatively the coordinative changes. Elsewhere, we have examined the experimental observations and interpretations made by Stetson in this chapter, and have offered our own (Kelso, J.A.S. et al. *J. Phonetics*, [1986, *14(1)*, 29–59]). There is remarkable evidence for phase transitions—rather abrupt changes in coordinative patterns that occur at a critical speaking rate—that reveal loss of stability in one pattern and the spontaneous emergence of another. We refer the reader to that discussion, for there is no need to repeat it here. Suffice to note that Stetson's methods may allow us to identify and differentiate patterns of coordination among the articulators. Moreover, an analysis of his work (op. cit) may reveal why the consonant-vowel syllable type is the core of all known languages, and why it dominates in the babbling of infants. But perhaps most important of all, we see (through these somewhat contrived experimental situations) how the process of producing speech influences phonetic content. Therein lies a hint that language evolves from dynamical processes—in contrast to formal, axiomatic schemes of linguistic development.

FUNCTION OF CONSONANTS IN THE LINKAGE OF SYLLABLES

Abutting (Linking) Consonants

The syllable is always incorporated in a breath group. If there are two syllables or more they are not only adjacent but connected in the breath group. The movements of the syllable pulses affect each other and their auxiliary movements may join. The arresting consonant of one syllable and the releasing consonant of the next syllable may be linked.

The tension-tenue-détente analysis of Rousselot led him to group the arresting (terminal) consonant of one syllable with the releasing (initial) consonant of the next syllable; these were made to constitute a single "group". On occasion the distinction between the two constituents was noted:

"If the two consonants are attached (s'appuyer) to a single vowel, as in *'psaume, p'tit, apt'*, their union is closer than it is if they are attached (s'appuyer) to two different vowels, as in *'aptitude'*." (72, p. 81)

If the group confined to a single syllable is called a "compound" consonant, the abutting consonants of two syllables may be called an intersyllabic pair. In case of abutting consonants it often happens that the arresting consonant of the first syllable and the releasing consonant of the next syllable are the same consonant repeated; this is the familiar "double consonant". It is of especial interest because the syllable division must take place during this double consonant. The process which divides the syllable also makes the consonant "double".

Sievers notes that the double consonant is different from a single consonant prolonged. He points out that when implosion-explosion occurs within such a double consonant, there is "discontinuity of expiration" and that the syllable division takes place between the doublets. (78, p. 191)

F. Josselyn, using Rousselot's methods for the study of Italian phonetics, discusses the peculiarities of the Italian double consonant, showing the increased length of the occlusion and the compensatory shortening of the preceding vowel. It is evident that the double consonant is very unlike the single consonant in duration and in function. (40, p. 227 f., Cf. 72, p. 78)

But Rousselot's analysis failed to differentiate the double from the single consonant. He states: "The initial and final consonants can produce only a single impression. That is the case also with a consonant between vowels pronounced without effort. But if the utterance of the consonant in this position has a certain force and an unusual duration, *two* consonants are heard, that of taking position (tension) and that of quitting position (détente). The length of the silence which separates the 'tension' from the 'détente' allows the ear to recognize the characteristic sounds which accompany first the closing, and second the opening of the vocal canal." (70, p. 993; 72, p. 50)

"A consonant prolonged becomes double" is Rousselot's conclusion, in spite of the work of Poirot which he cites. Poirot showed that both the pressure of the lips, and the pressure of the air behind the lips, have two definite maxima in the case of the double labials "*ap-pa*" and "*ab-ba*". (70, p. 1087)

Rousselot publishes a tracing of the Swedish "*pap-pa*" with a distinct depression in the middle of the "*p-p*", and points out the "*p* implosive" and the "*p* explosive". (72, p. 77)

He also publishes such tracings for the labial "*v*", but is certain that the other double consonants show no such maxima. (70, p. 351, 1087) Rousselots' apparatus could not respond to fluctuations at the rate involved, so that his experimental findings seemed to bear out the statement.

Rousselot's statement that a consonant between vowels, if prolonged, becomes double, is not adequate. The doubling depends on the occurrence of a second consonant stroke with a new chest pulse. In the phrase "I'm Ike", the "*m*" may be indefinitely prolonged without becoming double. In the case of "I'm Mike", the second consonant stroke and the entrance of the new chest pulse with this second "*m*" can be perceived. Neither Sievers nor Rousselot explain the greatly increased length of the double consonant or its influence on the preceding vowel. (94, p. 4 ff.)

Only a few English and French words contain true double consonants, but in many phrases the consonant is doubled. In English, "*up puppy; lob Bobby; topic* and *top pick; top egg* and *top peg; Otto ought to; hit him, hit Tim; I do, I'd do; this eye* and *this sigh; Z is Z; unknown, un-own;*

I owe none, I own none; *I'm Ike, I'm Mike*; *I lie, I'll lie*" are phrases in which the contrast between the double and single consonant is marked. In most cases the meaning depends on making the distinction. A careful English enunciation can distinguish between "*whole ode, hoe load*", and "*whole load*"; between "*thus E, the C, thus C*".

If records give proper details, one should expect to find two distinct consonant strokes which arrest and release the separate chest pulses of the two syllables; and there will be two distinct maxima of the air pressure in the mouth, as the first chest pulse is arrested and as the second chest pulse is released. This should be the form of the typical tracings of doubling consonants (Cf. Fig. 36).

Tracings of Double Consonants
(Special Form of Abutting Pairs)

The tracings of the various words and phrases containing doubled labials and doubled linguals show without question that the "double" consonant is actually two consonants. There are two distinct maxima in the curve indicating the movements of the lips or of the tongue. And the curve of the air pressure in the mouth also shows the ending of the one chest pulse and the beginning of the second. The pressure for the "double" consonant is a bimaximal curve, showing the arrest of the one syllable pulse and the back stroke of the chest muscles, before the increasing pressure for the release of the second syllable pulse.

The division of the syllable is to be seen 1) in the two maxima of the double articulation; 2) in the two maxima of the curve of pressure in the mouth (which mark the arrest of the one syllable pulse and the release of the second syllable pulse); 3) in the minimum chest pressure between the syllables (in the recordings which include a tracing of the chest pressure).

Fig. 34 shows the tracings of the phrase "*up puppy*" in which the first "*p*" is doubled, but the second "*p*", in spite of its orthography, is not doubled. The utterance is fluent enough to produce the complete double consonant; both the consonant curve and the air pressure curve show the two maxima. It is apparent that the pressure of the lips is greater for the arresting consonant.

Fig. 38 gives the tracing of a continuant, double and single, "*Z is Z*". The two maxima of the consonant curve are not so well defined as in an occlusive, but they are evident. The air pressure curve for the double shows the stress of the arresting consonant of the double.

Fig. 39, "*topic*" and "*top pick*", shows a sharp contrast between the single consonant and the double. The air pressure curve has the ordinary doubling form, but the maxima of the "*p*"'s in the double are separated, although the lips do not part.

Fig. 40, "*half pay*", shows a form precisely like the doubles preceding; the abutting consonants in this case are two different labials. It is plain that the two consonants of the "double" function precisely as do the two abutting consonants. Table I (Appendix XI: Table I; statistics and double consonants) gives summaries of the actual measurements of tracings of the various phrases recorded to show the contrast between the double and the single consonant. The attention of the subject was not called, however, to the fact

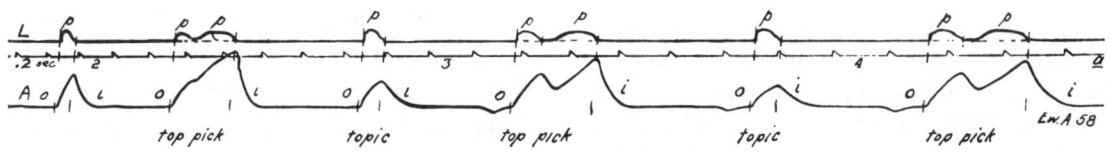

FIGURE 39. Single and Double Stop

Syllables: *top pick* and *topic*. (The tracing shows only the p and the p-p.)

L—Lip marker. The consonants of the double are very distinct though the lips are not parted during the double; the pressure between the strokes of *p-p* is very slight.

A—Air pressure in mouth. The curve shows the familiar doubling forms. The tube for the air pressure was so adjusted that it received little or no pressure during the occlusion of the *t* and *k*.

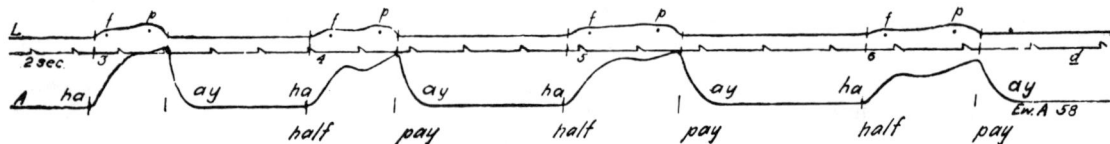

FIGURE 40. Abutting Consonants for Comparison with Doubles
Syllables: *half pay*.
L—Lip marker. Tracing of *f-p* cannot be distinguished from *p-p*. The two maxima are clearly marked.
A—Air pressure in mouth. The forms of the curves are very much like those of the double in *up puppy*, Fig. 34.

There is nothing in the detail of Fig. 40 to distinguish it from the record of a double consonant.

---

that the same consonant appeared as single and as double in each word or phrase; instead he was asked to say the phrase so that the meaning would be clear; he chose his own rate of utterance. In most cases the two maxima show in the curve of the consonant and also in the curve of the air pressure. It is difficult to record the very slight air pressure in the case of the "*l*" and nearly all the records are defective.

The difference in length between the single and the double consonant is pronounced, except in the case of the "*n*". The word chosen, "*unknown*", was not fortunate, as the single consonant occurs in the final position where there is a tendency to prolong the nasal consonant. Many of the recorded lengths of the single "*n*" are greatly in excess of the average value of the consonant as given by Rousselot, e.g., and as shown in other records. "*Unknown*" and "*un-own*" give comparable forms, but were used with only one subject.

It is to be noted that liquids and nasals like "*l, n, m*", and fricatives like "*s/z*", give the same type of doubles as do the occlusives "*t/d*" and "*p/b*". Compare Rousselot's records for "*v-v*" previously cited.

The subject S. sometimes substitutes a prolonged releasing consonant in the second syllable for a double. (Cf. Fig. 42.) It is probable that the series "*Otto ought to*" (A Fig. 47 d), and "*Topic, top pick*" (A Fig. 64 b, d, e), are of this type, but they have been included in the table.

Fig. 41 gives the distribution of the lengths of these double consonants. The curves represent percentages in order that they may be comparable and may on occasion be combined. Each curve is made up of a number of sub-groups of readings. The actual number of readings in each sub-group depends on the number of tracings available for measurement. To make certain that the chance variation in the number of readings of the sub-groups has not affected the result, the data of the curves has been computed in two ways: 1) The percentages of each sub-group were

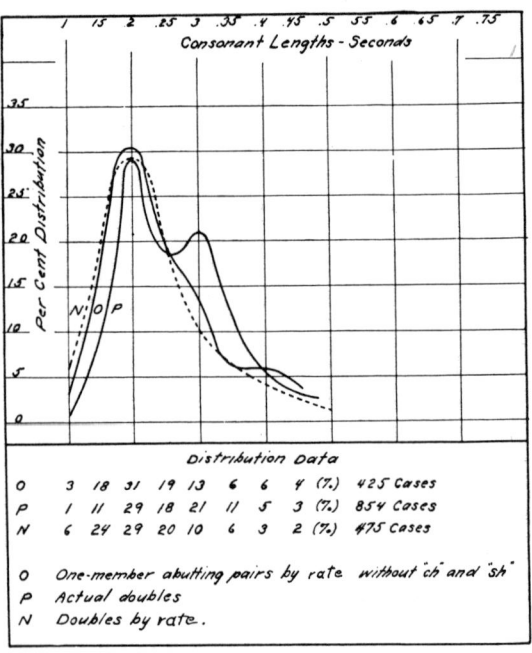

FIGURE 41. Distribution Curves of Doubles and Abutting Pairs
Comparisons of the distributions of the lengths of:
N—Doubles produced by increasing the rate.
O—One-member abutting pairs; consonants unlike, but produced by the same member, e.g. *half-pay*.
P—Actual doubles, e.g. *up puppy*.
The anomalous hump in the curve P, actual doubles, is due to a single group of syllables by the subject Ew.

computed, and the percentages averaged. 2) The actual readings of all the subgroups were added and averaged, and these averages reduced to percentages. In no case was there any significant difference between the averages of the sum of the percentages, and the averages of the percentages of the sums. (This applies to Figs. 41, 51, 65, 70, 107–110.)

The graph shows that some 29 per cent of all the cases of double consonants lie between the lengths 0.2–0.24 sec. There are very few indeed whose length is below 0.15 sec.; the distribution is much more extended above the mode .20–.24. There is a physiological limit to the rate at which the consonants may be spoken, and as speech always tends toward rapid rate, the lengths of the consonants cluster toward the lower limit. There is no assignable upper limit to the length of a consonant if a subject chooses to prolong it. The continuant may obviously continue indefinitely and the occlusion of the other consonants may be held indefinitely.

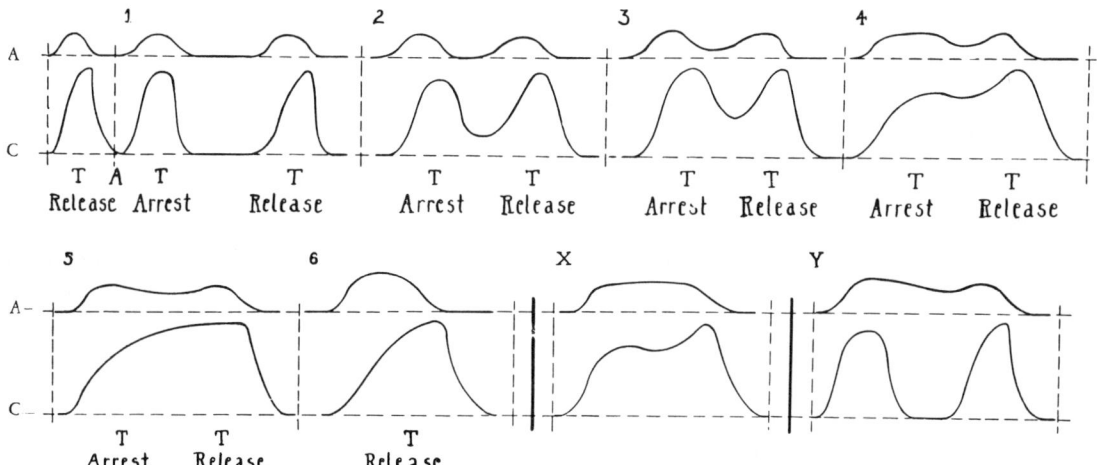

FIGURE 42. Curve Forms of the Doubling Consonants. Drawings based on the Tracings of Doubling and Abutting Consonants

The series 3–6 shows the usual progress when doubling occurs because of the gradual increase in rate of utterance.

1. The second consonant, arresting of *tat*, shows the normal rounded form of air pressure curve for a separate arresting consonant. The following consonant, releasing, shows the normal pointed form for the separate releasing consonant. Cf. Fig. 43, Syl. 3-4.

2. The mouth pressure curve does not fall to zero between the arresting and releasing consonant at the syllable frontier. The consonant tracing shows that the tongue barely remains in contact between the syllables; the consonant maxima are separate. Cf. Fig 43, syl. 5-6; Fig. 56, syl. 6-7, line *c*.

3. The maxima of the mouth pressure curve of the arresting and releasing consonants have fused; it is apparent that the curve is a combination of curves of 1 and 2. The tongue is in contact throughout the double, but the two maxima are well defined. Cf. Fig. 43, syl. 6-7; Fig 56, syl 8-9, line *b*.

4. A more advanced stage of the doubling process. The form of the mouth pressure curve is very common. Cf. Fig. 43, syl. 10-11.

5. The "convex-concave" form of mouth pressure curve; this is like the curve of a single releasing consonant very much prolonged. It is possible also that it be the combination of the curve forms of 1 and 2. Cf. Fig. 43, syl. 9-10, 12-13; Fig. 56, syl. 10-11, line *b*, etc.

6. Not a double but a stressed releasing consonant which frequently appears just after singling in a series at increasing rate. Both the form of the curve, and the length of the consonant show that it is single. In Fig. 47, syl. 8-9-10, such an emphatic releasing consonant has been substituted for a double. Cf. Fig. 81.

X. Doubling shows in the air pressure curve, but not in the consonant curve, Cf. Fig. 46.

Y. Doubling shows clearly in the consonant tracing, but the pulses of the mouth pressure tracing are separate. Cf. Fig. 44.

The distributions are most significant in showing the limits of the doubles. The modes are significant in that they show that there is a single set of causes at work, and that they probably appear in the several similar groups. The modes do not represent constants which it is important to determine. The distribution must be somewhat general; there are variations from subject to subject, dependent on variation in the subject's "repetition time".

Single consonants measured in the same way show a distribution much less wide; especially single consonants at high speed. Seventy-six single consonants from Rousselot show a mode below 10 sec. (72, p. 96 f.). (The measurements are not quite comparable but nearly so.) One hundred and ninety single consonants taken at random from a large group of tracings show a mode at .10–.14. On comparing the length of the double consonant with that of the single consonant, it is apparent that the double is about twice the length of the single consonant at rapid rate. Only a rough comparison can be made, for the processes measured are not the same; the tracing of the single consonant shows only the phase of contact with the opposing surface, while the tracing of the double consonant gives not only the phases of contact of the two doublets but also the back stroke between the doublets.

Since the movements of the articulatory organs are rapid ballistic movements, the minimum length of the double consonant should be in accord with the time limits of such movements. This means that the component consonants of the double at rapid rates should occur at the rate of some 8–12 consonants per sec., depending on the subject. The subject's maximum rate of uttering consonants will correspond to his "repetition time". This gives .20–.25 sec. as the minimum length of the double consonant, including the complete movement of both doublets. As the movement appears in the tracings, e.g. Fig. 34, it is apparent that the double form includes the beat stroke of the first consonant, the back stroke of the first consonant, and the beat stroke of the second consonant, but not the back stroke of the second consonant. This second back stroke to be added can be estimated. When a series of movements is running at maximum rate the beat stroke and back stroke are equal (Cf. Fig. 23). Therefore the double at rapid rates consists of three equal parts as recorded; the remaining back stroke will be one-third the length of the high speed double. When this third is added to the measurements of the tracings of the double consonants, the lengths agree very well with this theoretical value of .20–.25 sec.

There are a number of exceptions to the typical form of tracing indicated. Of 854 cases studied, 117, or 14 per cent, do not show the doubling form in the tracings, either in the mouth pressure curves or in the consonant curves; 41 per cent show the doubling in both mouth pressure and consonant curves; 69 per cent show the doubling in the mouth pressure curves.

The tracings of two different abutting consonants made by the same member, like "*f-p*" in "*half-pay*", "*m-b*" in "*humbug*", show precisely the same curve forms as do the double consonants. But it is evident that the two different movements are managed with more care by the subjects. Of 251 cases studied, 13, or 5 per cent only, do not show the "doubling".

In some cases the record of the pressure in the mouth is imperfect; in others the classification of the curve forms is uncertain. Only those pressure forms which show two obvious maxima have been classed as "bi-maximal" (bm). The convex-concave form (cc) may be the result of two chest pulses; indeed many of the records show that it does actually result from such a succession, but it has not been included in the list of "double forms" (Cf. Fig. 43).

The double consonant may take one of several forms which are typical also of the various cases of abutting consonants:

1. The consonant strokes are separate but the mouth pressure curve shows a definite doubling. Fig. 42. The intersyllabic interval is not long enough to permit the mouth pressure to fall.

2. Both the tracing of the consonant and of the mouth pressure show definite doubling. This is the common and, one may say, the typical form. Any of the records show such tracings (Fig. 42).

3. The tracing of the consonant is double, but the mouth pressure curves are separate; occurs when the interval between the syllables is rather long, but the subject keeps the lips or tongue in contact between the syllables (Figs. 42 and 44).

4. The tracing of the consonant movement shows a single consonant prolonged, but the

INFLUENCE OF THE PHONETIC UNITS ON EACH OTHER

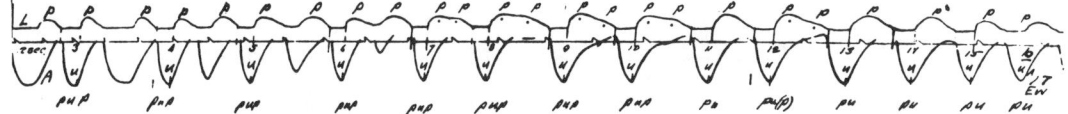

FIGURE 43. Doubling and Singling with Increase of Rate

Syllable: *pup pup* becoming *pu', pu', pu'.*

L—Lip marker. p remains separate syl. 6-7. 7-11 double forms; one single *p*, syl. 11. At syl. 13 singling occurs.

A—Air inside mouth. Doubling form appears, syl. 5–6, and is consistent with the consonant forms throughout.

mouth pressure curve makes it clear that there are two pulses. This "long consonant astride" is the form that Rousselot considered typical. In the tracings studied it is very rare, but it does occur with the subject S. who is inclined to substitute a single consonant movement for the double; this can easily be detected in his speech. Since the chest pulse may be controlled by the chest muscles alone (as in the syllable composed of a single vowel), it is possible that the shift from pulse to pulse takes place while the lips or tongue are in contact. It may be called a pseudo-double (Figs. 42 and 46).

5. Not a double at all, but a stressed releasing consonant at the beginning of the second syllable. It is listed here because in certain cases, to be discussed later, such a stressed, releasing consonant comes to take the place of a double in enunciation at rapid rate (Figs. 42 and 47).

In general, all the consonants function in the same fashion as releasing and arresting, doubling and abutting. There are some variations to be considered in the case of the continuants, especially "s"; these will be discussed later when the various abutting consonants are considered in more detail.

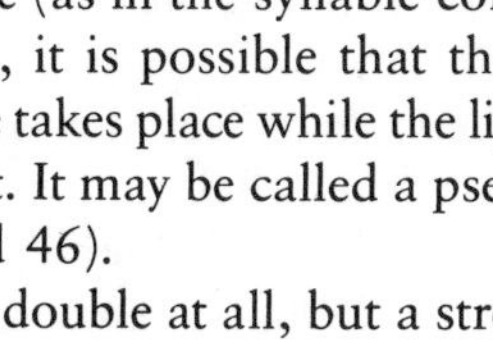

INFLUENCE OF THE RATE OF UTTERANCE ON ABUTTING CONSONANTS (INCLUDING DOUBLES)

In all these cases we have seen the properties of the "double consonant" as they appear in ordinary speech, and the properties of an abutting pair. What leads the two consonants to assume a more or less continuous form? If the two chest pulses are actually present, and if the abutting pair has actually the two functions of arresting and releasing the syllable movements, what causes the abutting? It is evident that if the syllables are spoken slowly in a word like "*unknown*", or in the phrase "*up puppy*", the consonants are separate. The rate of utterance is the thing which leads to the doubling of the consonants (Cf. Fig. 34).

The modification of the articulations is one of the most important aspects for study in experimental phonetics. The study of such changes reveals the speech apparatus at work. The two great causes of phonetic modification are changes of rate and of stress. And these two factors are both involved in rhythmic grouping.

Rate forces movements to coalesce or drop because the rate determines the duration of the individual movement in the movement series. The stressed syllables are most resistent to such changes. The syllables are more resistant than the consonants which are auxiliary movements and may be "dropped" (i.e. actually replaced by the faster, briefer chest movement of releasing or arresting).

The releasing consonants are more resistant than the arresting consonants because the

FIGURE 44. Double Consonant Forms with Single Pulses in Mouth

Syllables: *nas nas*..

T—Tongue marker. Double forms show that the tongue maintains contact with palate.

A—Air in mouth. The pulses are separate. Higher pressure for the continuant sibilant.

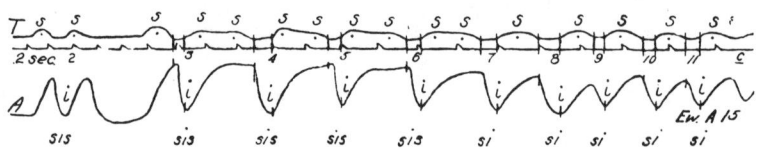

FIGURE 45. Double Consonant Forms with Single Pulses in Mouth

Syllables: *sis sis*..
T—Tongue marker. Well defined doubling forms 3-7. At 8 becomes *si' si'*..
A—Air inside mouth. Well defined doubling forms 3-7. At 8 becomes single form.

duration of the releasing consonant does not add to the syllable. The vowel is conserved with its syllable with the increasing rate; but it changes quality; less and less time is given in which to approximate the specific shape of the vocal canal. In English it is possible to note a regular series of reduced "values" of the vowel, which ends in shwa. With the increase in rate all vowels in unstressed syllables arrive at the common shwa.

Stress

Stress must affect rate; the stressed syllable is lengthened in the breath group. The breath group tends to maintain its rate and therefore the unstressed syllables within the group are shortened in compensation for the lengthening of the stressed syllables.

Stress affects the factors of the syllable on which it falls; all the auxiliary movements tend to increase in amplitude. Added breath pressure increases the intensity; increased opening of the jaw modifies the quality of the vowel toward the maximum opening of "*ah*". Added stress on the consonants increases the duration of the consonants. The stops tend to become continuants, since the increased air pressure breaks through the occlusion. A surd phase of a sonant appears; and the consonants tend to be aspirated, because of the accumulating mouth pressure due to the stress.

Extreme stress on the syllable leads to "Brechung", diphthongizing, common in languages with heavy word stress.

Rhythm shows the effect of rate and stress in the grouping of the syllables. It is fundamental to the character of the syllable that it appears as a factor in the rhythmic pattern. The breath groups are the phrases of the rhythm, and may appear as the phrases of a prose period, or as the lines ("verses") of poetic stanzas.

The method of gradually increasing the rate, and gradually decreasing the rate of a series consisting of a selected syllable repeated, shows the various types of modification of the factors of the syllable as the changing conditions throw them together or force them apart.

Any utterance consists of feet and of breath

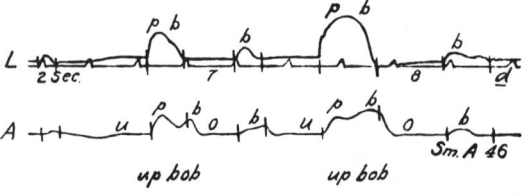

FIGURE 46. Double Consonant Forms without Separate Consonants

Syllables: *up bob*..
L—Lip marker. No indication of the double consonant, except the duration.
A—Air in mouth shows distinct pulses for each consonant.

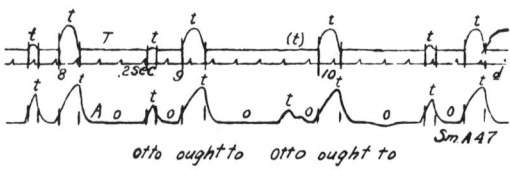

FIGURE 47. Single Long Consonant substituted for a Double Consonant

Syllables: *Otto ought to*..
T—Tongue marker. Single and "double" *t*'s distinguished only by duration.
A—Air in mouth. Forms are all of a single consonant; difference in stress.

INFLUENCE OF THE PHONETIC UNITS ON EACH OTHER

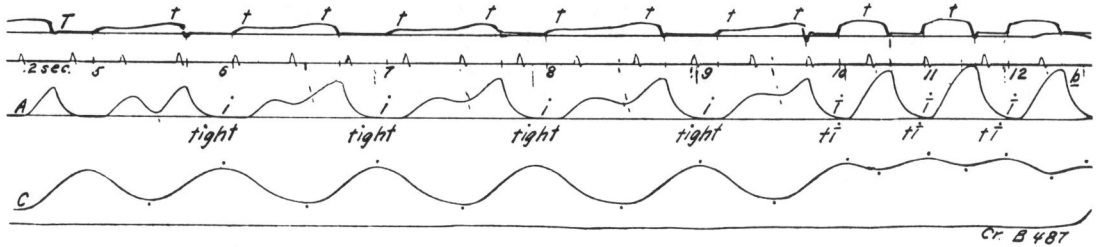

FIGURE 48. Doubling and Singling with Chest Pulses Directly from Trachea

Syllables: *tight tight . . ti' ti'*

T—Tongue marker. Double forms, syl. 5-10, when the arresting *t* drops.

A—Air in mouth. Doubles and singles follow the consonant forms.

C—Chest pulses from trachea. Pulses for each syllable, and breath group, are well defined, Syl. 5-10 show a separate breath group for each syllable. At syl. 10 a continuous indeterminate breath group appears, marked by the rise in pressure.

groups, and although the primary concern at this stage of the discussion is with the syllables and their factors, the types of foot and breath group involved are to be noted. The foot throughout is either a one syllable foot in each breath group, or it is a rapid succession of syllables in a breath group of indeterminate length. Such an indeterminate unit-group is common in music, as the trill or run, but such an indeterminate breath group of rapid syllables occurs in speech only in the unusual form of "patter". The breath groups each consist of a one-syllable foot, or of the rapid-series 'foot' in the breath group of indeterminate length (Cf. Figs. 48, 49, 50, 57, 59, 60, 61, 63).

These unusual forms of foot and breath groups are supplemented below with a detailed study of the various types of feet in breath groups of two to five syllables.

In order to study the influence of rate on doubling (abutting), tracings were made of a series of syllables like "*pup, pup. . . .*" in which the rate of utterance is gradually increased so that the syllables at first distinct, come closer and closer together. As the rate increases, the arresting consonant of each syllable doubles with the releasing consonant of the next syllable; "*pup, pup. . . .*" becomes "*pup-pup. . . .*". At a still higher rate of speed it is impossible to execute the prescribed number of consonant movements per sec., and the arresting consonant of each syllable drops; "*pup-pup. . . .*" becomes "*pu' pu'. . . .*". The whole series appears as: "*Pup, pup, pup pup pup-pup-pup-pup-pup-pu' pu' pu' pu' . . . .*".

It is possible to note the beginning of the doubling process, the rate at which it occurs, and

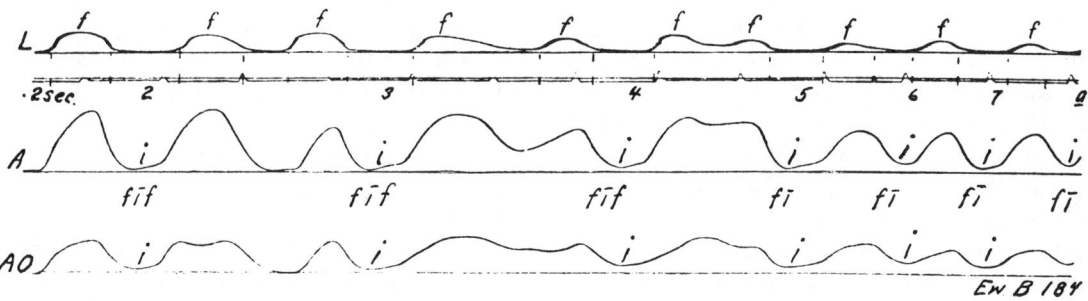

FIGURE 49. Doubles of Continuant Consonant with Increasing Rate

Syllables: *fife fife . . fi' fi' . .*

L—Lip marker. Single, separate forms, doubles, and singling forms.

A—Air in mouth. Follows the consonant forms.

AO—Air outside mouth. Follows closely the air pressure within mouth of continuant fricative.

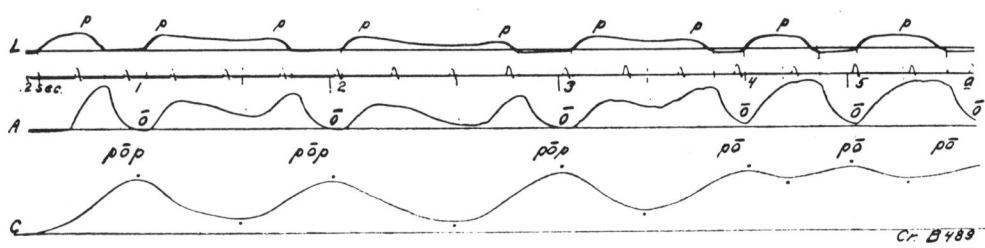

FIGURE 50. Doubles with Increasing Rate; Chest Pulses directly from Trachea indications.

Syllables: *pope, pope .. po' po' ..*

L—Lip marker. Typical single, double, and singling forms.

A—Air in mouth. Forms follow the consonant

C—Chest pulses from trachea. Breath group for each syllable, 1-4. At 4 a continuous indeterminate breath group appears.

the point at which singling begins when the arresting consonant drops.

Tracings of Double Consonants Produced by Increasing the Rate

The full list of syllables developed into series by increasing the rate is given in Appendix A.

The tracings of Fig. 43 show forms of transition from the series "*pup pup....*" to "*pu' pu'....*" produced by the increasing rate of utterance. There are the usual phases in which a stage of doubling, "*pup-pup....*", occurs before the arresting consonant drops and the series becomes "*pu' pu'....*". Both the tracings of the movement of the lips and of the pressure in mouth show the distinct abutting consonants in the doubling forms, and it is clear that there is a definite change in the coordination when the arresting consonant drops, and "singling" occurs. Rarely doubling does not occur at all. Instead, the arresting consonant drops abruptly.

Fig. 45 is added so that the doubling of a continuant like "*s*" or "*f*" can be compared with that of the occlusives. It is clear that the process is exactly the same, that the continuants function in doubling precisely as do the other consonants.

Fig. 49 shows tracings of the pressure outside and inside the mouth for continuants. The outside pressure runs high during the "*f*" or "*s*", but the mouth pressure has its maximum as usual during the consonants.

Fig. 48 shows the chest pressure tracings for occlusives with long vowels. It is to be noted that the rise in the chest pressure, marking the inception of the second syllable, occurs in the middle of the doublet, not in the middle of the releasing double consonant. Fig. 57 shows a single doubling form and has the striking rise in general pressure level which is usual with rapidly increasing rate; this leads to the vocalization of a releasing surd.

Fig. 41 gives the distribution of the lengths of such consonants doubled by increasing the rate. A comparison of the curve P with curve O shows that the general distribution of the lengths of these doubles, by increasing the rate, is very like that of the lengths of the actual doubles.

The rate at which doubling begins varies from 1–3.5 syllables per sec. It is apparent from curves d, e, in Fig. 51, that four-fifths of the series show the change from separate to double between the rates of 1 and 3 syllables per sec. And in no case do the consonants remain separate at a rate higher than 3.5 per sec. The doubles may continue from a speed of 2 syllables per sec. to a maximum rate of 4 syllables per sec., whereupon singling must occur with the dropping of the arresting consonant. Cases of singling may occur at as low a rate as 2.5 syllables per sec. The distribution of the rates at which individual series have singled, Fig. 51, "*f, g*", show a definite mode at 3.5—3.9 per sec. This indicates a tendency to jump to a considerably higher rate when the doubling ceases.

These "doubles induced by increasing rate" show all the varieties noted in the case of actual doubles. On occasion, type 5 (Fig. 42, 6, p. 87), appears just after doubling ceases with the increase of rate.

After a little practice in increasing the rate of utterance uniformly, the subjects usually produce

INFLUENCE OF THE PHONETIC UNITS ON EACH OTHER

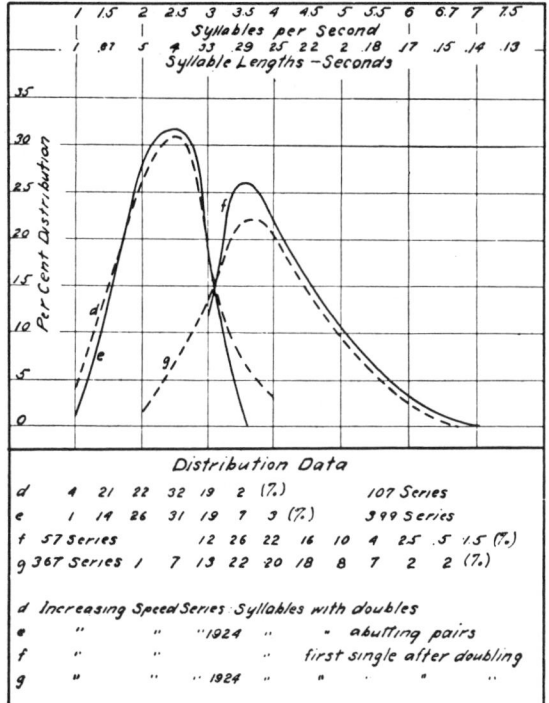

FIGURE 51. Distribution Curves showing the Rates at which "Doubling" and "Singling" occur when a Single Syllable is repeated at Varying Rates

"Doubling" is used of all cases in which two consonants come to abut at the syllable frontier; it includes the formation of the double consonant, *t-t*, as well as the abutting pair *d-t* or *p-t*.

"Singling" is used of all cases where the rate is high enough to cause the arresting consonant to drop, leaving the single, releasing consonant.

tracings with the doubling stage. Like the general group of one-member abutting pairs, only about one series in seven fails to show doubles.

Of 444 double consonants tabulated in series of this type, 124, or 28 per cent, do not have a clear indication of the bi-maximal curve in either the consonant or the mouth pressure tracings. This is a large fraction; but the mouth pressure tracings of liquids and nasals are often unsatisfactory, and the consonants "*ch*" and "*sh*" (English) double with difficulty. Of the labial forms, 80 per cent have a clear indication of doubling in the form of the curves. As in other cases, only those curves have been counted "bi-maximal" in which the two maxima are apparent.

There are two discontinuities in these series. The first is between the separate syllables, "*pup, pup*...." and the doubling form "*pup-pup*....". This is indicated by the closing up of the interval between the syllables, and by the double form of the consonant- and of the mouth-pressure-curves. The length of the vowels tends to remain the same throughout the series.

At the initial low rate of utterance there is no difficulty in enunciating the closed syllable "*pup*"; there may be an indefinite interval between the syllables. With a slight increase of rate, the interval between the syllables equals the interval between the consonants of the syllable, and the consonant movements are evenly spaced. The coordination may be schematized:

Cons.   *Arresting*   *Releasing*
Mvt.— beat str. back str.   beat str. back str.
Syl.
Mvt.—   back stroke   beat stroke

The syllable movement is arrested by the arresting consonant. Although the movements are not in phase, there is ample time for the beat- and back-strokes of the movement (Fig. 52).

As the rate increases, the movement of the arresting consonant comes to abut that of the releasing consonant and there is no longer time for the back stroke to leave the opposing surface; the consonants have doubled. The coordination may be schematized:

Cons.   *Arresting*   *Releasing*
Mvt.— beat str. back str.   beat str. back str.
Syl.
Mvt.—   back stroke   beat stroke

This involves two consonant movements (beat- and back-stroke) per syllable and the consonant movements are unevenly spaced; the abutting consonants are much closer than the consonants on either side of the vowel (Figs. 53, 54).

As the rate increases the movement, the second discontinuity, between the doubling form "*pup-pup-pup*...." and the singling form "*pu' pu' pu'*...." appears. The consonant movements will tend to become regular by dropping the arresting consonant; this will equalize the movements of the consonant, and the syllable movement, now with chest-arrest, will fall in line. The arresting consonant drops as the syllable becomes chest-arrested.

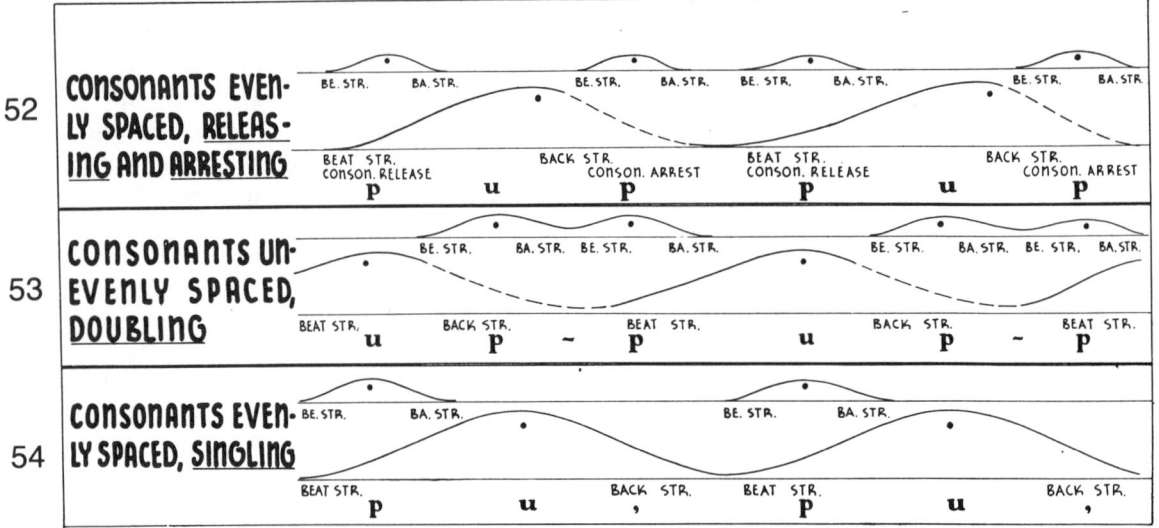

FIGURE 52. Relations of Consonant and Chest-pulse Movements
1. Consonants Evenly Spaced, Releasing and Arresting. There is space for the beat stroke and back stroke of the consonants; at the slow rate indicated, the consonants are evenly spaced, the releasing with the arresting.

FIGURE 53. Relations of Consonant and Chest-pulse Movements
2. Consonants group together in doubling forms as the rate is increased, and doubles appear. Uneven spacing of the consonants lowers the maximum rate.

FIGURE 54. Relations of Consonant and Chest-pulse Movements
3. Consonants are again evenly spaced as the arresting consonant drops and singling occurs.

The breath group of the separate syllables and of the syllables with doubles is a breath group with a one-syllable foot.

This second discontinuity is marked by the change in the consonant curves which again show a single maximum; the form of the mouth pressure tracing also shows the change from the bi-maximal, arresting-releasing type, to the simpler releasing form. At the speed of 4.–4.5 syllables per sec., this change *must* occur; the doubling of the consonant is no longer possible, for it entails 8 consonant movements per sec., a rate which is only possible when the movements are evenly spaced and, is at best, near the maximum rate for repeating a movement. There must be fewer consonants per syllabic.

And it is now apparent that the arresting consonant will be the one to drop. The arresting consonant is losing its function because the syllable movement is becoming chest-arresting. The arresting consonant is becoming a superfluous item in the syllable; it is off-phase, out of step with the syllable movement in that its beat stroke occurs with the back stroke of the syllable movement. The chest arrest is faster than the consonant-arrest. The consonant mechanism involves a column of compressed air, while the muscles in chest-arrest act directly on the ribs of the chest. At a rapid rate the movements tend either to get into step or to drop in order to simplify the coordination; therefore the arresting consonant will drop while the releasing consonant retains its position because it comes in on the beat stroke of the syllable. This tendency is very marked in all phonetic coordinations; the case has already been mentioned in which the series "*at, at*...." becomes "*ta, ta*...." as the rate increases (Cf. Figs. 26, 27 and 28). The phenomena are very striking in the case of abutting consonants involving two members (Cf. Fig. 59).

INFLUENCE OF THE PHONETIC UNITS ON EACH OTHER

It is to be said, however, that the arresting consonant does not always "drop" without a struggle. Often the movements of the arresting consonant fuse with those of the releasing; it is not a matter of mere omission. Tracings of series of writing movements, in which the rate is so rapid that "dropping" occurs, show that the amplitude of the movement crowded out is reduced because the beat- and back-strokes of the "dropping" movement come to overlap; a stasis may result; in the end the slight excursion, or the stasis, is absorbed into the back stroke of the coming movement.

In Fig. 55, I shows the beat actually present, but reduced in excursion, and becoming part of the back stroke of the coming beat. II shows the more advanced stage in which the beat appears as nothing but a slight inflection in the back stroke of the following beat. III shows the dropping beat represented by a stasis at the opening of the following beat. In IV the beat has disappeared but the back stroke of the following beat is lengthened. Such "dropping" of movements is very common in handwriting at rapid rate. It has played a part in the development of cursive forms, just as the "dropping" of phonetic movements has played a part in the modification of pronunciations.

There is likely to be a sudden increase in the rate of utterance when "singling" occurs; there is a definite physiological limit to the speed of doubling; but when the arresting consonant drops, there is nothing to prevent a rapid rise in rate (Cf. Fig. 51).

The breath group of these syllables with singled consonants is a continuous group of an indeterminate number of syllables, like the trill or run in music; an unusual form of utterance heard only in patter (Cf. Figs. 48, 50 and 57).

At a rapid rate in the series "*pu' pu'....*", the type of the consonant curve and of the curve of pressure in the mouth is invariable. The movements are perfectly regular, the phases are equal, and the movements exactly in step. The coordination may be schematized:

Arresting	*Releasing*	*Arresting*
back stroke	beat stroke	back stroke
back stroke	beat stroke	back stroke
chest-arrest		chest-arrest

The study of these tracings of double consonants, produced by increasing the rate, shows that the criteria of doubling are quite consistent. The rate at which doubling begins and ends, the form of the consonant curve which shows the combination of the doublets, and the bi-maximal form of the curve of mouth pressure during doubling, are all in accord. And the results agree with the characteristics of the actual doubles (ordinary words and phrases) as determined above (Fig. 54).

RESTORATION OF THE ORIGINAL FORM WHEN THE RATE DECREASES

The reverse processes occur if the subject is directed gradually to reduce the rate of utterance after reaching the maximum rate. If the form "*pup, pup....*" has been prescribed, as the rate rises it passes through the stages, "*pup-pup....*" and "*pu' pu'....*". As the rate slows again it passes from "*pu' pu'....*" to "*pup-pup....*" and finally to "*pup, pup....*". The subject is not aware that

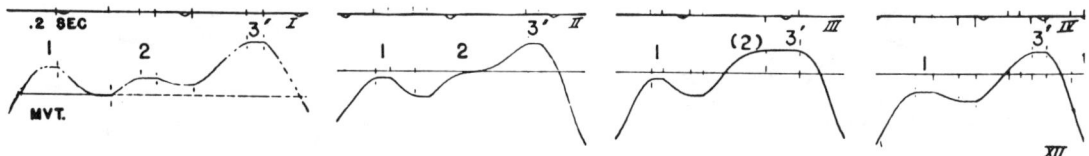

FIGURE 55. Writing Movements at a Rapid Rate showing Reduction and Elimination of a Movement

I. The three movements are quite distinct, though the beat stroke of 2 is small in extent.

II. The three movements are still apparent, but there is time for only a very slight beat stroke for 2, and the movement is evidently being fused with the stressed beat, 3'.

III. There is no longer a beat stroke for 2, but the plateau shows the fusing of the movements.

IV. The plateau has disappeared, 2 has dropped, and the series has become I 3'.

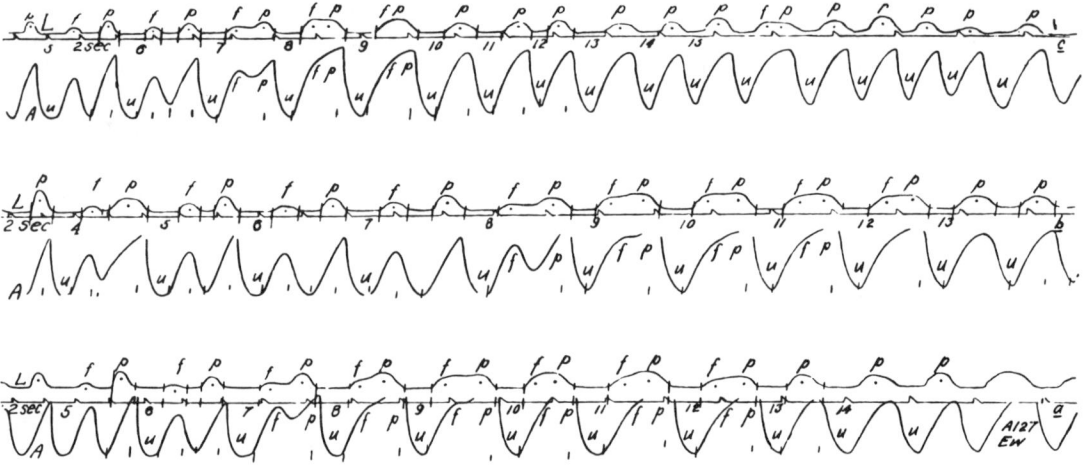

FIGURE 56. Abutting Consonants which Single as the Rate increases. The three Series were taken at the same Session

Syllables: *puff puff*..
L—Lip marker. The doubling forms of the *f-p* are distinct. The appearance of the doubles is rather abrupt in all cases.
A—Air in mouth shows the normal doubling forms.

Incipient doubling shows in the air pressure curves when it is not apparent in the consonant contacts. From the tracings alone this might be a simple record of *pup pup*..

he has doubled the consonants and then dropped the arresting consonant, reducing the syllable to "*pu' pu'*"; neither is he aware that he has restored the arresting consonant as the rate slows, and that he has finally come back to the original form prescribed (Cf. Figs. 26 and 28).

This restoration of the prescribed consonant, when the rate permits, is of importance because

the process of elimination and restoration is constantly going on under the ordinary conditions of speech. It is not the case that a consonant has actually disappeared because it is for the moment suppressed by the rate of utterance; it is in abeyance in the breath group, and will promptly reappear when the rate permits. Much survives in the movements of a language which is not

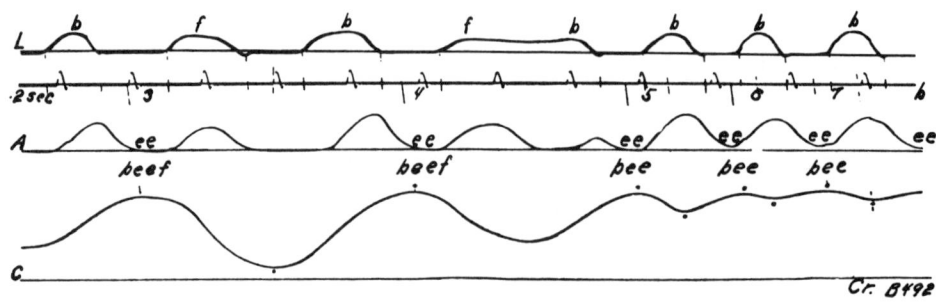

FIGURE 57. Abutting Consonants due to Increasing Rate; Stop and Continuant; Chest Pulses Directly from the Trachea

Syllables: *beef beef* .. *be' be'*
L—Lip marker. 4-5, the one abutting form.
A—Air in mouth. Typical forms.
C—Chest pulses recorded directly from trachea.

Syl. 1-3 show a single breath group for each syllable. Syl 5-7 show a continuous indeterminate breath group.

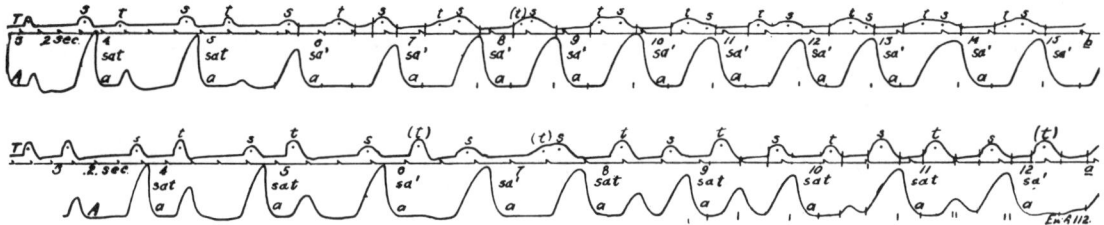

FIGURE 58. Abutting Consonants, "Doubling", Stop and Continuant

Syllables: *sat sat* . .

T—Tongue marker. The *t* stroke is rather weak at first. The *t* stroke in 7-8 does not function at all, but an abutting pair has developed and persists, syl. 7-15:

A—Air in mouth. In *b* the pulse is chest arrested after two feeble consonant arrests in 4 and 5. Although the tongue makes a definite stroke for the *t* of *sat*, the *t* does not function and has actually dropped. The subject is saying *sa' sa'.*

---

heard; the French aspirate "*h*" still has a place in the pronunciation, though it is seldom heard. One may expect then great freedom in modifying the prescribed consonant forms. When the rhythms compel rapid utterance the consonants may "double", or "single", and they may be shifted from one syllable to another, but as the rhythm and the rate revert, the original form will return. The subject has not lost the original pattern of the breath group, though it is freely modified by phonetic exigencies.

This restoration of the consonant forms, and later of syllable forms, will be treated when other series at increasing and decreasing rates are discussed, and also when the various stressed groups of syllables are considered. This tendency to restoration is important in all these cases; it is the great conservative factor in pronunciation (89, p. 46).

ONE-MEMBER ABUTTING PAIRS. TRACING OF ABUTTING CONSONANTS PRODUCED BY THE SAME ARTICULATORY MEMBER

When series like "*puf, puf*. . . ." and "*sat, sat*. . . ." are uttered at increasing rate, abbuting pairs of the form "*f-p*" and "*t-s*" result. Such abutting consonants are very much like double consonants; the two consonants are different but they combine under much the same conditions.

The list of syllables which were developed into series by increasing the rate of utterance is given in Appendix I, B.

Fig. 56 shows series of the syllable "*puf*. . . ." passing through the stages of "separate", "doubling", (= abutting) and "singling". Fig. 58 illustrates cases in which the doubling does not occur, and instead the arresting consonant drops at once. It is significant that the presence or absence of a consonant does not depend on the articulatory stroke, but on the function of the consonant. If the consonant arrests the chest pulse, it is audible; but if the chest pulse is chest arrested, the consonant movement does not make a consonant. A consonant may drop, although the articulatory movement is vigorous. And it is interesting to see that although it fails to function as an arresting consonant, the "*t*" movement may nevertheless combine with the "*s*" movement, and actually produce the stroke of a compound consonant "*ts*".

The lengths of such one-member pairs abutting with increasing rate are comparable to those of the doubles by increasing the rate, and to those of the actual doubles in ordinary words and phrases. Fig. 51, p. 93 shows the practical identity in curves, N, O, P.

The rates at which doubling takes place are practically identical with other abutting rates (Cf. Fig. 51, p. 93).

An inspection of the tracings makes it apparent that a majority of one-member abutting pairs have the doubling form clearly indicated in the consonant- and mouth-pressure-curves. Of 607 cases of front lingual pairs, like "*t-s, d-l, th-n*", etc., only 12 per cent do not show the characteristics of the arresting-releasing pair; 40 per cent show the characteristics in both chest pulse and

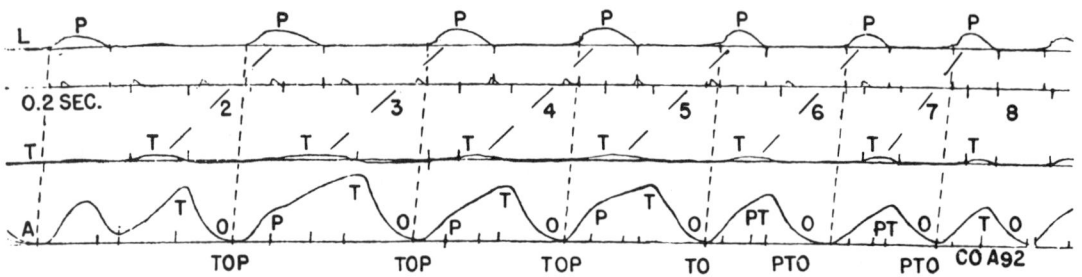

FIGURE 59. Two-member Abutting Pairs Produced by Increasing Rate

Syllable: *top top* . .

L—Lip marker. Well defined movements persist whether or not the *p* functions.
   In syllable 2 the contact is prolonged as the 'doubling' occurs. The arresting *p* finally coincides with the movement of the *t* as the rate increases.

T—Tongue marker. Contact of the *t* is prolonged as the 'doubling' occurs at syl. 2-3. Releasing *t* functions thoughout. Although the contact of the *p* is longer, the release of the *t* always occurs after the end of the *p* contact.

A—Air in mouth. Syl. 1-2 gives the typical round and pointed maxima of the arresting-releasing form. The forms of 2-3-4-5 show the two maxima. Syl 6, 7 have been labeled "*pt*" because they have not quite coincided. The limits of contact draw nearer and nearer together until at 7-8 they coincide.

The stage of doubling is nearly always more brief with two-member than with one-member pairs of consonants.

---

consonant movement; 76 per cent have the characteristic abutting form in the mouth pressure curve. Of 142 labial pairs, "*f-p*", "*v-b*" etc. only 4 per cent do not show the arresting-releasing form; 56 per cent show the characteristics in both air pressure and consonant movement; 90 per cent show the characteristic abutting form in the mouth pressure curve. This is a decidedly larger number than in the case of the double consonants produced by increasing the speed of utterance. It is possible that the two different consonants tend to preserve the two consonant strokes and the two pressure maxima. The difference in the force of the consonant strokes of the two components, and the difference in the mouth pressure of the two components show clearly in the tracings of such one-member abutting pairs.

Series in which the rate decreases from the maximum show the return of the "doubling" and finally of the original form. This is the tendency to reversion mentioned in connection with the doubling series, p. 85.

TWO-MEMBER ABUTTING PAIRS. TRACINGS OF ABUTTING CONSONANTS PRODUCED BY DIFFERENT ARTICULATORY MEMBERS

This method of study may be extended to abutting consonants of all types. When the arresting consonant is produced by one member, and the releasing consonant by another, the conditions are somewhat different.

Tracings were made of series in which such pairs of abutting consonants were produced by increasing the rate of utterance. "Top, top. . . .", in which the arresting consonant is a labial, and the releasing consonant a lingual, will illustrate the general form. Independent tracings of the lip movement and of the tongue-movement were taken, along with the curves of pressure in the mouth and in the chest.

A list of the syllables which were developed into series with two-member abutting pairs of consonants by increasing the rate is given in Appendix I, C.

Various types of two-member abutting pairs are shown in Figs. 59, 60, 61, 62 and 63; "*top, top*. . . ." shows the abutting of a labial occlusive with a lingual occlusive; the arresting "*p*" drops and the series becomes "*to' to*'. . . ." In Fig. 60 "*sam, sam*. . . ." shows the abutting of a continuant labial, the nasal "*m*" and the continuant lingual "*s*"; the movements are almost in step, and it is easy for the movement of the "*s*" to shift slightly so as to form "*sm*" and metathesis has occurred. In such cases the overlapping brings coincidence and then progresses to a point where the two movements slide *past* each other, as it were, into an easier compound consonant. In Fig. 61 the overlapping does not go beyond the stage

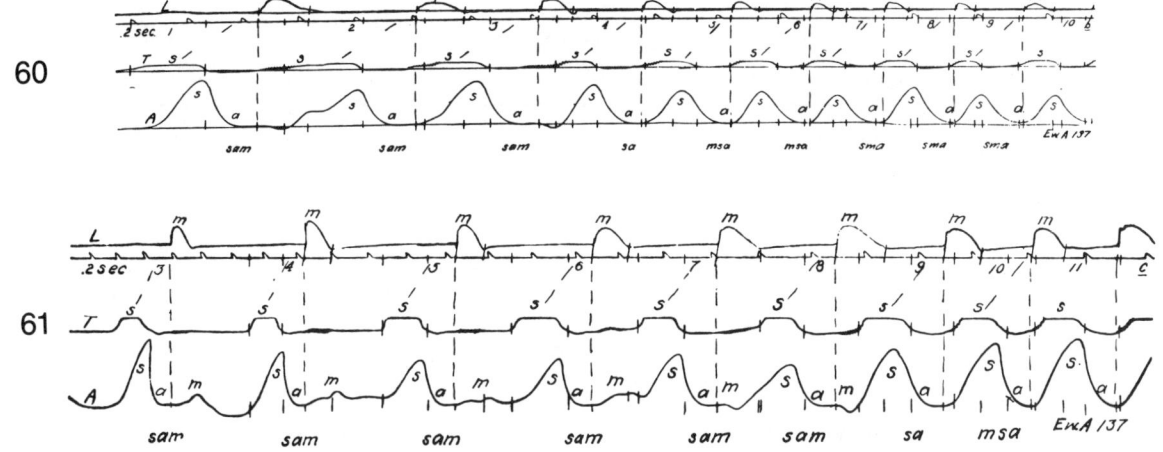

FIGURE 60 and 61. Two-member Abutting Pairs Produced by Increasing Rate

Syllables: *sam sam* .. with and without metathesis.

L—Lip marker. *m* movement persists thoughout.

Fig 60: the contact of the *m* begins exactly with that of the releasing *s* at syl. 5-6; thereafter the *s* contact leads. In doubling syl. 1-3 the contact of *m* is prolonged, stretching out to overlap the *s*.

Fig 61: The strokes are well defined and function as arresting consonant though syl 8, and as a factor in the releasing compound consonant *m*s thereafter; syl. 7-9 show the prolonging of the contact as the overlapping occurs.

T—Tongue marker. The tracing is affected by the vibration of the nasal *m*. This vibration shows that the *m* is present in all the releasing consonants.

A—Air in mouth. The continuant *s* and the compounds *sm* and *ms* do not give as sharp a fall to the releasing curve as does a stop.

The final result of the increased rate in the cases is not the dropping of the arresting *m* but its fusion with the releasing *s*.

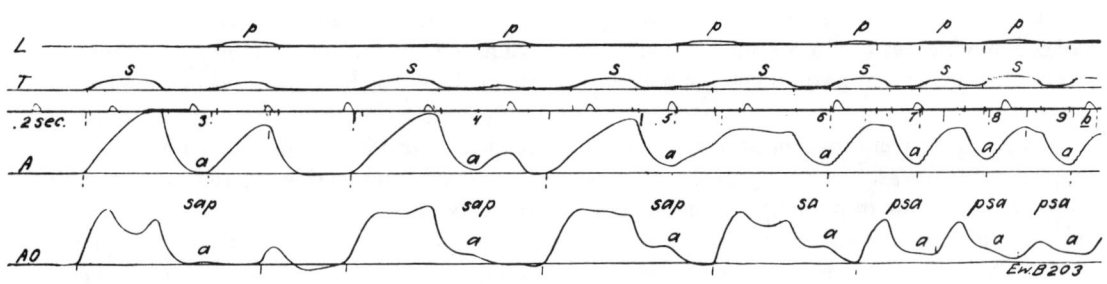

FIGURE 62. Abutting Consonants; Continuant with Stop

Syllables: *sap sap* ..

L—Lip marker. Contact grows shorter and lighter as the rate increases and overlapping and coincidence occur.

T—Tongue marker. Well marked doubling form syl. 5-6; thereafter the single releasing compound form *ps*.

A—Air in mouth. Doubling forms, syl. 5-6.

AO—Air outside. Varied in appearance because of the high pressure during the continuant *s*. Plateau of *s* becomes mere point as compound form appears, syl. 6-7.

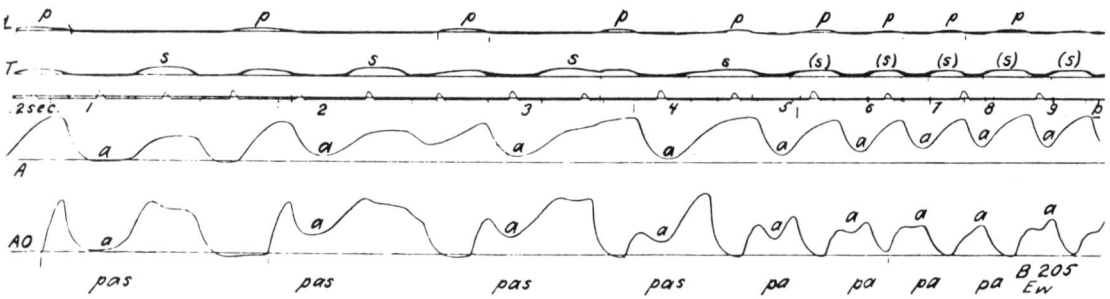

FIGURE 63. Two-member Abutting Pairs developed by Increasing Rate; Formation of Compound releasing Consonant

Syllables: *pas pas* ..
L—Lip marker. Contact grows shorter and lighter as rate increases.
T—Tongue movements. The *s* stroke is definite but the marker is also affected by the *p* contact of tracing above. Syl. 2-5 show the doubling form *s-p*; it is probable that from syl. 5-6 the form is the compound consonant *sp*; the *s* fuses with the following releasing *p* and does not drop outright.
A—Air in mouth. Doubling forms, syl. 2-3, 3-4, 4-5.
AO—Air outside. Plateau which marks the *s* becomes a mere point as the compound form appears, syl. 4-5.

of a releasing "*ms*". The forms in which "*s*" figures as part of a compound consonant may be counted normal. The phenomena of abutting in all these cases are very similar. The "*m*" is not easy to record and often shows negative pressure. The "*s*" usually shifts to form a compound releasing consonant in the next syllable. Figs. 62 and 63 show the abutting forms in the mouth pressure alongside a tracing of the outside pressure. The tracing of the outside pressure shows that the "*p*" stroke dominates in the compound consonant "*sp*", but that the "*s*" stroke dominates in the compound "*ps*".

The process of combination of abutting consonants in such cases is very interesting; the arresting consonant movement of one syllable and the releasing consonant movement of the next syllable quickly overlap and soon become simultaneous. (70, p. 949; 72., p. 81; 54, p. 108) Unless one of the components is a fricative (like the "*s*" in Fig. 60), the abutting pair does not persist more than a few syllables with any of the subjects; the arresting consonant disappears quickly as the rate increases.

When the arresting consonant shifts to the next syllable, the movement of the releasing consonant does not inhibit the movement of the shifting consonant; instead the movements tend to slip together, to fall into step, and it is apparent that the movement of the arresting consonant persists long after it has ceased to function in the syllable. It is a striking illustration of the tendency of the movements of speech to get in phase. The movement of the arresting consonant in the two-member combination can shift its position in the coordination to the next syllable without affecting the releasing consonant of that syllable; it actually slides into phase, so that the beat strokes of both consonant movements and of the syllable movement occur together; in reality, *both* consonants have the releasing position, but one of them does not function and cannot be heard. This persistence of the original arresting consonant as a movement in step with the releasing consonant is invariable. All the records of all the subjects show it. As the arresting movement shifts, so as to coincide with the releasing consonant of the next syllable, the pulse becomes chest-arresting; the form of the curve of the mouth pressure no longer indicates the end of the one syllable and the beginning of the next, for the pressure falls at the end of the syllable as in all cases of chest-arrest of the syllable movement. This illustrates a possible method of formation of such unusual sounds as the Slavic "*b* mouillé" reported by Rousselot (70, p. 605).

It is easier to see how the speaker retains the prescribed form in these two-member series than in the one-member series. Although the rate has forced the "dropping" of the arresting consonant,

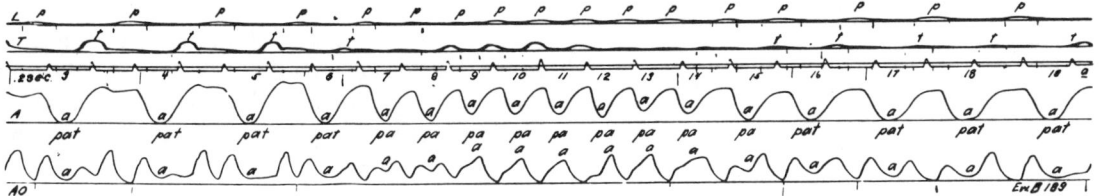

FIGURE 64. Two-member Abutting Consonants; with Increasing and Decreasing Rate, Arresting Consonant drops and reappears

Syllables: *pat pat . . pa' . . pat pat*

L—Lip marker. The *p* contact shortens during the rapid rate; little difference in intensity.

T—Tongue marker. Arresting *t* comes to coincide with releasing *p*; at syl. 11 they completely overlap, and the intensity of stroke diminishes.

Later, in syls. 16-17, the forms revert and the *t* is restored.

AO—Air outside. Although the *t-p* is double in the first and last syllables, there is considerable escape of air from the mouth between the *t* and the *p*. The first *pa' pa'* syllables show the mid-sag.

the consonant stroke is actually retained, but it coincides with the releasing consonant; they merely slide apart again as the rate reduces. Fig. 64 shows the restoration of the original prescribed form in a two-member series.

A comparison of the lengths of such two-member abutting pairs with the lengths of the one-member abutting pairs of consonants shows that the mode has a value slightly less than that of the one-member pairs (including doubles). Fig. 65 shows that the difference in the two distribution curves Q and R is not great; but it is probable that there is a slight difference in the play of the movements which makes the two-member pairs slightly shorter. The average of the 984 readings represented by curve R is .22 ± .04 sec. The minimum lengths of the two-member abutting pairs lie well within the limits of rate of two ballistic movements. Fig. 66 gives a comparison of the distributions of the lengths of doubles and of abutting pairs recorded in the second group with records in the first group. It is apparent that the distributions are practically identical.

The rates of the syllables in these series containing two-member abutting pairs, as given in the distributions of Fig. 51, p. 93, show that they agree very closely with those of the one-member pairs (*e* as compared with *d*).

There is no fundamental distinction to be made between the two-member pairs of abutting consonants, the one-member pairs of different abutting consonants, and the actual doubles; they all result from one and the same process. Combinations like "*bit-bit*" and "*fub-fub*" and doubles like "*pup-pup*" and "*sis-sis*" are all analogous. It is true that singling in the course of the two-member series does not mean that the arresting consonant stroke drops out; instead it shifts into the releasing position, in step with the next releasing consonant, and becomes functionless or fuses to a compound consonant. But the elimination of the arresting consonant in the two-member abutting pair, the shift of the arresting consonant series, like "*up-up*", to "*pu' pu'. . . . .*", are precisely like the processes of singling which appear in the series of doubles by increasing the rate, or in the series of one-member abutting pairs produced by increasing the rate.

These abutting consonants, made by two different articulatory members, cannot occur more rapidly than the abutting consonants made by a single member. In the playing of key-board and wood-wind musical instruments, and in many other forms of skilled movements, it is possible, by the use of two or more fingers in coordination, to attain a rate of 15–18 per sec. Nothing of the sort appears in the case of the consonants in speech; the number of consonantal movements which can be made by two different articulatory members is 8–12 per sec.; it is no greater than the number of consonants per sec. produced by one articulatory member.

This fact emphasizes the difference in type of coordination. In the case of the combined finger movements of typing or piano-playing, the separate pulses have their separate functions as beats in the process; each finger movement is an

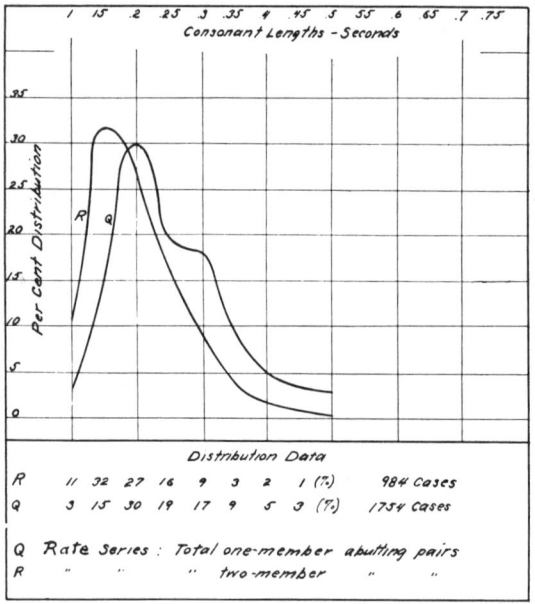

FIGURE 65. A Comparison of One-member Abutting Pairs (including Doubles) with Two-member Abutting Pairs

One-member pair consists of two consonants produced by the same member, either tongue or lips, *tut-tut, puf-puf, tas-tas,* etc.

Two-member pair consists of two consonants produced by different members, lips or tongue, *bus-bus, dip-dip, fuz-fuz,* etc.

---

independent movement. But the coordination of the consonants in utterance does not make them independent; they are auxiliary movements, only; they delimit the chest pulse, and in that function they can occur no oftener than required by the process of releasing or arresting the chest pulse. The finger movements in piano and flute playing give strokes which are individual elements in the rhythms; but no rhythms in speaking are built of separate consonants singly or in combinations—the rhythms of speech all have as units the syllables, the chest pulses, and never the consonants. This is fundamental evidence of the fact that the basic unit in speech is not the "sound", phoneme, but the syllable. The movements and coordination of speech are the movements and coordination of syllables in the breath group.

In the two-member pairs the abutting consonants seem to stretch toward each other (Fig. 67). The tracings of the contacts of the consonants show that they elongate, each in the direction of the other. This is part of the tendency of the movements to fall into step, to coincide. The first consonant stroke is held in anticipation of the one to come, and the second consonant stroke occurs early in order to fuse with the previous stroke. Like drops of liquid they tend to run together. Of 95 series taken at random, 72 show such "attraction" of the consonants. The average length of the consonants before doubling of the individual consonants is 0.17 sec. (214 readings). The average length of the individual consonants while doubling is 0.20 sec. (284 readings). The difference in these averages is significant, as the readings were made in pairs and in every case the value of the consonant before doubling was lower than the value of the consonant while doubling. Any influence of the increasing rate of utterance would work against this tendency to lengthen the consonants as they come to abut. Fig. 67 gives cases in which the "attraction" of the doubling consonants is very marked.

ASSIMILATION OF ABUTTING CONSONANTS

When the rate of utterance is high enough to produce abutting pairs of consonants, it often happens that the vocalization of the two consonants becomes alike. it is difficult to shift the vocalization within the pair at a rapid rate. In French the tendency is always to weaken the arresting consonant, because arrest by the intercostals first supplements and then supersedes the consonant arrest. Therefore the following releasing consonant is dominant and the vocalization of the releasing consonant prevails. The assimilation is said to be regressive, meaning that the arresting consonant takes the vocalization of the following releasing consonant. In English or German a stress on the first of the adjacent syllables reinforces the arresting function of the first abutting consonant; and the two consonants may not affect each other. Sometimes what might be an abutting pair is separated by a definite hiatus. Cf. "obscene, obtrude, blackboard". In other cases the first syllable is vigorously arrested and the vocalization of the arresting consonant affects the following, releasing consonant. The pronunciation of an English word like "absolution" varies with the rate of utterance from no assimilation to "progressive assimilation".

INFLUENCE OF THE PHONETIC UNITS ON EACH OTHER

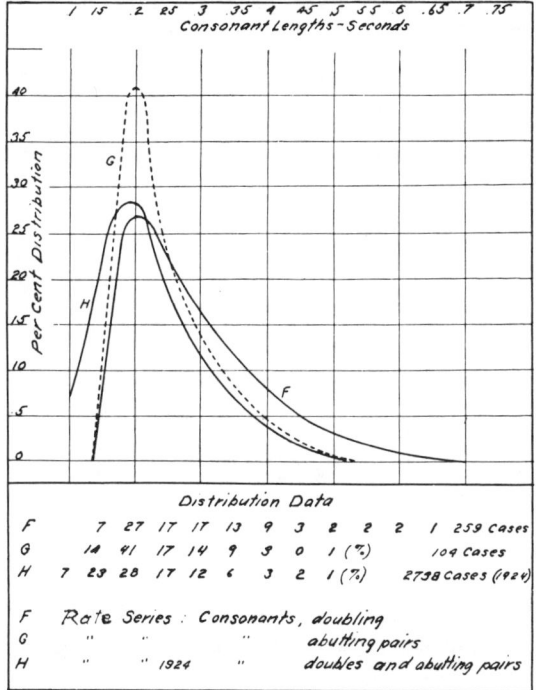

FIGURE 66.
Distribution of the lengths of doubling consonants produced by increasing the rate in a series, either of one member forms like *pu-pup* ..*pu' pu',* or *ted-ted* ..*te' te'* or two-member forms like *pet-pet* ..*pe' pe'.*

ASSIMILATION IN WHICH THE ABUTTING PAIR BECOMES A DOUBLE CONSONANT

In many languages the pair of abutting consonants becomes a double consonant: ad-similate = assimilate, ad-breviate = abbreviate, syn-logism = syllogism, etc.

Where but one member (lips or tongue) is involved, it is ordinarily said that it is easier to repeat the same movement than to make a different though similar, movement to the same bearing when the conditions of articulation are different. The repetition of one "sound" can be said to be simpler than the articulation of the two different "sounds". Where two members (both lips and tongue) are involved, it may be said that repetition of the movement of a single member is easier than movements of two different members (Cf. "applicate, immemorial, osservatore").

It is to be noted, however, in the case of one-member assimilations, as well as in the case of two-member assimilations, that actual experiment does not show the assimilation of "*d-p*" to "*p-p*", or "*b-s*" to "*s-s*" as a stage between the abutting of the consonants and the dropping of the arresting consonant. As the rate increases in a series like "*pad, pad....*" the double "*p-p*" does not always occur; the series may pass directly from "*pad, pad....*" to "*pa' pa'....*". So with "*men, men....*", the stage "*mem-mem....*" may not appear; the change may be from "*men, men.....*" into "*me' me'....*".

How then is the appearance of the doubled consonant in place of the abutting pair to be explained since it is a very common form of assimilation? With increasing rate there is a universal tendency to simplify by eliminating the arresting consonant; the restoration of such an arresting consonant is commonplace (Cf. Fig. 64).

But such restoration does not always occur. In the course of generations the rapid-rate pronunciation prevails; the sense of the original arresting consonant is lost. However, if the "short" vowel of the first syllable, the word stress, and the phrase rhythm persist, slow enunciation, especially with a pronounced stress on the first syllable, will force adventitious doubling (Cf. Fig. 95, 100, 101).

At this stage in the phonetic modification of the word, rapid utterance has eliminated the arresting consonant of the original pronunciation, but a slow, careful utterance substitutes a true double for the original abutting pair. In all languages, rapid utterance is to be distinguished from slow, careful utterance; as a rule, the standard orthography follows the slow, careful utterance (61, p. 4). It is often the case that such standard spelling prescribes double consonants which are seldom heard. At a later stage of phonetic modification, the double is no longer recognized in the actual pronunciation; it may or may not persist in the standard spelling. The Attic Greek shows a strong tendency to the omission of such doubles.

AN ARRESTING CONSONANT OCCUPIES THE INTERVAL OF A DOUBLE CONSONANT

It is possible to consider any arresting consonant as virtually a double, although it may not be

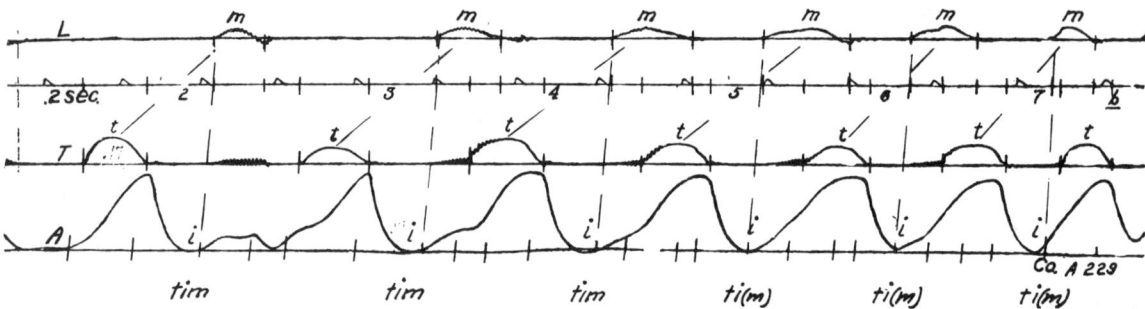

FIGURE 67. "Attraction" of the Consonant Movements as Doubling occurs in a series of Syllables with Increasing Rate

Syllables: *tim tim* ..
L—Lip marker. Syl. 4-6 show prolongation of contacts of the consonants.
T—Tongue marker. Syl. 4-6 show the prolongation of the contacts of the consonants as if they attracted each other. Sonance of *m* figures throughout record.
A—Air in mouth. Usual doubling and singling forms.

followed by a releasing consonant. In the case of a series of syllables with double consonants, the increase of rate forces the dropping of the arresting consonant. It cannot shift position and persist because the releasing doublet of the next syllable is produced by the same member. In the case of a series of syllables with two-member abutting pairs, the arresting consonant does shift position to become member of a releasing compound consonant, or to overlap the actual releasing consonant as a functionless consonant stroke. Likewise, in a series of syllables with single arresting consonants, as the rate increases the arresting consonant shifts to the unoccupied releasing position in the next syllable; and the shift occurs at about the same rate as does the dropping of the arresting doublet. The single arresting consonant has the position of an arresting doublet; the other doublet is represented by the zone of chest-release of the next syllable; when the rate increases, the arresting consonant slides into the releasing position like the arresting doublet of the two-member abutting pair. In all cases the arresting consonant disappears and a releasing consonant remains.

The graphs representing the distribution of single arresting consonants show the fact that there is no distinction between the "long" vowels and the "short" vowels in the matter of doubling. The long vowel can be shortened, but the short vowel cannot be lengthened. Since these changes occur at a fair rate of utterance, *all* vowels are actually of short duration.

The tendency of restoration of the original form is apparent in these series in which the single arresting consonant is affected by changing rate of utterance. When the rate is reduced, so that the original arresting form is again possible, the consonant shifts back to the arresting position; the original prescribed form is restored; later it will be obvious that the same thing occurs in stressed groups of syllables.

The distribution curves of the arrested syllables (Fig. 70), when compared with the distribution curves of abutting pairs (Fig. 63), show that the rate at which the change from arresting to releasing takes place is slightly higher than the rate for singling of a double. It is evidently easier to retain an arresting consonant than an actual double as the rate increases (Cf. Fig. 26).

Fig. 68 shows the mouth pressure and the chest pressure tracings for the phrase "*at E, at C*". The doubling form of the mouth pressure is apparent in "*at C*"; the maximum of the chest pressure occurs immediately on the détente of the double; the minimum occurs as usual during the releasing doublet. But in the case of "*at E*", the maximum of the chest pressure does not occur until .10–.20 sec. after the "détente" of the "*t*", and the minimum occurs at the détente.

Fig. 69 "*at E, at P*" shows the same contrast in the case of a two-member abutting pair, "*t-p*". In arrested syllables of this type, if the arresting consonant and the chest release of the next syllable are measured as a single interval, the duration corresponds to the duration of a double

INFLUENCE OF THE PHONETIC UNITS ON EACH OTHER   105

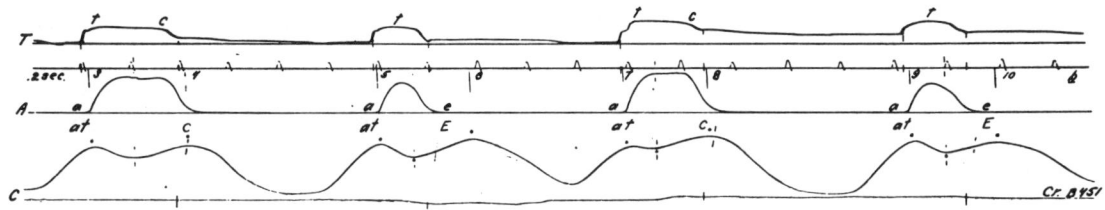

FIGURE 68. Contrast of the Double with the Arresting Consonant; Chest Pulses recorded directly from Trachea
Syllables: *At C, at E*.
T—Tongue marker. The variation in duration of the double and single consonants is clear, but the doubling form does not appear by chance.
A—Air pressure in mouth. Characteristic double and single forms.
C—Chest pressure direct from trachea. Division between the syllables shows in each case. For *at E* forms maximum pressure does not appear till well after the consonant—there is the necessary interval for chest release; for the *at C* forms the maximum appears immediately at the détente of the *C* as there is a consonant release.

consonant (Fig. 70). If the arrested syllable is repeated at increasing rate, the shift to a released syllable occurs at the same rate as the singling of a double consonant. If the rate is reduced, the consonant reverts to the arresting position at the proper rate (Cf. Fig 51, p. 93).

COMPOUND CONSONANTS: CONSONANT GROUPS WHICH FUNCTION AS A SINGLE CONSONANT

Two or more adjacent consonants may be classed as an intra-syllabic group when the group figures as a compound consonant in releasing or arresting the syllable movement, as contrasted with abutting consonants each of which has a different function in two different syllables. It is possible, of course, that a compound consonant figures as one of the abutting consonants.

In the group of the compound consonant the consonant movements are as nearly simultaneous as the nature of the movements combined will permit. Together they function as a single, arresting or releasing factor in the syllable and frequently they are so brief and so close together that they must contribute qualities, rather than distinct elements, according to the "law of discrete succession".

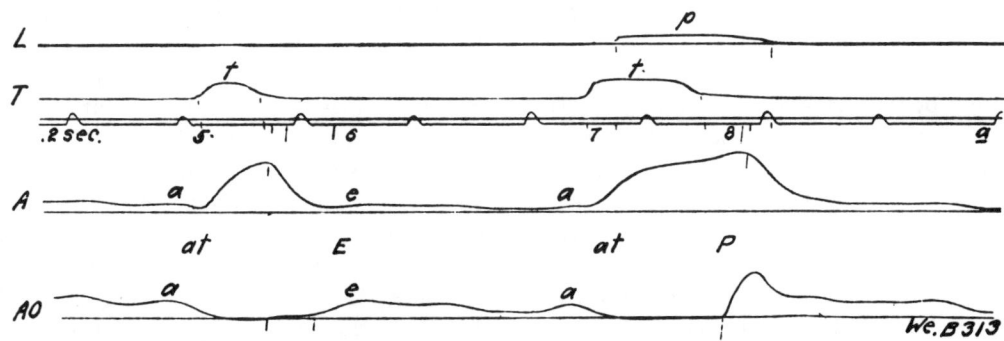

FIGURE 69. Contrast of the Two-member Pair of Abutting Consonants with the Arresting Consonant
Syllables: *at E, at P*.
L
T—Lip- and tongue-markers. Arresting *t* at *E*, is much lighter than in *at P*.
A—Air in mouth. Doubling form is well marked, syl. 7-8.
AO—Air outside. In *at E* the pressure drops to zero after the détente of the arresting *t*. The chest released *E* is indicated by the rise in pressure after the drop to zero. The forms after T and P are typical.

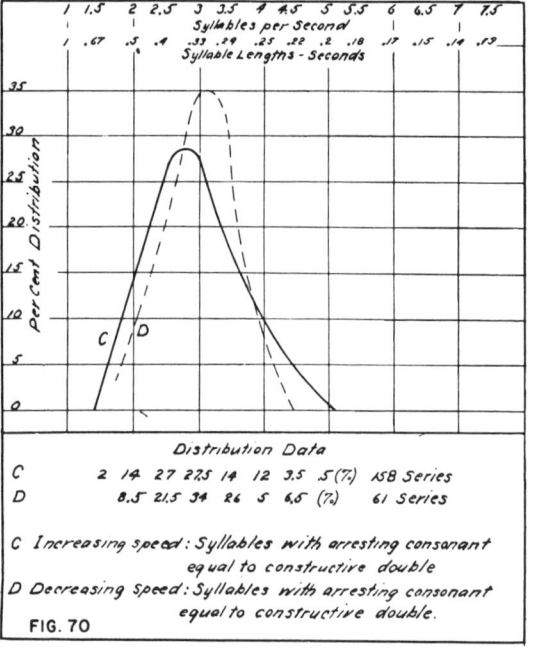

FIGURE 70.
Distribution of the Rates at which an arresting consonant shifts to releasing position and reverts; the syllables become released, and then revert. Cf. Fig. 26, 28.

The distributions are practically identical. It is probable that all the types of series, doubling and singling, would show the same values if the study had been made.

Rousselot's analysis of such intrasyllabic groups is masterly: If the consonants are produced by two different members, they are prepared together, and the movements of uttering them may be simultaneous—which is quite true of "*pla*" and "*fla*". In every case, at the moment when the first consonant is being articulated, the second is fully prepared. The two détentes follow each other more or less rapidly. . . . If the consonants involve the same member, there are two cases: 1) the articulation takes place at the same point, e.g. "*tla*"; 2) the articulations occur at separate points, e.g. "*kla*". In 1) a single initial movement is made for both and a slight deviation in the tracing marks the entrance of the second consonant; in 2) the movements are inevitably successive (70, p. 950).

The intrasyllabic groups differ somewhat according to whether their function is arresting or releasing, but there are certain features common to them all.

There is the group which is a compound consonant, and which has but the one consonant beat stroke; the primary quality of the group occurs at the beat stroke, the accessory qualities occur during the preparatory phase of the beat stroke, or during the relaxation phase, the back stroke. In such common groups as "*sp*", "*st*", "*sk*", the fricative occurs during the preparation of the beat stroke. In forms like "*ts*", "*tch*", "*dz*", "*ks*", the accessory sound occurs during the back stroke. It is often difficult to say whether the group represents a single "sound" or a combination; languages differ in their handling of many of these groups. The German spells a group "*tsch*", which the French spells "*ch*", and the English "*tch*". The English spells a group "*ts*" which the Polish represents by the single "*c*". The Greeks analyze the voiced occlusives into "*mp, nt, nk*" which other languages treat as simple sounds. The Greek sigma is possibly a simple sound but it can be represented by "*sy*" (*y* consonantal). The French "chuintantes", and some sounds certainly simple like "*s*" in many words, have passed through all the stages from distinct consonants combined, to a simple "sound". For methods of distinguishing simple and compound consonants in a given language (Cf. p. 111).

Such groups appear when certain series are uttered at increasing rate; instead of dropping, the arresting consonant fuses with the following releasing consonant. Thus "*tas, tas . . . .*" gives rise to "*sta, sta . . . .*". Such compounds appear in the releasing position. Compound consonants in the arresting position are also common, e.g. "*apt, apse, asp*", etc.

The series involving a fricative often results in such compound consonants when the rate of utterance is increased.

The compound consonants "*st*" and "*sf*" appear in Figs. 71 and 72; the process is apparent by which they are produced. Such compound consonants often persist as a stable releasing consonant and may be present at rapid rates, at 5–7 syllables per sec.

In the releasing form of the compound consonant, with an initial fricative component like "*v*" "*f*", and especially "*s*", the air pressure curve is apt to show a slightly prolonged and rounded

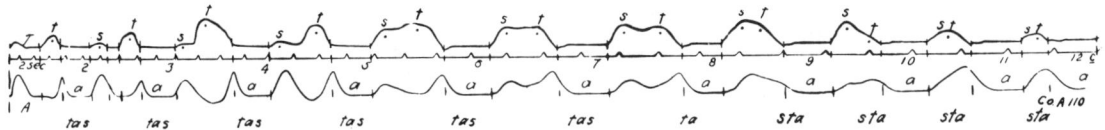

FIGURE 71. Development of the Compound Consonant *st-* in Series at Increasing Rate

T—Tongue marker. In the separate contacts of syl. 2 and 3, the releasing *t* stroke is much stronger than that of the arresting *s*, and this remains through the 'doubles' syl. 3-6; in syl. 6-8 the two tongue strokes are clearly marked and equal in force; up to that point the arresting-releasing form *s-t* persists; from syl. 8 to end of record, the consonant tracing shows various forms of the compound *st-*; in syl. 8-10 the strokes are fairly distinct, but in syl. 10-12 the releasing form prevails.

A—Air in mouth. Syl. 3-5 show separate pressures for the two consonants, though the consonants have combined in the tongue stroke. Cf. Fig. 44, p. 65. Syl. 5-8 show the normal arresting-releasing form; syl. 8-10 show disturbance of the coordination, and at syl. 10 the syllable pulse is chest arrested and the form *sta, sta* is established.

form "convex-concave" (Cf. Fig. 42). In some cases there develops an unvoiced preceding syllable and a bi-syllabic form results. This shows rarely in the records of these English-speaking subjects. But the history of the Romance languages shows this development of the preceding syllable, especially in the case of *s*, cf. "spiritus, esprit", etc.

The very common group of a stop consonant and a liquid is of a different type. The liquid (*l*, *r*) is so open a conformation that it permits the pulse of the syllable movement to begin, and although the liquid component involves a distinct stroke, this occurs during the beat stroke of the syllable. This type of liquid might be called an "internal consonant". Like the conformation of the vowel, the conformation of the liquid may be assumed *before* the preceding consonant is uttered and retained while the consonant is being executed; the conformation of the "*l*" or "*r*" does not interfere with the enunciation of the consonant; this is often the case with the vowel. Releasing groups with a liquid are very common, e.g. "*glide, crow, try, blow, pry*". For some reason "*tl*" and "*dl*" do not appear in most of the western languages.

In arresting groups the liquids figure as "internal consonants". Sweet long ago observed that the liquid continues the vowel, or rather occurs with the vowel. In a form like "*grilled*" there is no vowel to be heard save the two internal consonants "*r*" and "*l*". The nasals also appear as possible components of arresting groups e.g. "*hand, unkempt, Kampf*".

These compound consonants are to be distinguished from abutting consonants. In the phase "*a tall D told E*" the succession "*l, d*" occurs as an abutting pair in "*tall D*", and as a compound arresting consonant in "*told E*". In Fig. 73 the doubling "*l-d*" is indicated in the mouth pressure tracing, whereas the "*ld*" is a single

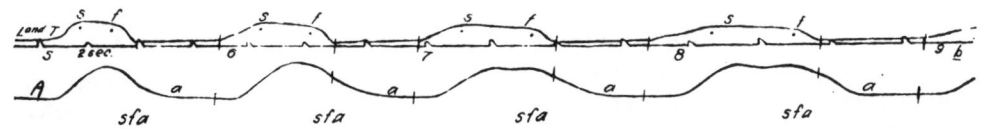

FIGURE 72. Groups *sfa*, as both Compound Consonants and as Abutting Consonants

Syllables: *sfa;* the rate of utterance is normal; there is no increase in rate.
L
T—Lip- and tongue markers. The two strokes are not clear; the group is ca. 0.40 sec.

A—Air in mouth. The forms show compound types with single maxima at syls. 5 and 6, but syls. 7, 8, and 9 indicate the form (*e*)*s-fa*. Such groups show the releasing-arresting form; it is marked in syl. 8.

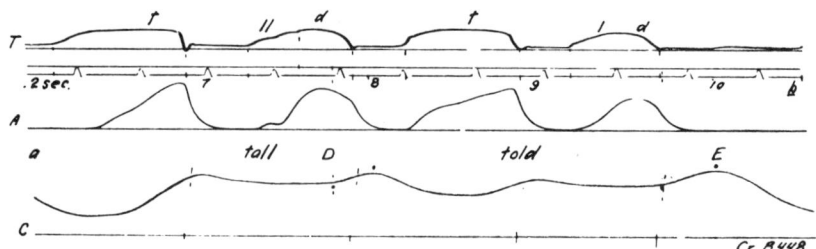

FIGURE 73. Comparison of the Compound Consonant and the Abutting Pair; Chest Pulses recorded from Trachea

Syllables: A tall D told E. Abutting pair l-d; compound consonant -ld arresting.
T—Tongue marker. Abutting pair, l-d, apparent arresting form; the releasing "d" of "l-d" contrasts with the arresting "ld" in the position of the maximum in the chest pressure in each case.

syl. 7-8. The compound consonant, -ld, is shorter, syl. 9-10.

There is also the compound consonant in which the components maintain their identity and each has its own beat stroke, but the beat strokes occur so close together that they fuse with each other in arresting or releasing the syllable movement. In the French pronunciation of "*pneumatique, psychologie, psaume*", in the Greek pronunciation "*bdellum, ptyalin, kteino*", and in the German pronunciation of "*Pfeil*", the two beat strokes of the beginning consonants are apparent; but a breath pulse does not occur between the strokes; there is little escape of air. (It is to be said, however, that tracings betray the fact that such groups often break up into a preliminary silent syllable followed by a voiced syllable; (Cf. Fig. 72). In English forms like "*lugg'd, act, apt*" (Cf. Fig. 74, "*apt*") and in the German "*Kampf*", the succession of beat strokes is obvious.

The grouping in time of the components of a compound consonant is very close; the group of two or three beat strokes often occurs in the interval of 0.08–0.10 sec. They are close enough to fuse in the syllable movement to a single rhythmic beat (32, p. 553; 84, p. 346).

The tracings of "*sfa*" in Fig. 72 illustrate the alternate forms of such groups. If the monosyllabic form is preserved, the two beat strokes of the consonants must occur close enough together so that they are part of one releasing movement. Although not quite simultaneous in these cases they must cluster on the beat-like "grace notes" or the components of a "broken chord" in music. Such compound consonants show a single form for the release of the chest pulse. But the pronunciation is often facilitated by breaking up the group into two abutting consonants; the first consonant becomes the arresting consonant of an adventitious syllable, and the second consonant releases the chest pulse of the original syllable. The word becomes bi-syllabic; "*ef-sa*", has developed. Sometimes the adventitious syllable is unvoiced but it shows clearly in the arresting-releasing forms of the air pressure curve (Cf. Fig. 72).

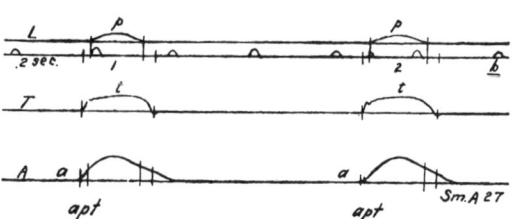

FIGURE 74. Compound Consonants in the Arresting Position in Series at Increasing Rate

Syllables: *apt apt* . .

L—Lip marker. The beat strokes of the p enter with the strokes of the t, but the p quits contact earlier.
T—Tongue marker. Prolongation of the t stroke after that of the p indicates that the t tends to become releasing.
A—Air in mouth. The rounded form of the arresting curve is apparent.

Record illustrates the fact that in a compound consonant the strokes of the components are as near simultaneous as possible.

INFLUENCE OF THE PHONETIC UNITS ON EACH OTHER 109

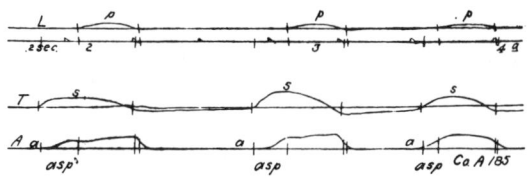

FIGURE 75. Compound Consonants in Arresting Position at Increasing Rate
Syllables: *asp asp* . .
L
T—Lip- and tongue movements. Throughout, the contact of the *s* precedes that of the *p*, but the ends of contacts come to be simultaneous.
A—Air in mouth. Syls. 2 and 3 show distinct releasing-arresting forms. In many cases the syllable *asp* is uttered with a single chest pulse, with a single arresting air pressure form. The two maxima and the sharp fall in pressure in the forms of syls. 2 and 3 indicate the pronunciation "*as-pe*, a bi-syllabic form; a syllable has been added. Syl. 4 shows the rounded form of an arresting consonant and indicates a true compound consonant *-sp*. This arresting form continues to the end of the record.

release is definite.

In the arresting form of the compound consonant, with an initial fricative like "*s*", the mouth pressure curve is rounded if no second syllable develops. But an unvoiced second syllable often occurs, the form becomes bi-syllabic and the characteristic arresting-releasing form appears in the air pressure tracing. This development of the bi-syllabic form is not as likely to occur with the fricative-occlusive arresting compound ("*asp*") etc., as it is with the occlusive-occlusive type like "*apt*". In all cases the consonant strokes tend to coincide if the true compound consonant occurs (70, p. 950). The development of the bi-syllabic form "*ap-te*" is marked by the prolongation of the contact of the second occlusive, and by the arresting-releasing form of the air pressure curves which indicates the two chest pulses. As the rate increases, such bi-syllabic forms cease, and at maximum rate the coordination shifts to a releasing consonant (Cf. Figs. 74, 75, 76).

With a liquid or a nasal as the first component of the compound consonant, the forms do not differ from that of the ordinary simple consonant. There may be a slight elongation and rounding of the air pressure curve. Increasing the rate of utterance shifts the coordination to the releasing position, and the compound consonant may simplify, losing its liquid component.

The releasing compound consonant composed of an occlusive, followed by a liquid, "*r*" or "*l*", is very like a simple releasing consonant. The "*l*" stroke permits considerable escape of air, but the

DIAGRAMS AND CHECK LISTS OF THE COMPOUND CONSONANTS

Syllable "*print*":

Releasing compound consonant				Arresting compound consonant		
Principal consonant	+ Internal consonant	VOWEL		Internal consonant	+	Principal consonant
P	r	i		n		t

Consonants can be prefixed to the principal stroke of the releasing compound consonant, and suffixed to the principal stroke of the arresting compound consonant. Thus the syllable may become:

Syllable "*sprints*":

Prefixed consonant	+	Principal consonant	+	Internal consonant	VOWEL	Internal consonant	+	Principal consonant	+	Suffixed consonant
s		P		r	i	n		t		s

The various two-component and three-component compounds are shown in the following table:

Releasing compound consonant:				Arresting compound consonant:			
	Prefixed consonant	Principal consonant	Internal consonant		Internal consonant	Principal consonant	Suffixed consonant
Syllable "*spry*"	s	P	r	Syllable "*rants*"	n	t	s
Syllable "*spy*"	s	P		Syllable "*rant*"	n	t	
Syllable "*pry*"		P	r	Syllable "*rats*"		t	s

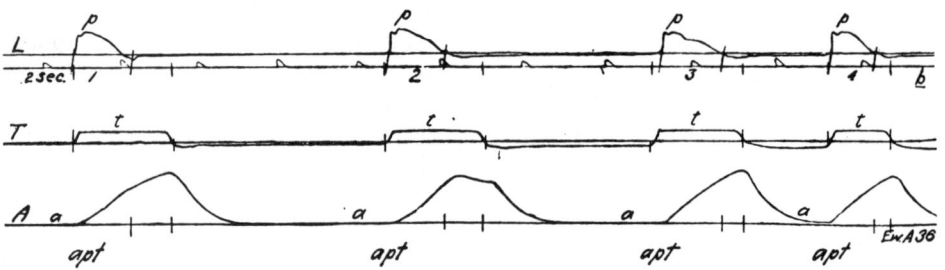

FIGURE 76. Compound Consonant in the Arresting Position in Series at Increasing Rate

Syllables: *apt apt* ..

L

T—Beat strokes of *p* enter with the strokes of *t*, but quit earlier. Prolongation of the *t* stroke after the *p* indicates a tendency to become releasing.

A—Air in mouth. Syls. 1 and 2 show the arresting-releasing form of the curve; the pronunciation has become "*ap-te*", bi-syllabic.

Consonants which may occur as principal consonants of a compound:

1. Any voiced or voiceless stop may have the principal stroke: p/b, t/d, k/g.
2. Voiced and voiceless continuants may have the principal stroke:
   a. Fricatives and sibilants: f/v, s/z, sh/zh, ch/j, th/th.
   b. Liquids and nasals: l, r, m, n, ng.

Consonants which may occur as internal consonants:

With releasing consonants: The semi-vowels w and y. "y" does not appear in the orthography; cf. "*tune*".

The liquids l and r are very common. (No nasals or s/z in English.)

With arresting consonants:

The liquids l and r give complete series.

The nasals, m, n, ng, give almost a complete series.

The voiceless s and sh with voiceless principal consonant; incomplete series.

Consonants which may occur as prefixed consonants:

The only prefixed consonant in English is

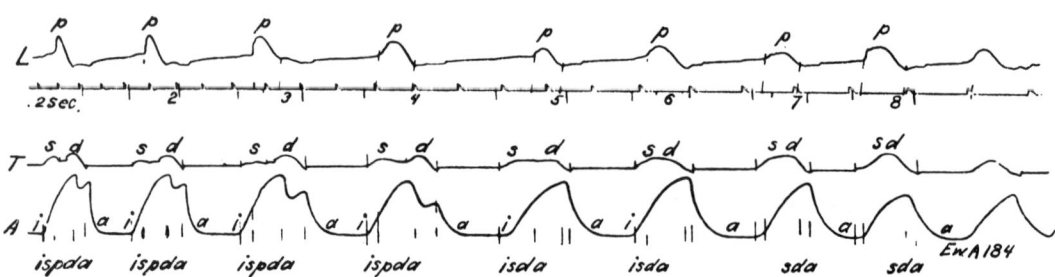

FIGURE 77. Abutting Consonants in which Doubling occurs across an Intervening Consonant, with Increasing Rate

Syllables: *ispda .. isda .. sda ..*

L—Lip marker. Lip stroke occurs throughout but does not function after syl. 4. *p* retains the arresting function in syl. 1, 2, 3.

T—Tongue marker. *s* and *d* are separate in syl. 1 and 2; adjacent in syl. 3, doubling in syl. 4, 5,; there is a single releasing consonant (compound?) in syl. 6, 7, 8.

A—Air in mouth. The arresting-releasing form appears in syl. 1, 2, 3, 4. As the double *s-d* shifts to the releasing coordination and becomes the compound *sd-*, the word becomes monosyllabic, and is marked by a simple releasing form in the air pressure curve. The series probably becomes *sda sda*.

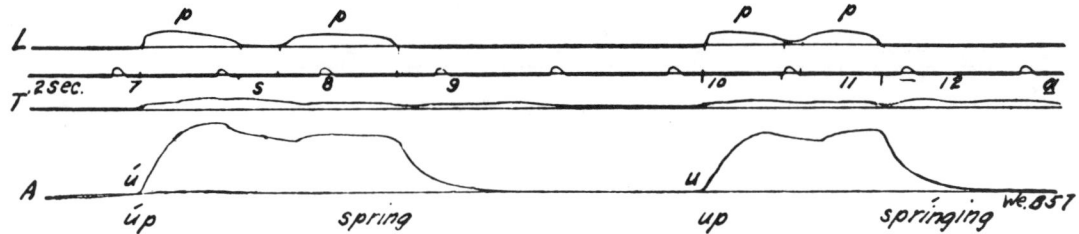

FIGURE 78. Compound Consonant Functioning as Releasing Member of Abutting Group

Syllables: *up'spring, upspring'ing*.

L—Lip marker. In *upspring*, syl. 7-8 with the stress on *up'*- the distance between the two *p* contacts is greater and the whole process takes more time than in *up'springing*, syl. 10-11. In syl. 10-11 the *p*'s approach a doubling form.

T—Tongue marker. Contact of the *s* begins with the arresting *p* and continues throughout the double.

A—Air in mouth. Forms are evidently doubling. Syl. 7–8 shows stress on the first doublet for the stressed *up'* and on the second doublet of the stressed *-spring'-*.

s, and only with voiceless principal consonants.

Consonants which may occur as suffixed consonants:

The t/d group which mark the past participle, e.g. "*passed, earned*".

The s/z group which mark the plural and the possessive, e.g. "*Alps, adds, Jim's*". (Obsolete st. second singular of verbs, no longer used.)

Cf. Appendix XII: Check List Compound Consonants in English.

The relation of the compound consonant and abutting consonants may be used to test a phoneme of a given language as to whether it is a simple consonant or a compound consonant:

1. If the compound consonant occurs before or after a heavy stress at the division of the feet, it becomes two abutting consonants. "The Lor-d is my shepherd....", "Thou prepareds ta table....".
2. The compound consonant cannot be doubled. "*Apse, apse....*" with increasing rate becomes at once "*sap,sap....*"; and finally the "*p*" drops.

TRACINGS OF BI-SYLLABIC CONSONANT GROUPS

Rousselot has shown that in the case of an elaborate consonant group like "*aptma*" the movements of the consonants "*p*" and "*m*" tend to fuse, in spite of the intervening "*t*" (70, p. 957). Tracings of such bi-syllabic groups uttered at increasing rate show that one-member abutting pairs tend to develop, across the intervening movement of the different articulatory member. This is a variation of the "doubling" process and illustrates the fact that when the consonant movement is repeated at a certain rate, whatever the accompanying movements, it takes on the "doubling" form (Fig. 77).

At the same time, such complicated groups are important for observation of the releasing and arresting of the consonants. It is not the case that a bundle of consonants is tumbled in "between two vowels". Instead, whatever the rate, the consonants are definitely grouped so that they act either as arresting or as releasing factors, either singly or as compounds. In the word "*aft-pa*" the "*f*" coincides with the "*t*" forming a compound in the arresting position; the "*t*" keeps its

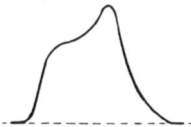

FIGURE 79. Diagrammatic Drawing of the "Inflected" Air Pressure Curve

There is a definite variation in the pressure, but the form is too brief to be a double. Figs. 61, p. 99 and 80, p. 112 show inflected curve with negative pressure due to same cause.

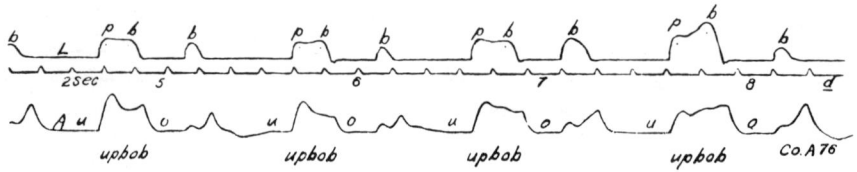

FIGURE 80. "Inflected" Air Pressure Curve in Series at Normal Rate

Syllables: *upbob*.
L—Lip marker. Usual forms. There is some variation in the intensity of the *p* and *b* strokes in the 'doubles'.

A—Air in mouth. Typical inflected curve appears in the arresting *b*'s. Indication of the same curve in doubling form in syls. 6, 7, 8. Cf. Fig. 61 p. 99.

definite arresting position until the word becomes monosyllabic; only then does it shift to the releasing position and become practically coincident with the "*p*". Mutatis mutandis, the same thing is true of "*s*" and "*p*" in "*isp-da*". In the words "*upspring*" and "*upspringing*", the "*p*" is the arresting stroke and the "*sp*" the releasing stroke throughout. But in the more rapid "*upspring*", the "*p-p*" may form a doublet over the intervening "*s*" (Cf. Fig. 78).

THE INFLECTED AIR PRESSURE CURVE OF THE SINGLE CONSONANTS

At first sight the inflected air pressure curve is like the "bi-maximal curve" of the double consonants and of other abutting pairs. But there is no difficulty in distinguishing the curve forms. The duration of the consonants involved is that of the single consonant (Cf. p. 48). Diagrammatic representation of bi-maximal and single consonant form (Fig. 79).

The inflected curve indicates a slight fluctuation in the air pressure in the mouth and is more likely to occur with nasals and with voiced occlusives like "*b*". It occurs in both the arresting and in the releasing positions in Fig. 80.

The reduction of the pressure is due to a rapid increase in the volume of the mouth, just as the mid-sag of the outside pressure is due to the change in mouth volume (Cf. p. 70). The experimental study of the process of voicing shows that this inflected curve is due to the increase of volume of the supra-laryngeal cavity when the sonant is produced. The mouth tube for sonants, and Rousselot's olive, used with nasals, tap the cavity behind the consonant occlusion and show this pressure variation. In one case Rousselot publishes a tracing of the air pressure in the mouth which is interesting because it shows the inflected form of the air pressure curve (35; 70, p. 496, Fig. 256b, p. 908, Fig. 588, *n*, p. 955, Fig. 641, *m*, p. 956, Fig. 642, *n*, p. 966, Fig. 652, general form of *n*, p. 967, Fig. 653, *n*, 3 cases, each a different subject; 72, p. 79, Fig. 71, *m*).

Chapter V

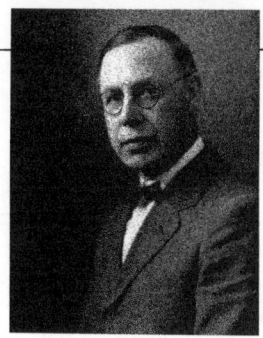

CLASSIFICATION OF PHONEMES

Editors' Remarks

Chapter 5 deals with taxonomic issues: On what basis should we partition speech units into natural categories? As always throughout the monograph, Stetson begins by using the *movements* of speech as a primary source of organization. In addition, he discusses issues related to the more traditional "features" of vowels and consonants. These issues of classification are far from resolved today. Descriptive systems for the vowel are still debated and characterizations of the sounds of the world's languages still produce "new" consonants and "new" features. Stetson's dissatisfaction with such "collections of symbols" is understandable, given his functional view of articulatory organization. The full complexity of spoken language defies description by a string of symbols and this chapter touches on some of the reasons for this. As Stetson says later in Chapter 8, "A language mechanism is an interrelated set of movements in which the various traits have their function; they are not isolated. The habit of describing the sounds and the rhythms of a language as if they were collections of independent peculiarities overlooks the fact that they are part and parcel of each other." In other, more modern terminology, we might say that the contents of language are not independent of the processes that realize language.

The development of the theory of the mechanism of speech determines the final classification of the phonemes. Classifications appear early, and those in current usage are not always consistent because they are based on various distinctions.

The classification of the phonemes must depend on the distinctions already made between the movements of the breath group, foot, and of the syllable. And the syllable is the basic movement which defines the constituent phonemes.

The first and fundamental distinction is between the vowel and the consonant. Although recognized by the ancient theorists, in cuneiform and in the early Semitic alphabet, some of the later notions fail to make the difference clear. Rousselot limited the opening-closing to the individual "sound", where Saussure had used it for the entire syllable. This left Rousselot without any fundamental definition of the syllable, and therefore of the consonant and vowel. Rousselot often assumes the syllable as an entity, and takes the contrast between consonant and vowel for granted, but his system of phonetics is defective at that crucial point.

Sievers introduced the notion of sonority as the basis for the syllable, which involved classifying the phonemes as to their "sonority" (Schallfülle, Schallstärke) and assumed that the phoneme of greatest sonority became the core of the syllable, and syllable formant. This was adopted by Passy, who supplemented actual sonority with "apparent sonority" and so accounted for the fact that Rousselot and others had been unable to show the differences in carrying power on which they depended for this sonority classification of the phonemes. Acoustic study of the vowels has left no place for the concept of "sonority"; it has no standing in the physics of sound. But under the label of "prominence" it still figures in many discussions as the basis for the consonant-vowel distinction. In one form and another it is recognized or assumed by the phonemicists (Cf. Bloch, Trager).

Physiological analysis of the mechanism of speech shows that the distinction between vowel and consonant is a matter of the difference of function in the syllable. The consonants delimit the chest pulse of the syllable; the vowels shape the vocal canal through which the chest pulse is emitted. On occasion the vocal canal may be shaped by a continuant consonant; a fricative which makes emission possible, like "*sh*...." or "*pst*", may act as a vowel; and "syllabic consonants (e.g., "*m, n, l, r, -ng*") are common in many languages.

The group of phonemes which are often thought of as on the border line, the "semi-vowels", "*w, y* (j)", are quite distinct in their function. When the closure of the vowel "*u*" is forced to the limit and quickly released the result is the consonant "*w*". The difference between consonant and vowel can be clearly noted in a series like "*oo, woo, oo, woo*". When the closure of the vowel "*i*" is forced to the limit and quickly released, the result is the consonant "*y*". The difference between consonant and vowel can be clearly noted in a series like "*ee, ye, ee, ye*".

The functional difference of vowel and consonant as constituents of the syllable, as characterized factors of the syllable, is an essential phase of the motor theory of phonetics.

CLASSIFICATION OF THE VOWELS

There are two common bases for the classification of the vowels: 1) The older, based on the position of the tongue. It is often used, and supplemented by indications of the position of the lips, is fairly adequate, though it is more complicated than 2) the classification based on the one cavity with the lips as orifice or the two cavities, anterior and posterior, which constitute a coupled resonator, with the blade of the tongue delimiting the orifice between the resonators, and the lips constituting the outer orifice. On this is based the two series of vowels:

1. From *i* to *ah*, with two cavities: in English, "*bee, pity, rate, yet, sang, bath*".
2. From *u* to *ah*, with a single cavity: in English, "*tooth, full, go, jaw, watch' ah*".

These are the cardinal vowels of English. They do not include the "dark-*e*" which is the minimum vowel opening, and is the lowest term to which a vowel can be reduced. In a language with a heavy word stress, like English, vowels are frequently reduced, so that a series by gradations from any cardinal vowel quality to this "dark-*e*", schwa, is possible.

The vowel is to be thought of as identified in part by the acoustic quality, its "value", and in part by a physiological shape which is defined by the movement of the tongue and of the jaw and lips. These movements are reciprocal, and there is a whole range of positions possible for the one vowel (Cf. Marichelle [51], and G. O. Russell [74]).

The range of positions for the one vowel is inevitable, especially in languages with arresting consonants, because the delimiting consonants determine the position from which and to which the vowel movement must be made. It is customary to refer to the vowel shape as a "position"; but in the case of most vowels in rapid speech, the vowel movement is continuous. There is no time for stasis in a "position".

In many languages the vowel has a "length" which is phonemic. Owing to the varying rates of utterance, the distinction proves to be between 1) vowels which may be prolonged, but which are often short, and 2) vowels which cannot be prolonged and which are always relatively short in duration.

English has a peculiar series of "short vowels" in which the arrest is entirely consonantal, e.g., "*pap, pep, pip, pup*". The chest muscles do not figure at all in the arrest. The familiar Continental languages have no such vowels.

The distinction between vowels which are arrested wholly or in part by the consonant has led to the familiar distinction of "tense" and "lax" vowels. If the arrest is due primarily to the consonant, the vowel is denominated "lax"; if the arrest is due primarily to the chest muscles, the vowel is denominated "tense". The muscles of the vocal canal are not concerned and are neither tense nor lax; the muscular tension which is present or absent is that of the intercostal muscles of the chest.

The tradition of a short and long contrast in quality may survive radical historical changes of the values of vowels. In English the popular sense has it that "*Pete*" is long and "*pet*" is short; that "*bite*" is long and "*bit*" is short; that "*bate*" is long and "*bat*" is short; that "*pope*" is long and "*pop*" is short; although the vowels are not now so related. It is an excellent illustration of the part that conditioning plays in determination of the relations of articulations.

The vowels of a language with pronounced word stress are subject to changes due to stress, and the consequent changes of rate. The prolongable vowels of a heavily stressed syllable tend to prolong, and in many cases to diphthongize, as in English. If the vowel is not prolongable when stressed, the arresting consonant or the intersyllabic interval are prolonged. In the case of unstressed vowels, the increase in rate makes for the reduction of the vowel toward schwa, and may even lead to the repression of the syllable.

Certain changes of vowels are due to accessory movements. The pure and nasal vowel qualities result from the closed and open position of the velum. In some languages whispered vowels occur in certain cases, due to the relaxation of the glottis. In the case of diphthongs, vowels may unite into double or triple compounds. It is evident that the change of the vowel-shape is slow enough so that the components are recognized. The components are often of unequal duration. If the diphthong is lengthened, the longer component is prolonged. Diphthongs arise by the serial fusion of two vowels, or by the effect of a vigorous stress on a simple vowel (Brechung). The umlaut is not a serial fusion but the modification of the value of a vowel by an element in the following syllable.

CLASSIFICATION OF THE CONSONANTS

The most obvious functional classification of the consonants divides them into the releasing and arresting consonants. In most cases the consonant can function in both capacities; but there are exceptions. In English "*w, wh, y (j), h*", are releasing only; while "*ng*" is arresting only, in function.

Since the consonant is a constriction, the closure may be either tight or leaky. The complete closure constitutes the stop (occlusive) and the partial closure constitutes the continuant. Continuants are often characterized as sibilant, fricative, liquid, nasal, depending on accessory movements and consequent noises. The complete closure of a stop when acting as an arresting consonant is sometimes affected by a heavy stress and tends in that case to become continuant.

The sounding of the vocal folds makes the familiar difference between the surd and sonant. This is not due to the direct action of the glottis, though this is often assumed. The subject speaking with an artificial larynx is able to control the surd-sonant distinction when the reed is always in position to speak, and the surd or sonant trait must depend on the manipulation of an air pressure above and below the glottis. In rapid speech this distinction in voicing often fails, but the difference in force between the surd and sonant persists. The distinction of fortis and lenis proves more fundamental than that of the voicing. (35)

In some languages there is a phonemic distinction between long and short consonants. But there is no such distinction in English, German or French.

The phonemic distinction between the single and the double consonant is often assumed to be a mere difference of long and short. But a study of abutting consonants shows that the double consonant is an abutting pair in which the members are the same consonant. This has been recognized by Swadesh (94), who speaks of the association of phonemic length of the consonant, in Finnish, e.g., as always associated with other movements.

Simple, compound, and abutting consonants are to be distinguished. The simple consonant of a language cannot be separated into components. The compound consonant also acts as a single characterized factor in the syllable, but it may be resolved into two, or, on occasion, three components. Abutting consonants are in no wise single. The abutting pair functions, the one as an arresting consonant in the preceding syllable, and the other as a releasing consonant in the following syllable. Their traits have been considered in detail.

In cases where the compound consonant occurs between feet, and the next syllable is without a consonant, the compound consonant separates into its components, and becomes an abutting pair. This may be used as a test of the compound consonant (Cf. p. 88).

The influence of the abutting pair on each other is often spoken of as assimilation. The voicing of the one often affects the other; on occasion abutting consonants assimilate as a double determined by the releasing consonant, (common in Latin and Greek; "assimilate, symmetry"). In some cases the two abutting consonants assimilate to a third form, thus the abutting pair "s: y" become the English "sh; t: y" become the English "ch" (Cf. Hudgins and DiCarlo [33], pp. 462–464). In many cases the arresting consonant drops, and the abutting pair is replaced by a single, releasing consonant.

Perhaps the most obvious way of indicating the characterized factor of the syllable is to name the member or members with which the articulation is produced:

Labial,
Labio-dental,
Lingual, front, blade, and rear,
Lingual-velar,
Guttural,
Glottal.

On occasion two or more regions are involved, and a consonant is nasalized, labialized, or palatalized.

The position and the extent of the area of contact is affected by the stress and rate of the syllables involved; and differs somewhat between the releasing and arresting forms.

Determining the traits and classes of the phonemes leads to the system of symbols whereby the characterized syllable factors are indicated. The great achievements in theoretical phonetics lie in these systems of symbols:

The cuneiform characters embodied a fairly complete list of the syllables of the language, but did not distinguish the syllable factors.

The Semitic alphabet used the releasing consonant to represent the syllable and was followed by the Greek and Sanskrit alphabets which represented all the factors of the syllable, and counted the vowel as the core of the syllable.

The Japanese syllabary derived from the Chinese syllables, under the influence of the Sanskrit, set up a simple series of kana for the syllables of the Japanese and constitutes one of the simplest and most systematic of the methods of writing. (Complicated in use by the employment of Chinese ideograms.)

In spite of its pretensions and the fact that it is the basis of "phonemics", the I.P.A. (International Phonetic Alphabet) is an unsatisfactory collection of symbols. It was thrown together when the problem of phonetics was believed to be the determination of a fixed position for each "sound", and speech was thought of as a series of such "sounds".

The breath group, rather than the syllable, has been the unit used consistently in I.P.A. transcriptions. As a convenience, some transcribers divide their transcriptions into words, though aware that there is no phonetic unit corresponding to the word. There is no provision for the syllable, hence the syllable factors are not distinguished. The fundamental differentiation of vowel and consonant is not recognized. There is no distinction between compound consonants with a single syllable function, and abutting consonants, which function in two different syllables. The I.P.A. fosters the use of a loose term like "consonant cluster".

In actual use the transcribers have not been consistent in making the I.P.A. symbol represent the phoneme. They have often represented the variants of a phoneme by different symbols; and they speak of a "broad" and of a "narrow" transcription. An I.P.A. transcription is worthless unless the reader is familiar with the phonetics of the language, knows its syllabification and the variants of the phonemes.

Rime, assonance, alliteration, vowel harmony signalize various resemblances of the consonants and vowels. They are all involved in prosody.

Rime is the most elaborate. It occurs on the stress of the breath group, and depends on the *difference* of the release of the two stressed syllables of two parallel breath groups (consonant contrasts with consonant, or consonant contrasts with chest-release) and on the *identity* of the vowel of the stressed syllables and of anything following the vowel (arresting consonant or following unstressed syllables). Since the breath group for rime must be of a regular rhythmic pattern, rime figures primarily in verse. Rime echoes from breath group to breath group and is one of the devices for constructing the stanza in verse.

tata' tata' tata' taba' (t ta),
tata' tata' tata' tada' (t ta).

The conditions of rime (including identical intonation on the rime) are well known; but its nature has never been fathomed. (83)

In many languages the stress on the individual syllable is phonemic. This is the word stress, so variable in incidence and therefore so difficult in English and Russian. In other languages the placement of the stress is optional and defines the breath group, but does not have phonemic significance.

The intonation in the western languages does not affect the syllable; but in many Asiatic and American languages it is phonemic, and characterizes the syllable. In the western languages it may set up contrasts, characterized phrases, and is roughly a type of over-all punctuation.

CHAPTERS 6, 7, and 8 EDITORS' REMARKS

We consider Chapters 6, 7, and 8 as a unit because these chapters address the nature of rhythmical grouping and its influence on syllabic structure. Stetson's aim is to show the process of syllable interaction in connected speech. Grouping, as Stetson sees it, is conditioned by stress patterns, rates of speaking, number of syllables in a breath group, and so forth, but it is ultimately expressed by the gestural behaviors originally identified in the rate scaling experiments.

Chapter 6 describes the effects of stress and rate on syllabic cohesion. There is still much research to be done here and Stetson offers some of the tools and techniques to do it. Chapter 7 presents the experimental study of a variety of rhythmical patterns. Chapter 8, a very short chapter, discusses differences between the rhythm of different languages and how sound changes can occur. On the one hand, "temporary" phonetic changes can occur which revert with restoration of rate and stress. On the other hand, so-called diachronous language change occurs as a function of "perturbations of the language mechanism" that have somehow had a permanent effect. One is tempted to speculate on these views of linguistic stability and change in light of recent debates in evolutionary biology regarding whether evolution itself is best described as gradual and accumulative or "punctuated" by long periods of stasis and relatively brief, discontinuous change. One suspects that Stetson might have jumped into this fray with both feet, but we shall refrain from doing so.

In these chapters, Stetson argues strongly for a "wholistic" view of speech in which the sounds and the rhythm of language are not independent. As his experimental observations suggest, the nature of the phonetic units we call phonemes, syllables, and so on, is determined by their place in larger rhythmical structures. It is the nature of this overall language mechanism that Stetson strove to understand, and upon which new attacks may be based.

Chapter VI

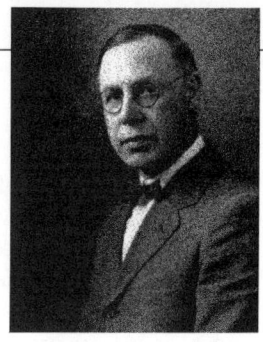

STRESS AND RATE AND THEIR RELATION TO THE SYLLABLE AND TO THE BREATH GROUP

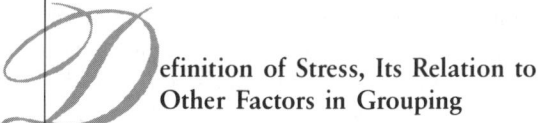

efinition of Stress, Its Relation to Other Factors in Grouping

The "breath group" is a division recognized by phoneticians of all schools. In the breath group in English the dynamic pattern which constitutes the "group" is made by the word stresses. That the syllables have varying degrees of stress, and that they are subordinated and grouped in rhythmic forms, has been commonplace since Aristotle. In poetry we have called the rhythmic unit-groups "feet", and have noted the regular patterns. Feet may also be observed in prose, following Aristotle, but the patterns are not regular.

There is still a difference of opinion as to what constitutes "word accent". There are many who insist that pitch may be the important factor. Ever since Mitford, in 1804 (cited in 76), there have been those who believe that change of pitch can produce an "accent". Also Coleman, cited with approval by Daniel Jones (11, 38), believes that accent is due to a turn in the pitch. The earlier advocates of this theory of pitch accent assumed a *rise* in pitch, but the experimental findings have made them fall back on some change in pitch, either rise or fall; so Abas (1), so Morris (55, 16).

It is only in the field of speech that "accent" has been assumed to be a matter of pitch change. A comparison with the conditions of accentuation in other rhythmic fields makes the notion very doubtful. In music it is apparent that a change of pitch cannot be the determining factor in "accent". It is possible to make abrupt pitch changes within a musical figure without changing the stress pattern; in fact such changes of pitch with an undisturbed stress pattern are commonplace. And if changes of pitch might in any circumstances determine an "accent", composers for the organ would certainly avail themselves of the device, because there is need of every resource for indicating stress at the organ.

It is not surprising that in speech changes of pitch should be noted at the stress; it is often the significant point in the group; and the heavy stroke of the accent involves the chest pressure and is apt to change the pitch because the laryngeal musculature is often affected by tensions in the other musculatures of speech. But if changes in pitch were in any way essential to word accent, it would be impossible to train the deaf mute to speak with a word accent, and impossible for the subject with an artificial larynx, or for one who whispers, to mark the word accent.

The logical analysis of sound as involving duration, pitch, and intensity, is responsible for the belief in pitch as an accentual factor; if duration and intensity affect accent, then why not pitch? But stress is not a matter of the properties of sound, it is a matter of the coordination and culmination of a movement. A movement must involve a stress, a pulse, and a movement must involve time, but a movement does not involve pitch. Rhythm is in no sense a matter of pitch; there is no rhythmic series however elaborate, no rhythmic grouping however complicated, which cannot be expressed without pitch. In speech all stress involves increased force of the syllable movement, i.e. of the chest pulse. This is Wundt's position:

Therefore the customary distinction between pitch accent and dynamic accent is mistaken. There is only one real accent and that is the dynamic or expiratory accent (106, p. 273).

MEASUREMENT OF INTENSITIES IN SPEECH

It is not an easy matter to measure the intensities of speech, whether they are conceived as intensities of sound, or intensities of expiratory force. If one were willing to assume that speech is a matter of acoustics, the measurement of the intensities of the series of acoustic combinations is difficult. The comparison of sounds at various pitches, of different vowels with varying acoustic patterns, of vowel sounds with consonant sounds, is the serious problem. The question is further complicated if it is assumed that duration and, pitch somehow figure in the "word accent".

Neither is the measurement of the expiratory force an easy matter. The commonest form of record has been of the pressure just outside the mouth; and this has been supplemented by occasional studies of the pressure changes in the chest during speech. The force of expiration is due to the contraction of chest muscles, but the flow of expired air does not depend on the contraction of the chest muscles alone; the flow of expired air is effected also by the conformation of the vocal canal. If the glottis and mouth are relatively open, the flow is large; if the glottis and mouth are relatively closed, the flow is small. Since the pressure just outside the mouth depends on the flow of expired air, tracings of that pressure are subject to correction for the articulation involved.

If the expiratory force is to be measured in terms of the pressures produced just outside the mouth, it is obvious that only artificial material can be used; it is impossible to handle the varying complexities of ordinary speech. The articulatory conformation must be the same from syllable to syllable if the changes in pressure are to correspond to the force of the muscular contractions of the chest. The pressure just outside the mouth will vary with the chest contractions if the conformation remains the same. But of course this outside pressure will drop to zero during any consonant occlusion, and such changes of chest pressure as occur during the occlusion are lost. The opening and closing of the mouth also introduces an artifact, the "mid-sag", already mentioned (Cf. p. 71).

It happens that some important changes take place during the consonant occlusion. The minimal chest pressure, marking the end of one chest pulse and the beginning of another, occurs during the releasing consonant, whether single or member of an abutting pair. Only in the case of a syllable with an arresting consonant does the pressure minimum show in the outside pressure; but it is often masked by the "mid-sag". To prescribe syllables with arresting consonants would only limit the experimental procedure; since the rate of syllables with arresting consonants cannot exceed three per sec. Such a rate would make it impossible to study the common rhythmic groupings for which the syllable stress is a primary factor.

Tracings of the pressure in the chest, taken directly from the trachea below the glottis, give definite indications of the chest pulses, both maxima and minima. As the tambour must be set to record pressures as high as 200 mm. water, the membrane cannot be very sensitive (Cf. p. 36). Variations of pressure in the mouth, due to the articulatory movements, do not affect the subglottal pressures because of the intervening glottis vent. The chest pressure tracings show very strikingly the groups of syllables. The continued slow expiratory movement which makes the grouping, maintains the pressure well above zero throughout the group (Fig. 18, 19, 20, 21).

It is possible to get direct records of the movements of the muscles in speech. The negative-pressure tracings show the variations of force in the expiratory pulses. Action-current records show the action of both the internal and external intercostals for the individual syllables, and the action of the abdominal muscles for the grouping movements of foot and breath group. (85, Figs. 5, 7; 91, Figs. 15–22)

STRESS AND THE RESULTING DYNAMIC FORM IN THE TWO-SYLLABLE, THREE-SYLLABLE, AND FOUR-SYLLABLE BREATH GROUPS

The breath group is composed of syllables grouped into feet. It is convenient to distinguish the types of feet in terms of the number of syllables.

Breath groups of a single one-syllable foot are presented in the studies of syllable modification: the one-syllable breath groups are shown at varying rates, the maximum rate of the simplest breath group is made apparent as well as the various connections between breath groups consisting of a single one-syllable foot. As the rate increases, such breath groups are succeeded by an indeterminate breath group (Cf. "patter").

In the two-syllable feet, the iamb and the trochee, there are but two degrees of force. But the dactyl shows not only small variations in the duration of the three component syllables, but also gradations in the force of utterance. The stressed syllable is merely the climax of the stresses of the dactyl (Cf. Fig. 81, 82).

Fig. 81 is an excellent example of the uniformity with which a subject often repeats a particular form of utterance. The extreme emphasis on the initial consonant is unusual, but is persisted through the three series of the sitting. There are slight differences in rate and a few small differences in detail but the identity is striking.

Like the organization of the foot, the organization of the breath group is due to a single movement of which the single syllables and the feet form apart, like the ripples on a larger wave. The notion of the stress as a single isolated peak rising from the plain, a mere marker for the breath group or foot, is inadequate. In reality, the primary stress is the climax of the single slow movement which underlies and constitutes the unity of the foot, and of the breath group. Compare studies of rhythm (83, p. 445–6; 84, p. 315). As the name indicates, it *is* a breath group in the sense that the inclusive movement is a movement of expiration, and therefore it appears in the tracing of the chest pressure, or in the tracing of the pressure variation just outside the mouth (Cf. Figs. 81, 82, and Figs. 100, 101).

Breath groups of a single one-syllable foot have been presented in the study of the syllables. A breath group may be constituted by a single foot of two syllables, trochee, or iamb. A study of the stresses of trochees and iambs shows that the subject seldom fails to mark the stress. The measurement of 23 trochees, "*te'tet, to'tot, ta'tat*", shows five reversals of the stress. The measurement of 29 iambs shows two reversals of the stress, 29 dactyls, from prescribed "*pup' up up*", show the normal stress in 25 cases (Cf. Figs. 83, 84). (Form B 5, 6, 7, 8, 9, sub. W. whispered series. Heights of outside pressure tracing measured and compared.) In none of these is the arresting

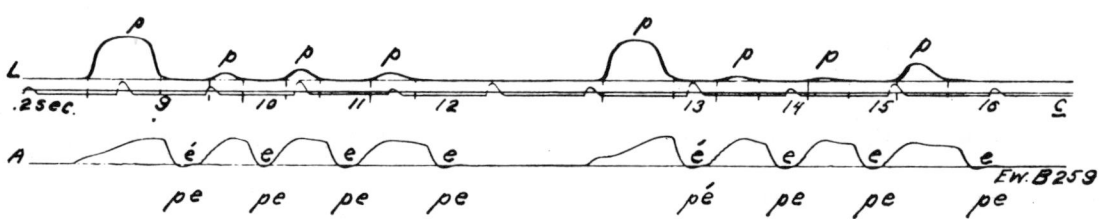

FIGURE 81. Exaggeration of the Initial Consonant

Syllables: *pe' pe pe pe*.

L—Lip marker. Heavy stress on the first syllable shows both in the length and the intensity of the consonant. Last syllable shows a slight secondary stress.

A—Air in mouth. Prolongation of the initial *p*; but there is no excessive pressure on the initial consonant.

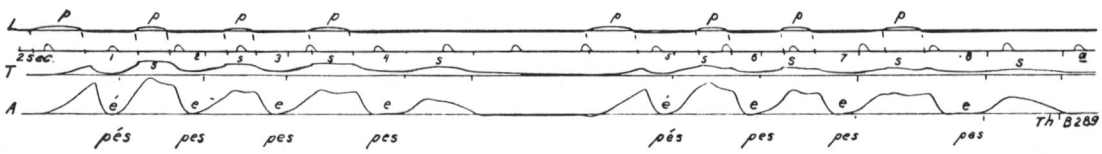

FIGURE 82. Stressed Group. Breaks up into Dactyl and one-syllable Feet

Syllables: *pes' pes pes pes.*

L

T—Lip- and tongue markers. Show the *sp* form, with exception of syl. 3-4 and 7-8 which seem like abutting pairs.

A—Air in mouth. Shows the stress on the first syllable, primarily in the *following* consonant; secondary stress on the last syllable. The doubling form is well marked at syl. 1-2, 2-3, 3-4, 5-6, 6-7, 7-8.

---

consonant of the first two syllables of "*pup' up up*" actually given; instead, the form uttered by the subjects is "*pu' pu pup*". Such modifications are very common; in the case of this dactyl it illustrates the tendency to eliminate abutting consonants and arresting consonants within a foot. A form prescribed as "*up' up pup*" vacillates between ⊥ _ x ⊥ and ⊥ _ x _. The double appears "*up pup-pup*" as essential to distinguish the word "*pup*", and this determines the division into two feet. (15 cases, B 353, 354 sub. W.) The same subject gave the series "*up' up up*" (alternating with the "*up' up pup*"). The result is "*u' pup up'*" sometimes with the primary stress on the initial and sometimes on the final. The arresting consonant, dividing the second syllable from the final, marks the division ⊥ _/⊥ . "*U'p up up*" may be uttered so that the separate words appear with an arresting consonant after the first syllable and with a double well separated between the second and third syllables, "*up, up-pup*". The forms "*pup up' pup*" and "*pup up pup'*" both result in a marked double between the median and final syllables; there is usually an intersyllabic space between the doublets (Cf. Figs. 83, 84).

The determining factors in such groupings are the stresses prescribed and the tendency to preserve the identity of the words. In English it is possible to make a distinction between "*up up up*" and "*u pu pup*" which would be impossible in French. But such distinctions are made by maintaining the arresting consonant as in "*up-up- up*" or an actual double as in "*up- up-pup*".

FOUR-SYLLABLE GROUPS

If a heavy stress is prescribed in a breath group of four syllables like "*te te' te tet*", the prescription is usually carried out. In 53 cases, three subjects, the prescribed stress is not given in 8 series.

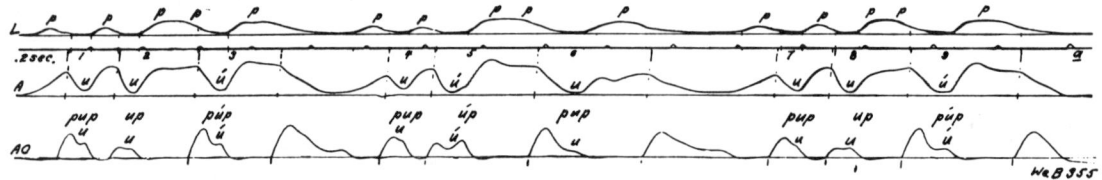

FIGURE 83. Stressed Groups showing Doubles between the Feet. Double does not depend on the Position of the Stress, but on Division of the Feet

Syllables: *pup up pup', pup up' pup.*

L—Lip marker. Indication of doubling, syl. 2-3, 5-6, 8-9. The final arresting *p*'s are prolonged and there is often indication of doubling, syl. 3.

A—Air in mouth. Double forms appear, syl. 2-3 before stress, 5-6 after stress, 8-9 again before stress. Syl. 3, 6 and 9 give indication of doubling in the arresting final consonant of that group.

Cf. Figs. 35, 37. Dynamics show very clearly in the culmination of force at the stressed syllable.

AO—Air outside. Double and final consonants only show the arresting form, Cf. Figs. 26 and 49. All other forms are actually releasing whatever the prescription. Dynamic culmination at the stress is apparent.

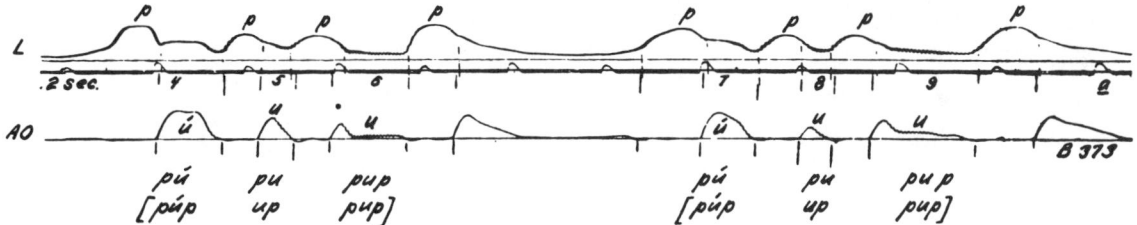

FIGURE 84. Changes of Prescribed Consonants due to Stress and Grouping. Dynamic Culmination at the Stress
Syllables: *pup' up pup* uttered as *pu' pu pup*.

L—Lip marker. The initial *p* is unvocalized, but there is marked vocalization of the median *p* of the trochee *pu pup*. The double prescribed between *up* and *pup* has been omitted. The prescribed arresting consonant of the initial *pup* has been shifted to the releasing position in the next syllable.

AO—Air outside. Dynamic culmination at the stress is apparent.

In 25 of the 53 cases, the primary stress is clearly on the second syllable; but it often happens that while the second syllable gets a definite stress, there is a heavier stress on the third or fourth syllable. There is a strong tendency to prolong and to stress the later members of such a series. No uniform pattern for the other syllables is apparent; the form is apt to open with an iamb, and doubling, "*te tet-te tet*", often appears; but the second unit-group may be a trochee or iamb; the iamb is the more common, repeating the first foot, and bringing stress on the final syllable. Such doubles, which appear when a single is prescribed, may be called "adventitious doubles"; they mark the division between the feet and often precede or follow heavy stresses (Cf. p. 81).

In the prescribed form, "*te te te' tet*" (short vowels), of 36 cases, three subjects, 33 have the prescribed stress; and it is obviously the primary stress in 24 cases. The exceptions are cases in which the grouping is "*te te te'/tet'*" and a heavy stress has been thrown on the final syllable. Here again adventitious doubles often appear, usually following the stress, marking the division. The grouping of the syllables is usually "*te' te/te' tet*", or "*te' te/tet' -/- tet'*"; but variants may appear in the first foot.

With long vowels the results are similar, __ _/_ __ __. In 63 cases, four subjects, 51 have the prescribed stress; it is easily primary in 36 cases, in others a heavier stress appears later.

With long vowels, __ _/_ __ __, 17 cases, two subjects, 16 show the primary stress on the prescribed syllable; the one exception has in

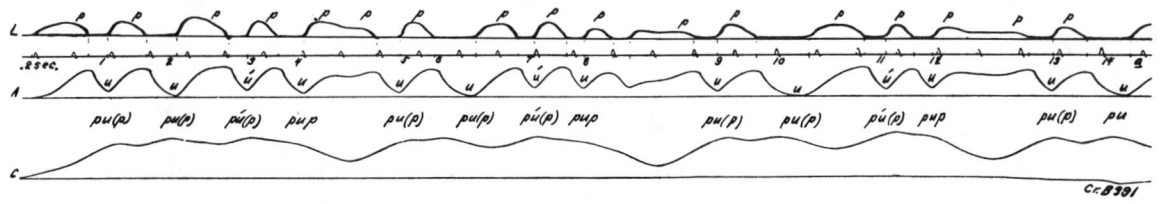

FIGURE 85. Stressed Group. Singling of Prescribed Doubles between Breath Groups. Chest Pulses recorded directly from Trachea.

Syllables: *pup pup pup' pup* actually uttered as *pu pu pu' pup-pu* etc.

L—Lip marker. Doubling forms between breath groups, syl. 4-5, 12-13. *p* at beginning of second foot of each breath group, syl. 2-3, 6-7, 10-11 is stressed and prolonged as if a double might appear.

A—Air in mouth. Doubles between breath groups, syl. 4-5, 12-13 are marked. Forms between the feet, syl. 2-3, 6-7, 10-11 might easily develop into doubles.

C—Chest pulses from trachea. Definite minima between breath groups over which consonant doubles. Slight indication of the two feet. The pulses of each syllable are marked.

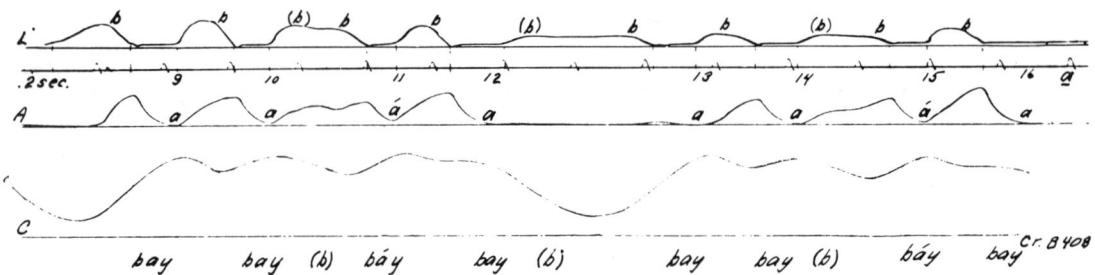

FIGURE 86. Adventitious Doubles in Stressed Group with Long Vowels; Chest Pulses recorded directly from Trachea

Syllables: *bay bay bay' bay* uttered as *bay bay b- bay bay b- bay*.

L—Lip marker. Well defined doubles, syl. 10-11, and 14-15. Double also appears between the groups, syl. 12-13.

A—Air in mouth. Well marked doubling forms, 6-7, 10-11, 14-15, but the pressure is not maintained between the breath groups, syl. 12-13.

C—Chest pulses directly from trachea. Division of the group into sub-groups (feet) is marked. Doubling occurs across this division.

addition a heavy stress on the last syllable. The unit-groups are very like those of the four-syllable groups with short vowels. Adventitious doubles are not likely to appear; though they are found in some cases (Cf. Figs. 86, 87).

When the group of syllables is as long as a series of four, the tendency to break up into two feet is apparent; there is a tendency to put a heavy stress on the final syllable of the breath group. Although all of the four subjects are English-speaking, there is a pronounced tendency to prolong and to stress the last syllable of the four-syllable group.

Abutting consonants (doubles) and arresting consonants appear only between feet; within the feet an arresting consonant is dropped. It makes little difference whether doubles are prescribed; either "*tet tet tet' tet*" or "*te te te' tet*"; the feet are likely to be separated by a double (adventitious when the single consonant is prescribed) and only the releasing consonant appears within the foot in any case.

A sentence like "*Lil' 'll lie low*" gives the same forms as the four-syllable group. But with no stress prescribed, the results are more varied. The main stress falls in 11 of 15 cases on the first

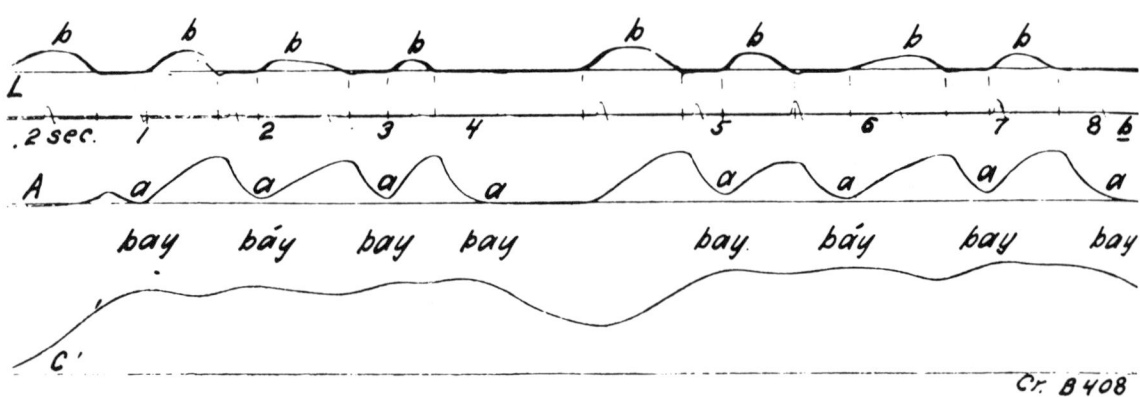

FIGURE 87. Stressed Group without Doubling; Chest Pulses directly from Trachea

Syllables: *bay bay' bay bay*.

L—Lip marker. Single consonants.

A—Air in mouth. Single consonants.

C—The sub-groups (feet) are not defined.

syllable, 3 times on the second, and once on the third syllable. There seems to be no tendency to stress the last syllable with the one subject uttering this particular phrase.

The five-syllable phrase, "*pop up a pop up*", as uttered by a single subject (W.), has a definite climactic stress on the penultimate "*pop*". But the form is not a dactyl "*pop' up a*" plus a trochee "*pop' up*", instead, the form is ⊥ / ⊥ _ / ⊥ _, with a definite arresting consonant marking the initial syllable "*pop*"; this avoids the form "*po pup*" and keeps the identity of the two words "*pop*" and "*up*". In 17 of 19 cases the primary stress falls on the penultimate syllable; the secondary stress occurs sometimes on the initial and sometimes on the second syllable of the group. No heavy stress falls on the final syllable; the grammatical subordination of the word prevents it. (In strictness, the syllables which may be compared are the initial and the penultimate syllables, "pop", and the second and final syllables "up"; the vowels are not otherwise comparable. Cf. Fig. 113.)

"*Runnin' 'n' neighin'*" also gives a five-syllable group, but it is impossible to say more than that it is easy to utter it in a single "breath group". The long vowel in "*neighin'*" is not comparable with the short vowel of "*runnin'*" (Cf. Fig. 111).

THE SEPARATING AND CONNECTING OF SYLLABLES AS A RESULT OF RATE*

The device of increasing or decreasing the rate of uniform series of syllables makes it possible to study in some detail the types of connection and of division which depend on rate. The rate of a series is an important factor in grouping for several reasons. In the first place, the absolute length of a group has limits, so that increasing the number of syllables in a group increases the rate of the component syllables. This is apparent in the studies of Rousselot, et al., who note the decrease in the length of syllables when something is added. In the second place, speech tends always to a rapid rate and the increasing rate of

---

*Cf. p. 89

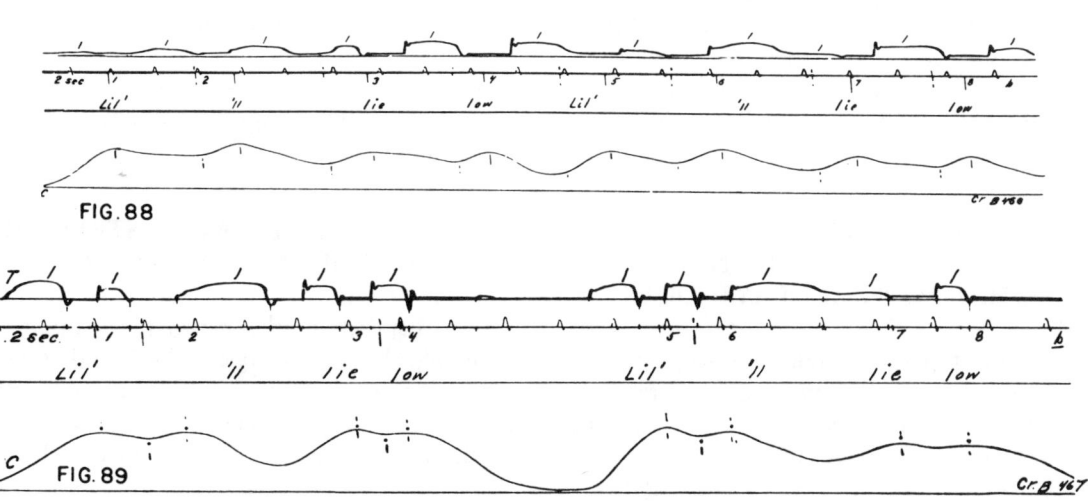

FIGURE 88 and 89. Consonant Functioning as Syllabic Consonant. Contrast in grouping of Syllables of the same Phrase. Chest Pulses recorded directly from Trachea

Syllables: *Lil' 'll lie low* Differently grouped.

T—Tongue marker. The l's are very distinct, except the single double, syl. 6-7; the second member of the double is much weaker as is usual with doubled l's.

C—Chest pulses direct from trachea. The syllables are given with well defined pulses; there is a slight indication of the division butween the two phrases, syl. 4-5. In Fig. 89 there is a division of each phrase into two-syllable feet.

In both records the maximum chest pressure does not occur during the *l* but *between* the consonants during the vowel; the rise in pressure is due to an independent chest pulse and not to the constriction of the vocal canal.

a rhythmic series, with long and short syllables, will modify the short syllables while the long syllables are still unaffected by the rate. And finally, increasing the rate of utterance will throw together into larger unities small groups which are ordinarily uttered separately.

As the rate of a uniform series increases, the adjacent syllables begin to group together; this shows in the formation of "doubles" or "abutting consonants" between the syllables having both releasing and arresting consonants (Cf. Fig. 90).

If the syllables in the series have only releasing consonants, the change is apparent in the chest-pressure tracing (Cf. Figs. 26, 28, 50, 57). If the syllables in the series have arresting consonants, the intersyllabic space disappears. A second type of grouping occurs at still higher rate when the arresting consonant drops from the abutting pair, or shifts to the releasing position. In these uniform series in which the rate is gradually increased or decreased, the indefinitely long breath group developed is artificial and unusual, and corresponds to the trill or run in music; such prolonged breath groups very seldom occur in actual speech. In the earlier part of such syllable trains, the syllables each have a breath group; as the consonants single the syllables have a long breath group of an indeterminate number of syllables; an unusual form of utterance except in "patter" (Cf. Figs. 40, 41, 42).

FUNCTIONS OF DOUBLING AND SINGLING IN THE GROUPING OF SYLLABLES

The same types of connection seen in these uniform series with increasing rate are to be found in syllables uttered in ordinary groups. When the individual feet (of one, two, or three syllables) are uttered separately, an intersyllabic interval occurs between the feet or breath groups, during which the chest pressure goes down to zero. When this space closes up, and an abutting pair or an arresting consonant remains, the linkage indicates the connection of one foot with another in a breath group. A two-syllable breath group composed of two single-syllable feet connected by a double is represented by $\_ x \_$. A four-syllable breath group composed of two iambs connected by a double is represented by $\_\_\perp x \_\_\perp$. It often happens that subjects actually regroup into larger phrases what were intended to be separate breath groups. This shows in the development of the abutting form between such prescribed groups. Fig. 85 is a case in which breath groups are accidentally connected by abutting pairs.

In such cases it is *not* necessary that the double occur either at the beginning or the end of the stressed syllable; doubling may occur between two stressed syllables (Cf. Fig. 85). As it often happens that the stress begins or ends the group, it is frequently the case that the abutting pair occurs just before or just after the stress.

"Singling" occurs when the connection is so close that the syllables involved form parts of a foot. When "*bub -bub*" becomes "*bu' bub*", the breath group of two monosyllabic feet $\perp x \perp$ has become the iamb $\_\_\perp$.

FUNCTION OF THE WORD STRESS IN THE GROUPING OF SYLLABLES

In actual speech another factor plays a part in grouping. As already stated, the "word stress" figures in the organization of the foot and breath group. The stressed syllable is in general lengthened; this prolongation of the stressed syllable

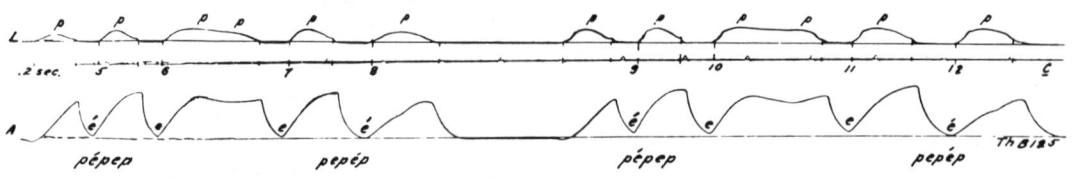

FIGURE 90. Doubles between Unstressed Syllables, at the Division between Feet
Syllables: pe' pep pe pep'.
L—Lip marker. Doubling forms, syl. 6-7, 10-11.
A—Air in mouth. Well marked doubling forms, 6-7, 10-11.

may appear as a pause after the beat-stroke, as in the iamb and anapest, $\_\_\angle$ and $\_\_\_\angle$. In the case of the trochee, the pause may appear before the beat stroke. Often the prolongation of the final member of the group masks the lengthening due to the stress, and the two syllables may be of approximately the same length. This relation of length and stress has been considered at some length by the rhythmists. (Cf. Riemann, 65.)

One might expect that the prolongation of the stressed syllable would naturally appear in a "double" (abutting pair) before or after the stress. Such doubling can occur, however, only when the stressed syllable occurs at the beginning or end of the foot. Thus a double may precede the trochaic stress in a series $\angle\_\_ x \angle\_\_ x \angle\_\_$; and a double may precede the dactylic stress in a series: $\angle\_\_\_ x \angle\_\_\_ x \angle\_\_\_$. And also a double may follow the iambic stress in a series $\_\_\angle x \_\_\angle x \_\_\angle$. But in a mixed series like $\angle\_\_ x \_\_\angle$ the double neither precedes nor follows the stressed syllables (Cf. Fig. 90).

If the stress is fixed, then the feet are formed to accommodate themselves to these stresses. In such cases the nature of the vowels sometimes figures in the formation of the feet and breath groups.

If the forms are trochaic or dactylic, the heavily stressed syllable is not prolonged; the slightly increased length of the stressed beat stroke appears in the preparation of the blow. Therefore there will be no double (abutting pair) following the trochaic or dactylic stress, however heavy the word stress. Indeed, a very heavy stress may lead to a "reduction" of a single median consonant to be discussed later. If the vowel of the preceding syllable is short, doubles are likely to appear before the stress, and so mark the division of the feet. If the vowel of the preceding syllable is long, a single consonant will not be doubled (a prescribed abutting pair may appear, however).

In the case of iambic (including anapestic) feet, the syllable receiving the stress must be somewhat prolonged ("apogogic accent"). This increased length is due to the heavier blow of the stress. If the syllable involved has a "long" vowel (i.e. a vowel that can be prolonged), the increased force of the stress shows in the increased length of the chest pulse, and the vowel is somewhat longer. If, however, the stressed syllable of the iamb has a "short" vowel (i.e. a vowel that cannot be prolonged), the increased chest pulse meets the obstacle of the arresting consonant. The consequent truncation of the blow results in the prolonging of the occlusion of the arresting consonant which provides for the increased length of the beat stroke as well as of the back stroke of the syllable pulse. The heavy stress on the iamb may force the single, releasing consonant of the next syllable into the arresting position, and the consonant may double. This is the "adventitious double". If the shift from the releasing position to the arresting position occurs without repeating the consonant, the result is an "arresting consonant" which marks the limit of the foot.

Neither the feet (one-syllable foot, iambs, trochees, dactyls) nor the larger breath groups are necessarily words. The identity of the word is lost in utterance. The breath groups of the phoneticians constitute the larger groups; sub-groups are the feet, within these breath groups; but none of them need coincide with words. The tracings of chest pressure during speech show these groupings surprisingly well. One finds not only the breath groups indicated but also the various feet within the breath group.

It is natural to think of the "long" and "short" syllables as important in the construction of rhythm forms, and the consequent organization of breath groups. A little study of the tracings shows that one difference between the "long" and the "short" vowels of English is the possibility of prolonging the "long" vowel, if the syllable is to be lengthened. The "short" vowel is one that cannot be prolonged if the syllable is lengthened; the prolongation must occur in the arresting consonant or the intersyllabic interval (Cf. Fig. 91). This distinction appears again in the differentiation of "tense and lax" vowels. When the syllable is arrested primarily by the consonant, the vowel is said to be lax. But if the syllable is arrested in part by the chest muscles, the vowel is counted "tense". Thus the attempt to prolong an English "short vowel" destroys its quality; in such cases the syllable is arrested in part by the chest and the vowel becomes tense. In calling or in singing, the prolonged syllables are always arrested in part by the chest, and an arresting consonant may become superfluous (88, p. 155).

On the other hand, it is always possible to shorten the "long" vowel wherever the rhythm

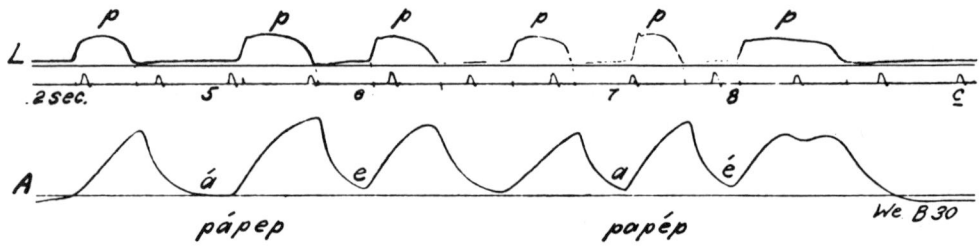

FIGURE 91. Stress causes Shortening of Long Vowel. No Lengthening of the Short Vowel

Syllables: *pa' pep, pa pep'*.
L—Lip marker. Spacing shows that syl. 5, *pa*, is long, while syl. 7 *pa* is short. But the spacing of syl. 6 and 8 show that -*pep* unstressed and stressed are of the same length as to vowel; the increased length of syl. 8 is obtained by prolonging the arresting *p*.
A—Air in mouth. Prolongation of arresting *p* in syl. 8 is apparent.

demands; in consequence we may find "long" vowels shorter than the "short" vowels. With a "short" vowel the elongation appears in the arresting consonant or in the intersyllabic interval. This is apparent in the series with changing rate with long and short vowels, and is exemplified in the study of the stressed groups which will be handled later. When the short syllable receives a heavy stress, there is a tendency to close the syllable with an arresting consonant; the heavy stroke runs into the releasing consonant stroke of the next syllable and so converts it into a double consonant. Since the syllable movement is arrested by this obstacle, the increase in force cannot lengthen the emitted pulse. Thus in the case of a closed syllable (i.e. with consonant arrest), increase of stress will not greatly lengthen the vowel; the coordination between the pulse of the consonant beat stroke and the arresting back stroke of the pulse is automatic (44, p. 311; 45, p. 258; Cf p. 127).

The increase of stress means that the moving member reaches the obstacle with a higher momentum. The contraction of the negative muscles, therefore will be correspondingly greater, and the back stroke of the arresting consonant will take a correspondingly longer interval. If the arresting consonant is a continuant, the consonant will be prolonged (Cf. Fig. 82). If the arresting consonant is an occlusive, the back stroke (or the equivalent relaxation phase) will take a correspondingly longer time. This will appear as a "pause" (intersyllabic interval) after the syllable. At the end of the group, the occlusion may be without détente (Cf. Figs. 91, 92, 94).

In the phrase "To be or not to be", Bell notes such a long pause, i.e. the relaxation phase of the vigorous "t" of the "not" (2, p. 78). It happens

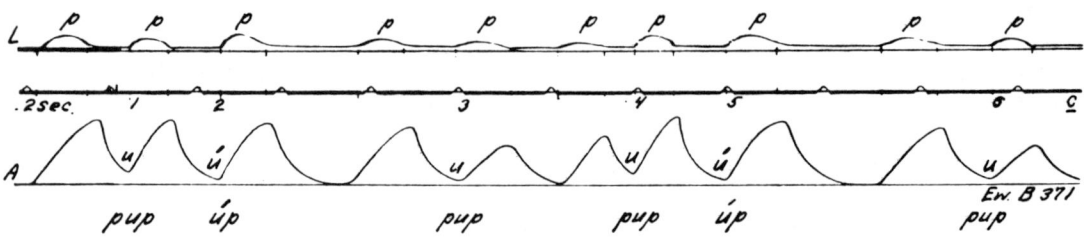

FIGURE 92. Separate Consonants in lieu of Double Consonants. Dynamic Culmination of the Group at the Stress

Syllables: *pup up' pup*.
L—Lip marker: *p* contacts are distinct throughout.
A—Air in mouth. Marked division between syl. 2 and 3 and between 5 and 6. No possibility of the doubling form.

in this example of Bell's that the long pause occurs in the midst of a double consonant.

The incorporation of a releasing consonant, the elongation of a "long" vowel in the open syllable, the incorporation of both a releasing and arresting consonant in the syllable with a short vowel, are all comparable to the agogic and apogogic stress of the musical note (65).

In music the stressed note is preceded by a slight pause and is slightly lengthened by the stress. In the case of the stressed note, additional time is required to prepare for the heavier stroke and additional time is required to take up the momentum of the stroke and prepare for the next stroke. In the case of the stressed syllable in speech, the preceding consonant is drawn in to assist in the preparation of the heavy stroke, and if the vowel is "short", the following consonant is drawn in to assist in the arrest of the heavy stroke. The increase of the interval just before the chest pulse of the stressed syllable makes the beginning of the stressed stroke always an available place for a consonant in rapid utterance. If the vowel of the stressed syllable is short the end of the stressed syllable is also an available place for a consonant. It is not so much that the consonant can be tolerated at the beginning of all stressed syllables, and at the close of stressed syllables with short vowels, but rather that they are needed in the releasing and arresting coordination of the syllable movement.

It is possible to offer an explanation of the influence of the double consonant on the preceding vowel, so patent in the study of Italian phonetics by Josselyn. When the consonant is doubled, the preceding vowel is closed. The first consonant of the double becomes the arresting consonant of the preceding syllable. The closed syllable with an arresting consonant is short in duration—that is the inevitable limitation of the syllable with unassisted consonant arrest. E. W. Scripture quotes Meyer's measurements of Wanger's records showing that a consonant is lengthened after a short vowel which is the reciprocal effect on the consonant; the arresting consonant is likely to be more vigorous than the releasing consonant and its occlusion is really part of the syllable (76).

Chapter VII

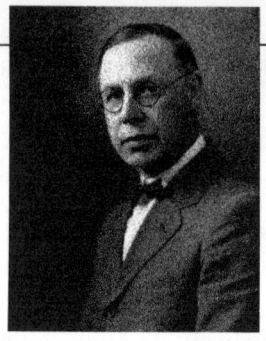

THE BREATH GROUP IN ENGLISH DEPENDENT ON THE STRESS PATTERN OF THE WORDS

The basis of the rhythmic organization of the "breath group" in English is the stress pattern of the words, although the word as such does not appear in the breath group. In some languages the word stress is fairly variable, and several accentual patterns are possible for the syllables of a given phrase. But in English there is little "déplacement de l'accent"; the rhythmic pattern is determined by the fixed word stresses. The rhythmic pattern is composed of feet; the etymological and grammatical connections of the words determine the grouping of the syllables about the stress in the foot. If every other syllable is stressed in the series the feet will consist of iambs and trochees, with transition made by an occasional one-syllable foot and by a compound form:

_ ⊥ / _ ⊥ / _ ⊥ _ / ⊥ _ / ⊥ _ / _ ⊥ / _ ⊥
iamb iamb iamb- trochee trochee single iamb iamb
           trochee

The third foot is a combination of the iamb and trochee, which is only a transitional form. (When repeated, this "amiphibrach" becomes a dactyl.) If every third syllable in the series is stressed, various combinations may appear:

⊥ _ _ / ⊥ _ _ / ⊥ _ _ / ⊥ _ / _ ⊥ / ⊥ _ _ / _ _ ⊥ / _ _ ⊥ _ _ / _ ⊥
dactyl dactyl trochee iamb anapest anapest- iamb
                                  trochee

_ _ ⊥ / _ _ ⊥ _ _ / ⊥ _ _ / ⊥
anapest- dactyl dactyl single (= dactyl catalectic)
dactyl

_ ⊥ _ / _ ⊥ _ _ / ⊥ _ _ / ⊥ _ _ / ⊥
iamb- iamb- dactyl dactyl single
trochee dactyl

Other more irregular patterns are presented of course by the word stress of ordinary speech. The choice of the grouping will depend on the syntax, and also on the presence of abutting consonants between the syllables. Doubling will tend to occur between the feet and neither doubles nor any other form of abutting consonants are likely to appear within the foot. A decided increase in rate may work further changes by eliminating certain unstressed syllables. Changes of that type will be considered later.

The larger groups, the breath groups, and often component feet are marked off by low points in the chest pressure. Every foot has its stress, and every breath group has a dynamic climax as its primary stress. The unity of the breath group is constituted by a slow movement of expiration of which the minor movements of feet and syllables form parts like the partials of a sound wave.

EXPERIMENTAL STUDY OF GROUPS OF SYLLABLES

The Group of Two Syllables

Rousselot has made observations on the group of two syllables (68). There are several possible groupings of two syllables in a breath group:

1. The iamb, $\_\,\bot$.
2. The trochee, $\bot\,\_$.
3. The separation into two one-syllable feet, $\bot\,/\,\bot$.

Types 1 and 2 occur when there is a single consonant between the syllables, and the stress is not heavy. Type 3 occurs if there is an abutting pair of median consonants.

In case the first syllable is heavily stressed, there are several possibilities:

1. A single median consonant is doubled, and type 3, $\bot\,/\,\bot$, occurs.
2. The median consonant (a) vocalizes, (b) reduces, (c) drops.

This occurs when the first syllable is heavily stressed and the group is uttered at rapid rate.

DISCUSSION OF THE IAMBIC GROUP

The average length of 234 iambs was 0.56 sec. (range 0.41–0.67 sec.). The stressed syllable is usually longer than the unstressed. The stressed syllable occupied ca. 60 per cent of the total duration (range 55–73 per cent).

If the rate is normal, median abutting pairs become single releasing consonants. It happens, however, that the resulting single consonant is often a hybrid form in which partial vocalization appears if the arresting doublet is a sonant and the releasing doublet a surd. If the abutting consonants are retained, a breath group consisting of two single stressed syllables, $\bot$ x $\bot$, develops, and the rate is slowed. The grouping is no longer that of an iamb; it has become a breath group of two one-syllable feet (Cf. Figs. 93, 95).

No cases were observed of "adventitious doubling" of the single median consonant in a two-syllable group with the stress on the second syllable; there is no tendency of such a group to divide under heavy stress into two single, stressed syllables.

The elimination of a syllable does not occur in the case of an isolated iamb, no matter how rapid the rate of utterance, nor how emphatic the stress. In larger groups, phrases, the median iamb is subject to reduction; the short unaccented syllable tends to "telescope", leaving the releasing consonant of the syllable in some cases. This abbreviation is evidently the result of vis a tergo; if there is material preceding the unstressed syllable, it is first compressed and then forced out. We shall consider the cases of "telescoping" and of elimination of the unstressed syllable of the median iamb as we come to them in breath groups of three and four syllables.

DISCUSSION OF THE TROCHAIC GROUP

The average length of 207 trochees was 0.61 sec. (range 0.37–0.81). The two syllables, stressed and unstressed, are usually of about the same duration. The stressed syllable occupied an average

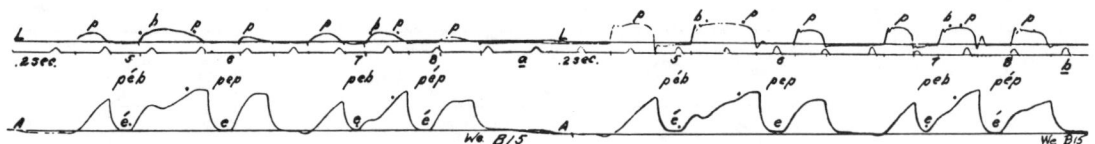

FIGURE 93 a and b. Doubling Form Marking the Division of Breath Group into two one-syllable Feet
Syllables: *peb'pep, peb pep*.
L—Lip marker. Abutting pair shows, a, b, syl. 5-6; the single consonant in the iambic foot is just as marked, a, b, syl. 7-8. Form *peb'pep* is given as two one-syllable feet with a double at the division.
A—Air in mouth. Doubling form well marked, a, b, syl. 5-6.

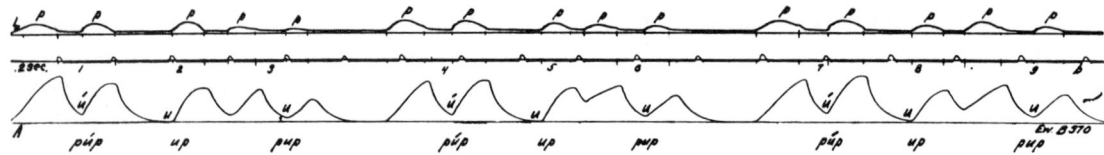

FIGURE 94. Separate Consonants in lieu of Double Consonants. Dynamic Culmination of the Group at the Stress
Syllables: *pup'up pup.*
L—Lip marker. *p* contacts are distinct throughout.
A—Air in mouth. Syl. 2-3 shows that the two syllables are separate; 8-9 and 5-6 represent stages in the development of a double; the rate is not quite rapid enough to complete doubling.

of about 50 per cent of the total duration (range 41–59 per cent). The fact that the unstressed syllable is the last syllable tends to prolong the trochee; this is more apparent in final trochees in larger groupings, but it has some influence in isolated trochees. A heavy stress on the trochee tends to lengthen the stressed syllable. Both these tendencies have been noted by Rousselot.

It is interesting to note that the average length of the isolated trochee is slightly longer than that of the isolated iamb. In larger groupings, of which trochees and iambs are constituents, no such difference in the average length is apparent.

If the rate is normal, abutting median consonants reduce to single or compound consonants. In this the reduction is somewhat like that of the iamb. One may say in general that all abutting consonants between the constituent syllables of a foot are reduced to single or compound consonants, and in every case it is the releasing consonant which persists. Cf. the series in which the consonants double with increasing rate. The rate of the elements in the foot is responsible for the elimination of the arresting consonant of a median abutting pair.

REDUCTION AND ELIMINATION OF THE MEDIAN CONSONANT OF THE TROCHEE

The iamb which stands alone is not subject to modifications which abbreviate the syllables, but this is not the case with the trochee. If the trochee it uttered very quickly, or if a heavy stress is put on the first syllable, internal modifications occur.

The median consonant of the trochee, the releasing consonant of the unstressed syllable, is 1) "reduced", 2) vocalized if a surd, 3) finally eliminated. The "reduction" means that the contact of the consonant becomes much briefer and the stroke to the opposing surface much lighter, and the pressure in the mouth for the consonant becomes much less. Much the same thing is to be seen in all series of syllables at very rapid rate. A heavy stress on the trochee increases the rate of the unstressed syllable, for it leaves less time for the unstressed syllable.

At the same time, the consonant becomes a sonant if it is a surd. It has been assumed that an inter-vocalic consonant is vocalized because that means less effort (10). But the fact is that

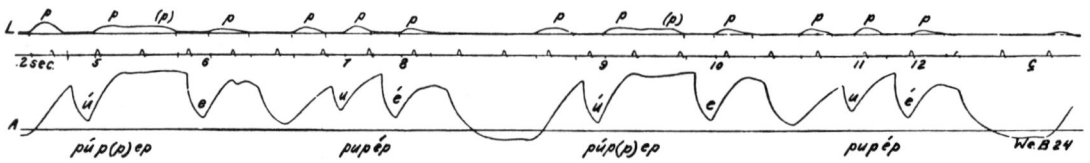

FIGURE 95. Stressed Group, Introduction of an Adventitious Double
Syllables: *Pu'pep, pu pep'pu'* becomes two one-syllable feet.
L—Lip marker. Doubles at syl. 5-6 and 9-10 are well defined.
A—Air in mouth. Doubling forms between feet are apparent, syl. 5-6, 9-10.

the vocalization is inevitable; the consonant occlusion grows less and less, and breaks the flow of air through the glottis for a shorter interval. It is not a sudden process as Fig. 96 shows. It is easy to see that the vibration of the vowel creeps into the occlusion and finally runs quite through it; the closure of the consonant becomes so brief that it does not interrupt the flow of air through the vocal folds.

When the contact has become so brief, there is little rise of the mouth pressure, the consonant functions almost not at all and the syllable movement becomes practically chest released. Since the median consonant stroke no longer functions it may disappear entirely, as a consonant stroke is certain to do if it has no part to play in the syllable movement. The median consonant of the trochee has dropped. The two vowels tend to fuse and a single syllable with a modified vowel results.

If the vowel of the unstressed syllable is extremely short, and if the trochaic median is sonant, especially if it is a continuant, the median consonant stroke may fuse with a final consonant, while the second syllable movement fuses with the stressed chest pulse. Thus *"debit"* if heavily stressed and rapidly uttered becomes *"deb't"*, which soon loses its internal consonant and becomes *"de't"*. *"Tes'et"* becomes *"tes't"*, which persists because the two arresting consonants fuse to a compound consonant, *"st"*. Some 50 cases occur in a total of 207 trochees studied.

Sometimes the reverse process takes place, and a syllable like *"elm"* or *"help"* opens into a trochee and becomes *"elum, helup"*—as often in dialectic English.

The causes of this reduction, vocalization, and elimination of the trochaic median consonant are to be found in the rate at which the unstressed syllable is uttered. If the first syllable is heavily stressed, the arrest must occur before the release of the unstressed syllable is possible. The releasing consonant has to occur in the very brief syllable at such a rate that the blow is very swift and therefore very light. If the unstressed syllable is not closed, the reduction process does not occur as readily.

If the subject takes the opposite way out, giving time to pronounce both syllables adequately, in spite of the heavy stress, the result is two feet, each of one syllable; and the breath group becomes ⊥ x ⊥ . In this case the abutting consonants persist if present; and a single consonant

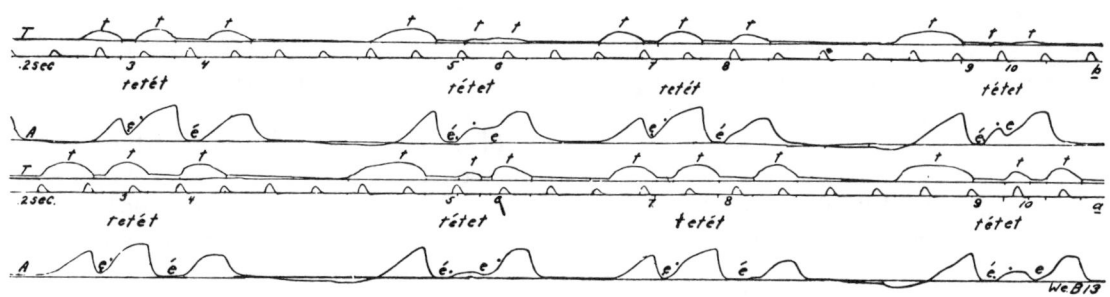

FIGURE 96. Reduction of the Median Consonant of the Trochee. Iambs for Comparison
Syllables: te'tet, te tet'.

T—Tongue marker. In iambic feet, introduced for comparison, the median consonant is of the same intensity as the other; though it may be slightly shorter. The trochaic feet, *a*, syl. 9-10, shows a well marked median consonant, though it is rather lighter than the intitial final consonants. Others show various stages of reduction and syl. 9-10 shows barely visible contact. In *b*, syl. 5-6, the median consonant of the trochee has fused with the final.

A—Air in mouth. In all cases the pressure for the trochaic median is decidely reduced. In all cases the median consonant is more or less vocalized; the contact becomes so brief that there is no stasis in the air flow. This is a common stage in the "reduction" of the trochaic median consonant.

A dot just above the tracing indicates the beginning of end of vibration.

is likely to be doubled (Cf. Figs 93, 95). It is much easier to terminate the heavily stressed syllable with an arresting consonant, therefore the consonant is shifted to the arresting position; this would involve at best a "pause", if the second, the unstressed syllable, is to be chest-released. It seems easier to repeat the consonant, and the result is the "adventitious double". Adventitious doubling is much more likely to occur if the preceding vowel is short. A heavy stress, then, may cause the prolongation of a "long" vowel; but a short vowel with a heavy stress demands an arresting consonant.

The peculiarities of the "long" and "short" vowels are well demonstrated in forms like "*totet*" in which the stress is thrown alternately on the first and second syllables, forming a series of alternating trochees and iambs, "*to'tet, to tet*'; *po'pop, po pop*'; *debit, debate*". In such cases the "long" vowel shortens when unstressed; but the "short" vowel does not lengthen when stressed. Instead, the short vowel is followed by a double or an arresting consonant which gives the syllable its rhythmic length (Cf. Fig. 91).

The simple grouping, the re-grouping, and the actual position and function of the abutting consonant pair (including the double), is remarkably well shown in these two-syllable breath groups. The trochee illustrates the process of dropping the trochaic median consonant, and also of dropping a syllable by fusion. And the trochee furnishes the first illustration of the "adventitious double" marking the division of the breath group into two one-syllable feet.

RELATIVE DURATION OF THE IAMB AND THE TROCHEE

The iambs and the trochees are of much the same average length; at maximum rate the trochee can be shorter than the iamb. The average of these two-syllable groups, .56–.61 sec., is much higher than the average length of the one-syllable feet into which the two-syllable breath group is divided on occasion. The average length of 717 one-syllable feet, when initial, was 0.26 sec. (range 0.18–0.50 sec.). The average length of the 657 one-syllable feet, when final, was 0.31 sec. (range 0.20–0.44 sec.). While the average length of the one-syllable feet overlaps the shorter of the iambs and trochees (Cf. ranges pp. 131–132) it is easy to see that the distribution is quite distinct. But it is to be remembered that temporal equality is not to be expected of spoken rhythms. Minimum time intervals for movements are important because they condition the form of the movement and may compel profound phonetic changes. But the wide variation in time intervals longer than the minimum has no particular rhythmic significance.

Breath Groups of Three Syllables

There are a number of feet which may appear in the three-syllable breath group:

1. ⊥ / ⊥ __   2. ⊥ ⊥ / ⊥   3. ⊥ / ⊥ / ⊥
   sing. trochee   sing. iamb   sing. sing. sing.
4. ⊥ __ / ⊥   5. __ ⊥ / ⊥   6. ⊥ __ __
   trochee sing.   iamb sing.   dactyl
7. __ __ ⊥   8. __ ⊥ __
   anapest   "amphibrach"

Of these breath groups, 1, 2, 4, 5, have each two feet, they are varying combinations of iamb or trochee with a one-syllable foot; 3 consists of three one-syllable feet; 6 is a dactyl; 8 is a similar form with the stress on the median syllable. Group 8 is a form which occurs only in isolation; a series of such amphibrachs would reorganize into the dactylic form 6. If all the syllables involved were closed syllables, the feet would be indicated by the doubling and singling of the consonants.

In breath groups of three syllables, certain characteristics due to the length of the group are apparent. The initial one-syllable foot of such a breath group is shorter than the final one-syllable foot. There is a tendency to prolong the final element of such a breath group; and as the expiratory movement of the breath group has rather definite limits, the earlier members of a breath group tend to become shorter and shorter as the breath group increases in length. This appears in the case of the iamb and the dactyl. The initial iamb or dactyl of a breath group is shorter than the final iamb or dactyl.

The pronounced tendency to prolong the last syllable of a series is apparent in these three-syllable breath groups, and is often the factor which determines the grouping. If the series is continuous, $\perp \_ \perp / \perp \_ \_$ etc., the dactyl may be preserved. But a group of three syllables, with the stress on the first syllable, is likely to drop into the form $\perp / \_ \perp$ or the form $\perp \_/ \perp$. And the prolongation of the last syllable is likely to give the three-syllable breath group, with stress on the median syllable, the form $\_ \perp / \perp$ rather than either $\_ \_ \perp$ or $\perp / \perp \_$.

The presence of doubling consonants and of long vowels will be determining factors in the breath-group organization. Thus "*ex'quisite*" = $\perp$ x $\_ \perp$; but "*exquisite thing*" = $\_$x$\perp\_$x$\perp$. With a pronouncedly short vowel in the final syllable, "*harmony*" has the characteristic dactylic form; but "*harmonize*" becomes $\perp \_ / \perp$.

In the three-syllable breath group, both the iambic and the trochaic unstressed syllable may be elided as the rate is increased. The iamb has a pronounced difference in the length of the two syllables, and if it occurs in succession at rapid rate, the rate may be too fast for the occurrence of the short syllable. If the original form gives an arresting consonant to the unstressed syllable, this will drop early, of course, leaving the unstressed syllable with releasing consonant only. At a higher rate the unstressed syllable stroke is fused with the following stressed chest pulse, but the releasing consonant may persist by shifting to the arresting position in the preceding syllable (Cf. Figs. 97, 98, 99). Thus "*beautiful*" becomes "*beaut'ful*"; "*business*" has become "*bus'ness*"; "*plentiful*" becomes "*plent'ful*"; "*laboratory*" becomes "*lab'ratory*".

In case the syllable preceding the eliding syllable of the iamb already has an arresting consonant, the releasing consonant of the syllable becomes functionless; it must either fuse with the releasing consonant of the stressed syllable or drop. In a form like "*institute*" becoming "*in'stute*", the median consonant of "*nst*" fuses with the releasing "*t*" (Cf. Fig. 99). In "*hospital*" becoming "*hostel*" the "*p*" does not fuse with the following "*t*" and therefore the "*p*" drops; so the "*b*" in "*presbyte*r" becoming "*pres'ter*" (Cf. Fig. 77). In "*abdicate*" becoming "*ab'cate*" the "*d*" drops, although the "*b*" and "*c*" are not formed by the same member.

It is worth noting that in these cases, with a continuant like "*s*", an intersyllabic sound does not develop. In the form "*instate*", if one attempts to prolong the syllables, one finds that the "*in*" can be prolonged by continuing the "*n*", but the "*st*" is given very briefly as the releasing consonant of "*state*". Such a prolongation of a syllable often occupies the time of the elided syllable, but it is not an equivalent, in the phonetic sense that the continued sound *becomes* a syllable. Instead the fact is that something like the same length is maintained for the rhythmic foot. This is the explanation of "*epenthèse*", discussed by Rousselot (70, p. 989). The transitional "sound" which develops as "*teneru*" becomes "*tendre*" is not the equivalent of the syllable. Actually, the releasing consonant has become "*dr-*" and the

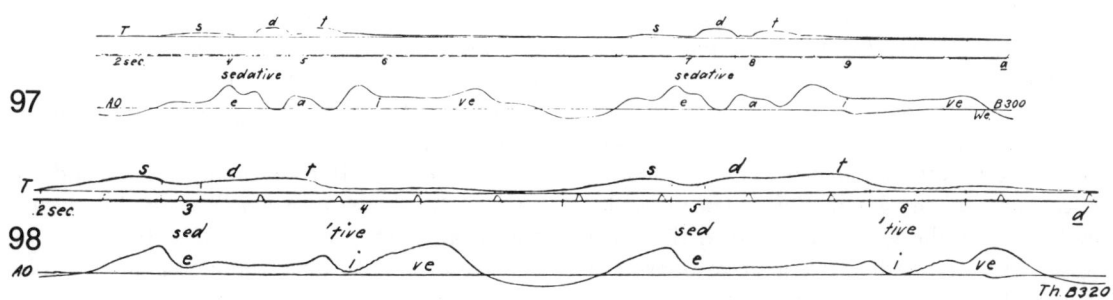

FIGURE 97 and 98. Telescoping of the Iamb

Syllables: *sedative*, slow careful utterance, $\perp / \_ \_$.
   T—Tongue marker. S, d, t are clearly marked; the s shows the lighter pressure and longer contact.
   AO—Air outside. Three distinct syllables with releasing consonants in Fig. 97 reduced to two syllables in Fig. 98; the length of syllables indicates breath group $\perp / \_ \_$. The longer syllable, *se-*, shows the mid-sag. The *-ive* is well marked in the outside pressure.

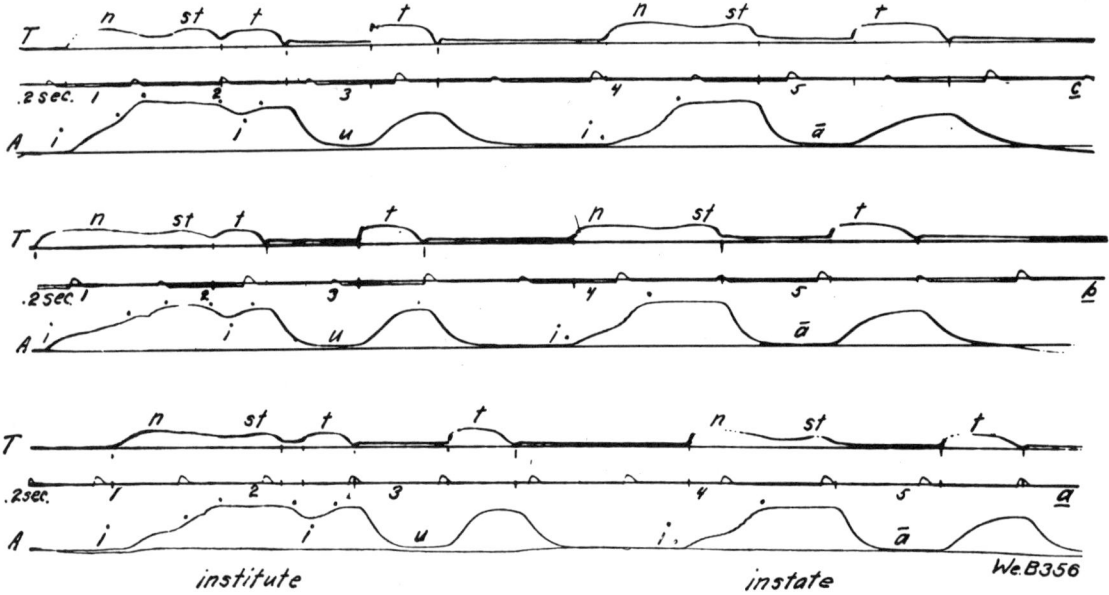

FIGURE 99. Abutting Consonants in which one of the Members is a Compound Consonant

Syllables: *institute, instate.* Cf. Figs. 97, 98.

T—Tongue marker. Doubling forms clearly marked. Form with heavy stress on the first syllable, *institute*, has a decidedly longer double than the form *instate*. Form of the abutting pair *n − st + t* shows that there is a decided tendency to iambic telescoping; the word tends to become *inst'ute*; it is sometimes so uttered.

A—Air in mouth. Doubling form marked, syl. 1-2, 4-5 throughout. The pressure on the *n* is very slight. In every case there is little drop of pressure for the *i* of syl. 2, though the vibration of the vowel is to be seen. The tendency to telescope, eliminating the iambic unstressed syllable, is apparent.

A dot just above the tracing indicates the beginning or end of vibration.

---

increased length means that the two syllables represent the same rhythmic foot that the three syllables did before.

Rousselot suggests the steps whereby *"cabitale"* (*capitale*) becomes *"ca-b-tal"* with *"b"* explosive; then *"cab-tal"*, *"b"* implosive; then *"capital"*, *"b"* surdifies, then *"cha'tel"* with the implosion still apparent and finally *"chetel"* in which the implosion has disappeared (70, p. 977). The analysis is good, save that the function of the consonant has not been noted; there can be no "explosive" (releasing) function for the *"b"* when the syllable *"-tal"* has the releasing *"t"*. And the same causes which force the arresting consonant out of the syllable *"cha-"* must prevent the formation of a hiatus at the close of the syllable; were there room for the hiatus there would be room for the arresting consonant. The problem of a single releasing (explosive) consonant functioning as a syllable is treated below. The steps would be:

"cabitale (capitale), cab-tal, chatal, chetel".

The surd between two vowels often becomes a sonant, as noted in the example cited by Rousselot above. This is the usual transformation of the trochaic median which has previously been discussed (Cf. Fig. 96).

Rousselot assumes that in the case of a syllable with *"e muet"*, the consonant alone may sometimes figure as the syllable when the *"e muet"* drops; *"la femm' se l'va"* shows the elision of the *"e muet"* after *"m"* and after *"l"*, and yet the syllable *"fe-"* of *"femme"* is not closed, nor the syllable *"se"* preceding *"l'va"* (70, p. 981). In such cases it is of course impossible that the consonant alone become a syllable; a chest pulse is essential to a syllable. But it is possible for the compound releasing consonants *"mse"* and *"lva"* to develop as the releasing consonant of each syllable, and the lengths of the rhythmic feet are adjusted as suggested above.

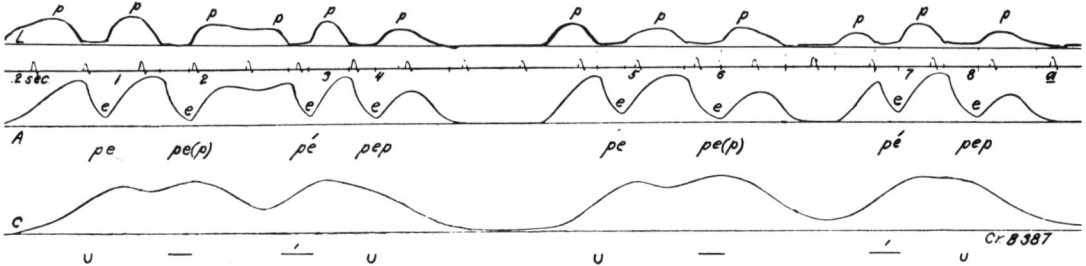

FIGURE 100. Adventitious Double between Feet before the Stress; Chest Pulses recorded directly from Trachea
Syllables: *pe pe pe'pep* uttered *pe pe(p)pe'pep.*
L—Lip marker. The doubling forms are obvious, except syl. 6-7 in which the adventitious arresting consonant is separated from the releasing consonant following.
A—Air in mouth. All doubling forms are obvious except syl. 6-7 where there are separate pressure forms for the arresting and releasing consonants which have not doubled.
C—Chest pulses from trachea. Division between the feet is marked, and also dynamic variations due to the stress. The feet and the breath groups are clearly indicated in these tracings; the chest pressure drops to zero only between breath groups. (This is common in all recordings of the sort.)

The Breath Group of Four Syllables

The group of four syllables presents a wide variety of combinations of the feet. The dactyl may be preceded or followed by one-syllable foot, the iamb or the trochee may appear in various successions with one-syllable feet, and trochees and iambs may occur together as initial or final. Combinations of trochees or iambs with dactyls are the only groupings which are not represented in the four-syllable breath group; and they would give no new arrangements of stressed and unstressed syllables, or of combinations of syllables with single consonants and with abutting pairs (including doubles). All possible modifications of the syllables are to be found in these four syllable breath groups.

The tendency to prolong the final feet of a breath group appears on comparing the trochees and iambs:

Initial	trochees	.48 sec.	370 cases
"	iambs	.48 sec.	225 cases
"	one-syllable	.28 sec.	717 cases
Final	trochees	.61 sec.	207 cases
"	iambs	.58 sec.	102 cases
"	one-syllable	.31 sec.	657 cases

These four-syllable successions develop series of feet between which abutting pairs are given full value, or between which adventitious doubles appear.

The adventitious double develops in the four-syllable breath group as it does in the three-syllable breath group. It usually occurs just *after* a heavy stress, but it may also ocur just *before* a heavy stress. If the vowel of the preceding syllable is "short", the pause during which the heavy stress is prepared may be occupied by a double. The alternative would be a hiatus after the chest-arrest of the short vowel. In 130 four-syllable breath groups, four subjects, adventitious doubles occur in 47 cases.

The Elision of Syllables, Modification and Contraction in Four-Syllable Breath Groups

The four-syllable breath groups offer a good field for the study of the tendency to drop syllables. There are two processes by which the four-syllable breath group is reduced to three syllables, reduction of the trochee and the telescoping of the iamb (Cf. Figs. 100, 101, 102, 103).

Since the adventitious doubles appear before and after the stress for reasons given above, and since the fusion of the syllables of the trochee must involve the stressed syllable, and since the telescoping of the iamb occurs just before the stress, it is easy to formulate a general rule that the various modifications of the consonants and syllables will appear just before and just after the

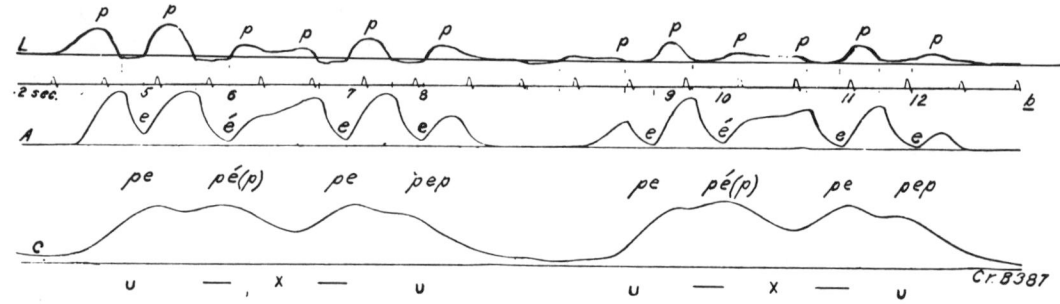

FIGURE 101. Adventitious Double after the Stress; Chest Pulses recorded directly from Trachea
Syllables: *pe pe'pe pep* uttered *pe, pe(p) pe pep*.
L—Lip marker. All doubling obvious.
A—Air in mouth. All doubling obvious.
C—Chest pulses from trachea. Division between feet is marked. Feet and breath groups are clearly indicated in these tracings.

stressed syllable. As the stresses may be in several patterns, this means that adventitious doubling, persistence of abutting consonants, telescoping, and fusion may appear between syllables 1 and 2, between 2 and 3, and between 3 and 4. It is only the initial and final syllables and consonants which are not affected.

Here, as elsewhere, abutting consonants, long or short vowels, long with the prescribed stresses, determine the precise series of feet developed within the four-syllable breath group.

It is convenient to schematize the changes in both consonants and syllables which occur in a series of syllables grouped in various types of feet, when the rate is increased. It is easy to see that in the case of the trochaic series, and of the iambic series, that all arresting consonants finally drop with the increase of rate; and that the releasing consonants of unstressed syllables drop also. The unstressed syllables invariably drop with the increase of rate. The stressed syllables and their releasing consonants persist, whatever the rate (Cf. Figs. 104, 105, 106).

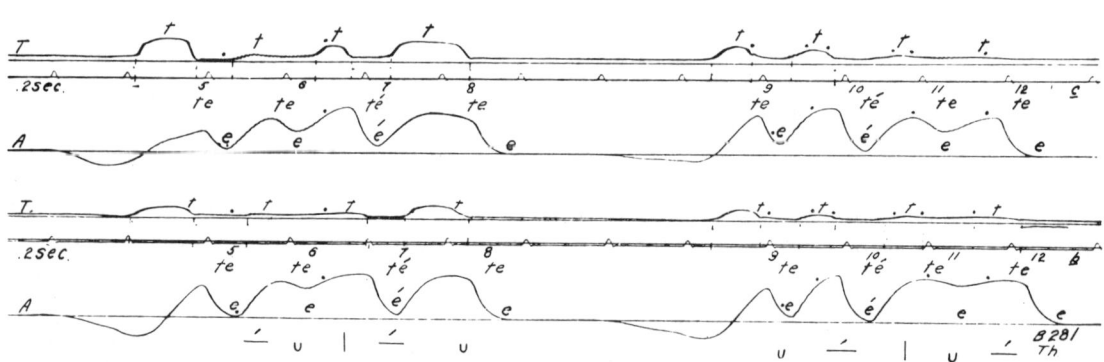

FIGURE 102. Stressed Group. Iambic Telescoping, Trochaic Reduction
Syllables: *te te te'te, te te'te te*.
T—Tongue marker. Although the *t* of the iambic short syllable, *b, c,* wyl. 11 is doubling with the *t* of syl. 12, they are of the same force. But the *t* of the trochaic short syllable, *b, c,* syl. 6, is less in force than either the *t* of syl. 5 or 7. Vocalization is apparent throughout the trochaic median consonant.
A—Air in mouth. Pressure of the arresting consonant in the iambic telescoping is as high as that of the releasing consonant, *b, c,* syl. 6-7. Vocalization is apparent throughout the trochaic median consonant.
A dot just above the tracing indicates the beginning or end of vibration.

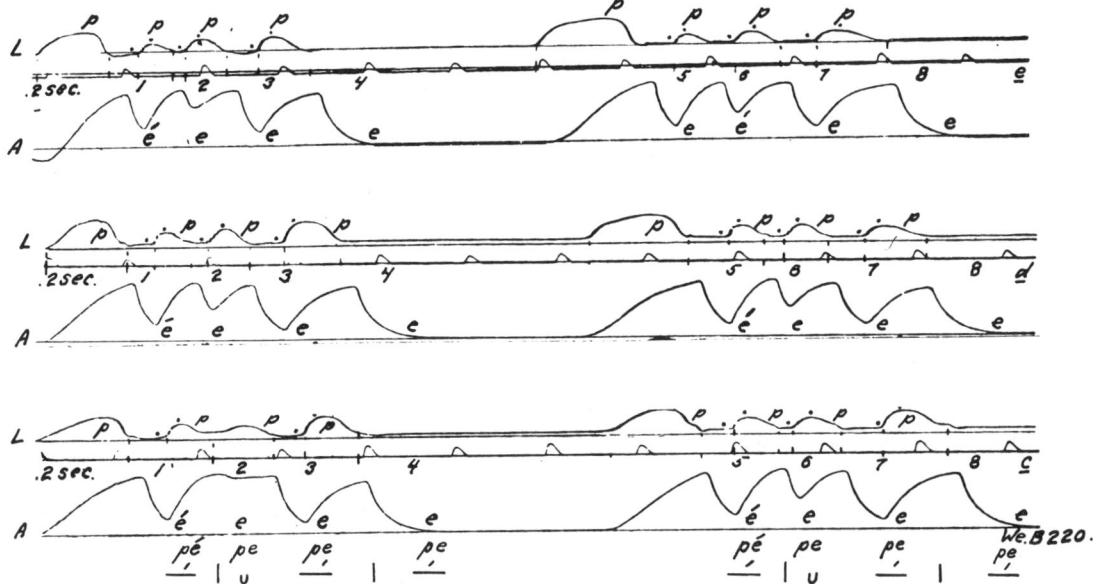

FIGURE 103. Iambic Telescoping. Stressed Group

Syllables: pe'pe pe pe.
L—Lip marker. c, d, e, syl. 1-2-3, happen to form a series in which the stages of telescoping appear; in e the p's are distinct; in d they are adjacent though the vibration shows that the vowel still sounds; in c the true doubling form appears; the vowel is not longer heard.
A—Air in mouth. In d and e, syl. 1-2-3, the pressure indicates the tendency to eliminate the syllable, but a complete double is not present. In c the doubling form appears; the unstressed syllable has been eliminated and only the consonant remains which has become the arresting consonant of the preceding syllable.

A dot just above the tracing indicates the beginning or end of vibration.

Comparison of the Abutting and Single Consonants of Stressed Breath Groups with the Abutting and Single Consonants of Series Developed by Increasing the Rate

Distribution curves of the consonant lengths make it possible to compare the lengths of doubling and singling consonants when produced by increasing the rate in artificial series, and when produced in the course of uttering the various stressed groups discussed. In Fig. 107 the curves I and J represent the distribution of the lengths of double and abutting consonants in the various stressed groups studied; they show that the double and the abutting pair are one and the same thing. The limits of distribution of the double and the abutting pair and the mode of the distributions of the measurements of duration are practically the same.

In Fig. 108, curve K represents the distribution of the lengths of all the doubles and abutting pairs recorded in 3101 cases. Curve M represents the distribution of the lengths of the doubles and abutting pairs in stressed groups recorded in a series of 705 cases. It is apparent that the distributions are practically identical, and that the process of doubling in the stressed group is precisely the process in the artificial series of syllables with changing rate. The curve L represents the distribution of 231 cases of arresting consonants. They are added to show that while the process of arrest with pause is nearly the same, there is a slight difference; the arrests with pause are slightly longer than the actual doubles or abutting pairs.

The rates of utterance in stressed groups, and of syllables in series with changing rate, show much the same common form; so do the consonant lengths just discussed. In Fig. 109, the curves A, B, are composed of d, e, 506 series, and of

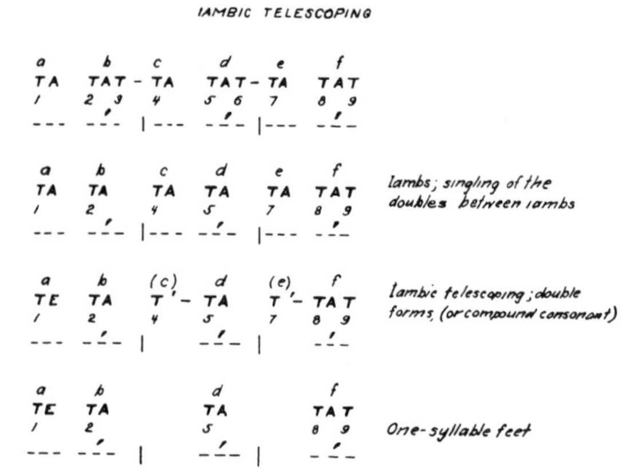

```
            IAMBIC TELESCOPING
  a    b    c    d    e    f
  TA   TAT- TA   TAT- TA   TAT
  1    2 3  4    5 6  7    8 9
  ---  --'- |--- --'- |--- --'-

  a    b    c    d    e    f
  TA   TA   TA   TA   TA   TAT       Iambs; singling of the
  1    2    3    4    5    6 7       doubles between iambs
  ---  --'- |--- --'- |--- --'-

  a    b   (c)   d   (e)   f
  TE   TA  T'-   TA  T'-   TAT       Iambic telescoping; double
  1    2    4    5    7    8 9       forms, (or compound consonant)
  ---  --'- |    --'- |    --'-

  a    b         d         f
  TE   TA        TA        TAT
  1    2         5         8 9       One-syllable feet
  ---  --'- |    --'- |    --'-
```

FIGURE 104. Iambic Telescoping, Diagrammatic Form

Syllables: *ta tat'-ta tat'-ta tat'* becoming *te ta'ta'tat'*.

Stages of elision in a series of the iambs as the rate is increased.

In the second line the doubles between the feet have disappeared.

In the third line the syllables *c* and *e* have telescoped, i.e. only double consonants remain, arresting the syllable *d* and releasing the syllable *f*. Introductory syllable is not affected.

In the fourth line the rate has eliminated the arresting consonant of the doubles, and only the syllables *a*, *b*, *d*, *g*, remain; *b* and *d* have become open syllables. Introductory syllable is not affected save that the vowel is reduced.

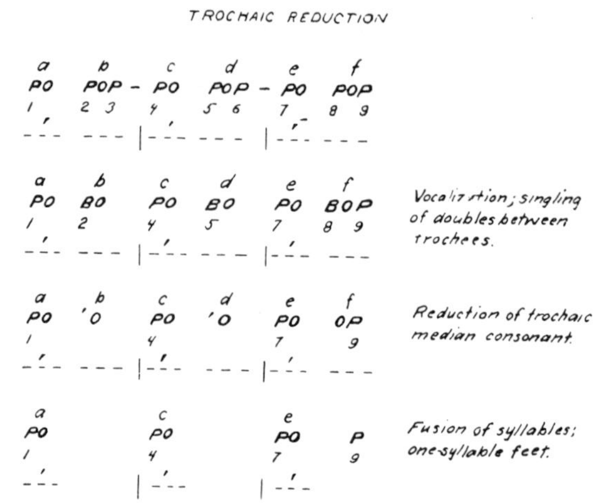

```
            TROCHAIC REDUCTION
  a    b    c    d    e    f
  PO   POP- PO   POP- PO   POP
  1    2 3  4    5 6  7    8 9
  ---  --- |--- --- |--- --'-

  a    b    c    d    e    f
  PO   BO   PO   BO   PO   BOP      Vocalization; singling
  1    2    4    5    7    8 9      of doubles between
  ---  ---  |--- ---  |--- ---      trochees.

  a    b    c    d    e    f
  PO   'O   PO   'O   PO   OP       Reduction of trochaic
  1    4    4    7    7    9        median consonant
  --'- --- |--'- --- |--'- ---

  a         c         e    
  PO        PO        PO   P         Fusion of syllables;
  1         4         7    9         one-syllable feet.
  --'-     |--'-     |--'-
```

FIGURE 105. Trochaic Reduction, Diagrammatic Form

Syllables: *po'pop- po'pop- po'pop'* becoming *po'po'pop'*.

Stages as the rate is increased of the elision of the unstressed syllable from the trochee, in a series of three trochees.

In the second line the doubles between the feet have disappeared; the median consonants, which become very brief, are vocalized if originally surd.

In the third line, the median consonant has been eliminated but the syllables remain.

In the fourth line the syllables have fused and a series of one-syllable feet remain.

---

f, g, 424 series, thrown together from Fig. 51. C represents the distribution of 96 cases in which a prescribed double in a stressed group has been uttered as a single consonant (due to the influence of the grouping of the syllables). The syllable lengths have been reduced to rates. It is apparent that the distribution is practically the same, i.e. the single consonant which appears in place of a double in a stressed group is as near to the doubling rate as possible, and therefore is very like the single consonant which appears just after doubling in the series at increasing rate.

Fig. 110 shows the curves A, B, which summarize the distributions of rates of syllables determined in "series at increasing rate"; curve *a*, which gives the distribution of the rates of syllables in stressed groups which have double or abutting consonants; and curve *b*, which gives the distribution of the rates of syllables in which a single consonant was prescribed. The distribution of the rates of syllables with doubles and abutting pairs in the stressed groups coincides with the distribution of the rates of syllables in the series with increasing rate. But the syllables with a single consonant, which does not take the place of a prescribed double, but which is single according to prescription, are decidedly faster than the syllables with a single consonant which represents a double. The distribution is symmetrical and represents a normal distribution between the limits of the rates of syllables with a single consonant, from 3–7.5 syllables per sec. There is no tendency to keep as close as possible to the rate of doubling.

These comparisons of the lengths of the doubles and abutting pairs, and of the rates of syllables with double consonants and abutting pairs, show that on the one hand, the rate of utterance will determine the form as "doubling" or "singling". On the other hand, the prescribed form of "doubling" or "singling" in stressed groups of syllables will determine the rate of utterance of the syllable in question. The form

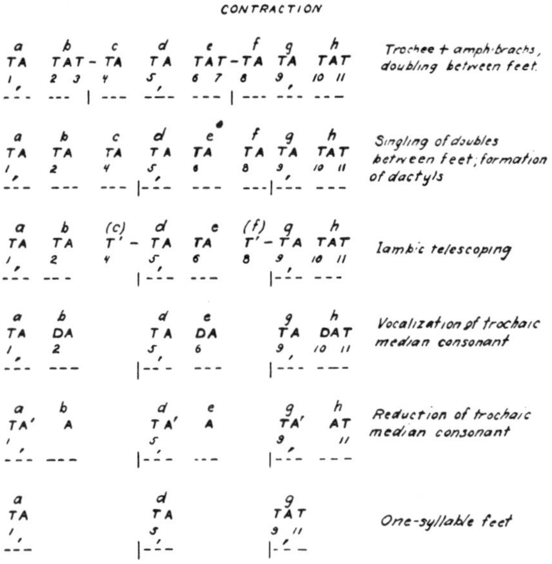

FIGURE 106. Contraction by both Iambic Telescoping and Trochaic Reduction. Diagrammatic Form
Syllables: ta'tat- ta ta' tat- ta ta'tat.

Changes as the rate is increased from amphibrach to dactyl; iambic telescoping; trochaic reduction.

The second line shows the singling of the doubles and the formation of the dactyls.

The third line shows the iambic telescoping which reduces the dactyls to trochees.

The fourth line shows the vocalization of the reducing trochaic median consonants.

The fifth line shows the trochaic median consonant eliminated.

The sixth line shows the entire series reduced to three one-syllable feet.

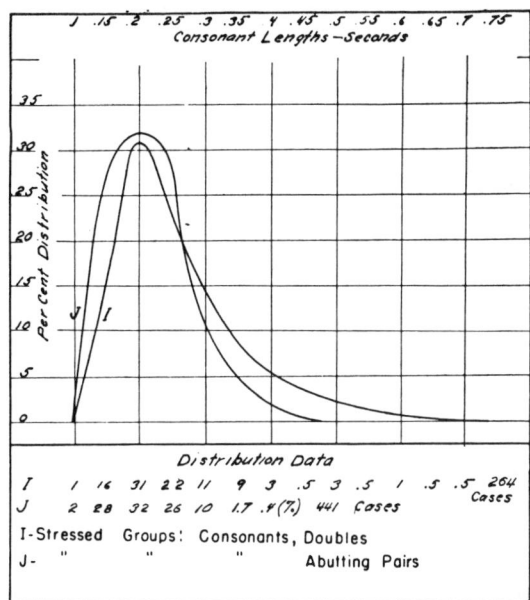

FIGURE 107. Distribution of the Lengths of Abutting Pairs, including Doubles, as they appear in Stressed Groups of Syllables
The distributions prove to be practically identical.

of doubling or singling and the appropriate rate of utterance go together.

Reversion to the Prescribed Form when the Rate and the Rhythm Permit

The tendency to restoration, to reversion, after a phonetic modification, plays a part in breath groups of syllables with a stress (arranged in rhythmic feet) just as it does in series in which the rate changes (Cf. p. 95). The prescribed consonants and syllables may be profoundly modified by the rhythm and the consequent rates; but the original form is still with the subject, and appears whenever the conditions will permit. Therefore stem forms remain through the varying modifications which result from the addition of suffixes and the shift of the stress. In forms like "*sled*", the "*d*" is arresting; in "*sled-ding*" an adventitious double might appear as the spelling indicates, but this is very seldom the case; instead, the arresting "*d*" becomes the releasing consonant of the next syllable, and the syllables are really "*sle-ding*".

In forms like "*adverti'sing*", and "*adver'tisement*", the "*s*" reverts from the releasing to the arresting position when the abutting pair "*s-m*" is produced by adding the "*-ment*". Shifting the stress often changes the division of the syllables, and often leads to the elision of syllables. The American pronunciation "*lab'oratory*" ($\perp$ / $\_\_$ $\perp$ / $\perp$ $\_$) leads to the dropping out of the short of the iamb, leaving "*lab'ratory*", with an abutting "*b-r*". The British pronunciation "*labora tory*" ($\_\perp\perp$ / $\_\_\_$) tends to the dropping of the short syllable of the iamb, "*labor'at'ry*", and finally to reduction of the trochaic median, leaving "*labor't'ry*", three syllables.

Breath Groups of More Than Four Syllables

It is possible to get an unbroken series of five syllables; the phrase "*runnin' 'n' neighin'*" may be given in a single series, as in Fig. 111. And of

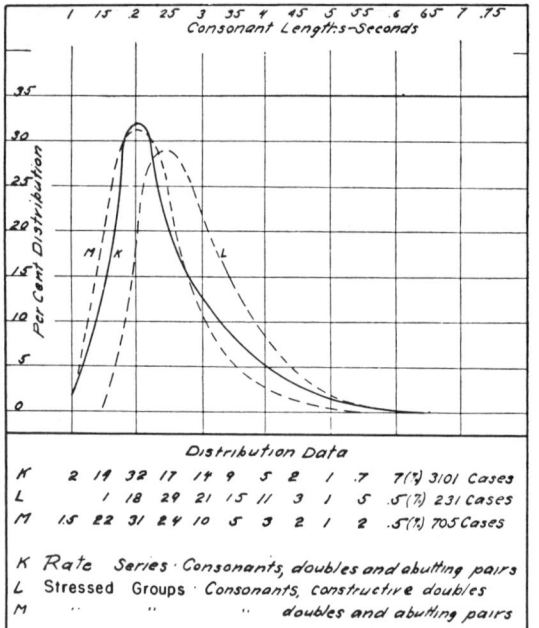

FIGURE 108. Distribution of 1) Lengths of Doubles and Abutting Pairs, and 2) Arresting Consonants with Pause as compared with Doubles and Abutting Pairs developed by Increasing the Rate

It is apparent that the distributions are the same with the exception of the arresting consonants which show a slightly longer form than the abutting pairs.

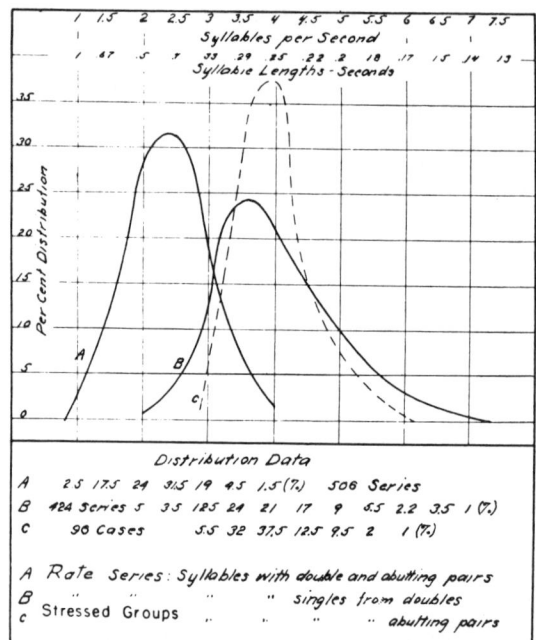

FIGURE 109. Distribution of the Lengths (and Rates) of Syllables

Data show sharp difference between single and abutting consonants.

course any series of syllables repeated with increasing rate gives a long series of connected syllables without break. But such unbroken series are not the usual breath groups; instead, one has a breath group which may continue indefinitely. It is much like the trill or rapid run in music, which may consist of an indefinite number of notes with no definite stress organization save the initial stress in the series of rapid, uniform notes. In such a series, the first indication of grouping will be the formation of simple feet (one-syllable, trochee, iamb, dactyl) which breaks the series into groups of one, two, or three syllables. Two, three, or possibly more of these feet may combine into a breath group, indicated by the subordination of the pauses (pressure minima), by the linkages (abutting consonants), and by the dynamic structure of the larger breath group. Such feet of five or more syllables are not common, but they may occur in certain forms of "patter". A series like "*Zeep Ope will be pope*" is likely to be given as two distinct breath groups, "*Zeep' Ope' / will' be pope'*". The form "*Zeep Ope will be pope*" ($\perp / \perp \_\_ / \perp$) is possible; but the form "*Zeep Ope will be pope*" ($\_ / \perp \_\_ / \perp$) results in "*Zee pope 'll be pope*" in which both the "*p*" of "*Zeep*" and of "*ope*" have become releasing consonants. "*Zeep Ope 'll be-p ope*" is also possible; the arresting form of "*Zeep*" is imitated by "*be-p*" in the second breath group (Cf. Fig. 112). In verse, series of six, eight and more syllables in a breath group are common, but it is usually the case that lines of more than four feet (eight to twelve syllables) are broken by a cesura. In prose, the longer breath groups may not be as long as in verse.

The prescribed formula "*pop up' a pop' up*" was uttered so as to make an interesting variation of the five-syllable breath group. The subject gave it "*pop' / up' a / pop' up*", with a primary stress on the final "*pop' up*". In 18 of the 19 cases measured the primary stress occurs on the final foot. In 10 of the 19 cases, the initial one-syllable foot "*pop*" is marked off by an arresting consonant, the adventitious double

THE BREATH GROUP IN ENGLISH DEPENDENT ON THE STRESS PATTERN OF THE WORDS 143

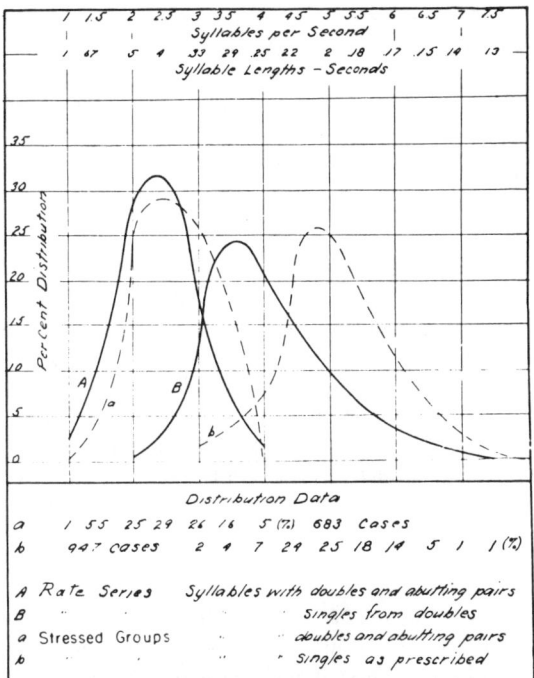

FIGURE 110. Distribution Data Collected for Comparisons
The distributions of the forms produced by changes of rate are in general shorter than the distributions due to change of stress.

"*pop-pup*" is avoided to keep the verbal "*up*" quite clear (Cf. Fig. 113).

Of course many phonetic changes of the consonants are not included in these processes of dropping the arresting consonant, of doubling and singling, and of reducing the trochaic median consonant. The changes involving aspirates, soft gutturals, nasals, semi-vowels, and liquids are often not of this group of changes. The influence of vowels on each other, and of consonants and vowels on each other, has not been considered in detail. Syllables are eliminated by other processes than iambic telescoping and trochaic reduction.

It will not be difficult, however, to devise series in which such elements are brought together, and it may be possible by changing the rate and the rhythm to produce in the laboratory the changes which occur in the history of a language.

Influence of Stress and the Syllable Movement in the Modification of "Sounds"

The quality of the sounds of the vowels may be affected by the stress. Even in French it is possible that the stress may produce slight differences in the vowels. Rousselot and Laclotte note changes of the vowels from open and closed to median qualities when the vowels become atonic: "*á*" (fermée) becomes "*a*" (moyenne) in *bas de soie*; "*é*" (fermée) becomes "*e*" (moyenne) in "*bonté de coeur*"; "*ó*" (fermée) becomes "*o*" (moyenne) in "*cotelette*"; "*oe*" (fermée) becomes "*oe*" (moyenne) in "*feu de joie*". (72) In every one of these cases the elision of the "mute *e*" leaves a consonant in the arresting position for the syllable in question. They are all cases of the elimination of the unaccented syllable of the iamb with the resulting abutting pair formed when the syllable telescopes. "*Bonté d(e) coeur, bas d(e) soie, cot(e)lette, feu d(e) joie*".

In English the shifting of the stress modifies the vowels profoundly. Note the "*i*" of "*ad'vertise, adver'tisement*"; the "*a*" in "*profane, profanation*"; the "*a*" in "*circulate, circulatory*"; the "*y*" in "*analyse, analysis*". The syllables which do not have the primary or secondary accent tend toward "dark *e*". The sense of the quality of the vowels persists and the proper vowel reappears in derivatives and in calling and singing.

This change of vowel quality with the change of stress is a matter of rate of utterance of the syllable. There is not time enough for the vowel movement to occur in normal fashion. The English "dark *e*" and the "mute *e*" of the French is merely the vowel reduced to its simplest and briefest form; it is the vowel "sound" produced when there is the least movement possible from the neutral position. The "dark *e*" is even briefer than the "short" English vowels.

If the syllables are chosen and the stress prescribed so that the unstressed vowels cannot reduce to "dark *e*", the maximum rate of utterance is much slower. "*Tee' too tay....*" can be repeated at a maximum rate of 4.5–4.8 syllables per sec., "*La' pee yo....*" at a maximum rate of 6 syllables per sec., while "*ta ta'....*" (becoming "*te ta'....*") can be repeated at a maximum rate of 8–10 syllables per sec.

The relation of the word stress to the quality of the vowel has been built into an elaborate system in the Hebrew. Possibly it is rather artificial as we have it now, but it undoubtedly represents something of the ancient practice. Vowels in syllables with the stress are systematically lengthened; vowels preceding the

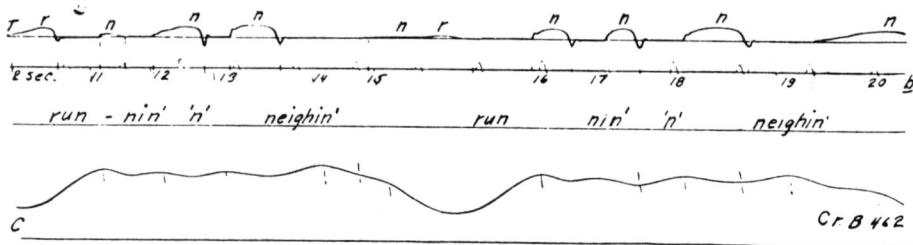

FIGURE 111. Syllabic Consonants as Syllables; Chest Pulses direct from Trachea

Cf. Fig. 88 and 89

Syllables: *runnin' 'n' neighin'*.

T—Tongue marker. The *n*'s and the *r*'s shows distinct strokes; there is no indication of doubling in the *n* series.

C—Chest pulses from trachea. The five syllables constitute a breath group; there is no clear indication of feet. Each of the syllables has a distinct pulse.

The maximum of the chest pressure does not appear during the *n*, but *between* the consonants; the rise in pressure for the syllable is due to an independent chest pulse and not to the constriction of the vocal canal. The chest pressure is maintained throughout the breath group. The syllables are represented by maxima in the pressure curve.

stress are regularly reduced to "dark e", the schwa. The vowel is a more variable factor to the Semite, because of the variations of the vowels of the stem in the course of inflection.

The effect of the actual movements on each other has been carefully described by Rousselot (consonant and vowel, vowel and consonant, vowel and vowel, consonant and consonant). The inflectional changes bring together various articulations, and the elision and modification of syllables in the course of historical changes subject phonetic movements to the influence of each other. Spelling and printing can only delay such changes, they cannot prevent them. In general the movements of speech are shaped by rapid utterance. Rhythm and stress will be preserved and the phrase must be comprehensible; but with these reservations the influence of mere velocity

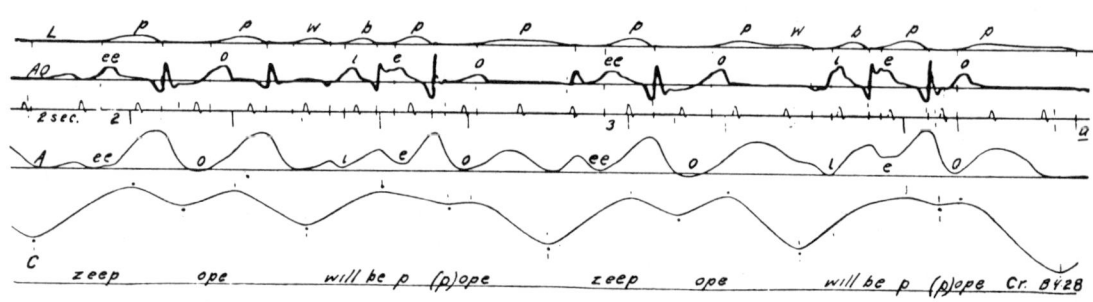

FIGURE 112. Syllables forming Feet and Breath Groups

Syllables: *Zeep ope will be pope.*

L—Lip marker. *P* and *w* show much the same contact. In breath group 2 the *p*, *w* do not abut, but in breath group 3 the abutting *p-w* appears.

AO—Air outside. The *o*'s have the characteristic form following an arrested syllable. The syllable *be(p)* is a good example of the outside-pressure tracing in a syllable with releasing consonant.

A—Air in mouth. The arresting *p*'s show the highest mouth pressure. Pressure for the *w* is very weak.

It is apparent on comparing the tracings that the *l* and the *b* coincide (doubling-singling) so that there is only a single consonant.

C—Chest pulses directly from trachea. The pulses for the syllables: *Zeep, ope, be,* and *(p)ope* are well defined, and the breath groups separate into two feet. In breath group 2 the syllable *will* has been entirely dropped (iambic elimination); in breath group 3 there is some slight indication of the syllable *will.*

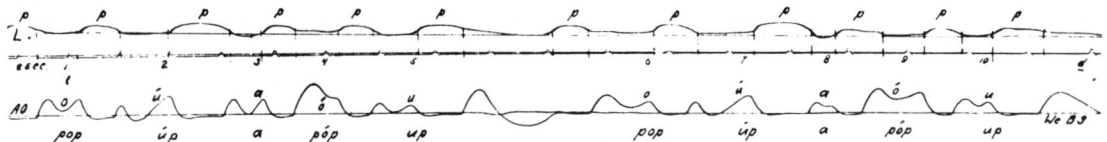

FIGURE 113. Grouping of a Stressed Group of Five Syllables

L—Lip marker. Forms as usual.
AO—Air outside. Syl. 1 has the usual releasing form with mid-sag. Syl. 2 shows the drop to zero after the arresting *p* of *pop*. In syl. 4 the stress shows in the form, but it is pronounced *po' pup*, not *pop'up*; there is no arresting form in the tracing of syl. 4. Syl. 7 has a form which indicates that the preceding *p* is arresting and that syl. 6 was made "*pop*". But the form of the vowel in syl. 9 is that of *po'* and it is obvious that syl. 9, 10 run *po'pup*. Vowel forms like those of syl. 1, 4, 6, 9, 10 indicate that the preceding consonant is releasing; vowel forms like those of syl. 2, 7 are typical of an arresting consonant immediately preceding.

The dynamic form indicates that the stress on syl. 4 and 9 is the culmination for the whole five-syllable breath group.

---

will dominate. It is a general law of language that all phonetic coordinations shape themselves by and for the maximum rate of utterance.

Generalizations have been made on the reciprocal influence of "sounds". There is a "law of assimilation" whereby the movements tend to become alike; "law of prevision", whereby movements are prepared in advance as in all fields of skilled movements; the "law of economy" whereby only the movements necessary for the given "sound" occur; the "law of fusion" in the case of two contiguous vowels. (72)

All such generalizations must finally be referred to the skilled movements involved. The word stress and the syllable movement play an important part in such reciprocal modifications. The back stroke of the releasing consonant must occur during the syllable and must modify the vowel. The preparation and beginning of the beat stroke of the arresting consonant must occur during the syllable movement and must modify the vowel. The patterns of Visible Speech show the vowel modifications in acoustic detail; the back stroke of the releasing consonant opens the vowel cavity and produces modulatory changes which indicate the place of the consonant constriction and the consonant's influence in the beginning of the vowel. The patterns of Visible Speech show that the beat stroke of the arresting consonant constricts the vowel cavity producing modulatory changes which indicate the place of constriction and the consonant influence on the end of the vowel. The consonant movement must be inferred and the detail of air pressures and the syllable pulse cannot be read in the Visible Speech recordings, but the consonant overlap and its consequences in the vowel are well shown for the first time (10). The back stroke of the arresting consonant may occur during the intersyllabic interval, or it may modify a following initial vowel. Since a releasing consonant in the next syllable may separate the back stroke (détente) of the arresting consonant from the next syllable, there may be no influence.

Consonants occur in juxtaposition in two cases: compound consonants in which the fused consonants function as a single releasing or arresting factor; abutting consonants in which each member has a different function in a different syllable.

The simplest fusions in compound consonants are those in which a continuant becomes the preparation or the back stroke of an occlusive, e.g. "*stay, play*". The mechanism of voicing is dependent on the articulatory organs and on the breathing apparatus, and changes of voicing are difficult in the very brief interval of the compound consonant; therefore the group of components tends to be voiced or unvoiced. (35)

With the abutting consonants the conditions are quite different, for members of the pair belong to different syllables. In many languages "assimilation", the influence of one abutting consonant on the other, is very common.

If the differences of stress and of length of syllable are not extreme, the releasing consonant is the dominant movement, and the arresting consonant is modified toward the releasing consonant. This is the rule in Greek and Latin, and in French. As the rate of utterance increases in a fairly uniform series of syllables, the arresting consonant must be uttered very rapidly just before the releasing consonant of the next syllable. A similar movement, or an identical movement, can be given in sequence more rapidly and certainly than two different movements.

But the Teutonic languages, with heavy word stress, series of "short" vowels in stressed syllables, and great variety in length of syllable, show much less assimilation. The changes of the abutting pair are not always in the direction of the releasing consonant. This is not due, as Sweet quaintly suggests, to an English "striving for distinctness"—there is too much against that idea—but to the function of the arresting consonant in a stressed syllable with "short vowel". Passy calls attention to the frequent "progressive assimilation" in English and German, as in the English "observe". (61) On occasion the form of the movement of the arresting consonant holds over to the releasing consonant. But as Passy indicates, the assimilation is not invariable. "*Observe*" may be compared with "*subserve*", in which there is no assimilation.

The words "*blackboard*" and "*flagpole*" have a secondary stress on the second syllable and the syllables remain distinct. When the two consecutive stresses are lost in rapid utterance, all sorts of changes are possible, as "*forehead*" (*for'ed*), "*forecastle*" (*fok'sl*), "*boatswain*" (*bos'n*), "*blackguard*" (*bla'gard*).

Nothing has been said of the influence of habit, "association", in modifying phonetic movements. It is certain that this factor plays an important part.

Chapter VIII

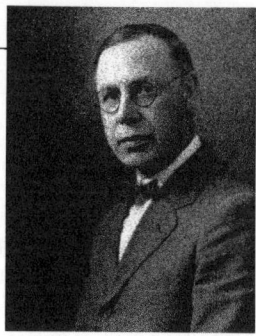

RHYTHM AND THE CHARACTERISTIC UTTERANCE OF A LANGUAGE

The rhythm is certainly one of the most fundamental characteristics of the utterance of a language, and is often most difficult for a foreigner to acquire. The play of the word stresses, the rhythmic grouping of the breath groups and phrases, the differences in the length of the syllables are all difficult, and all-important for a good "accent". And it is not the case that one can first master the "elements" of the pronunciation, the "sounds", and then set them in the rhythm. It is easy to see, that the rhythm "has a vital, underlying influence on the details of utterance. The word stress often determines the function of the consonant as arresting or releasing and also determines the syllable in which the consonant shall function. The rhythm at a rapid rate determines the slurring or the full pronunciation of syllables. In the end the rhythm guides the phonetic changes which every language is undergoing.

Sweet takes a practical view of the subject of stress- and pitch-accent in the early I. E. languages. He is certain that what happened in Greek was not that a pitch accent was replaced by a stress accent—which would be impossible for a variety of reasons—but that the early I. E. accent involved the essential stress factor along with a pitch factor; the pitch factor was lost but the essential stress factor remained.

Since the stress increases the tension, it is natural that the increased chest pressure, compensated by an increased tension of the vocal folds, raise the pitch. Thus a rise of pitch as a result of tension is a by-product. The stress may fall, however, on a syllable with a low pitch because of the intonation pattern, and especially at the end of the declarative phrase.

The Romance languages and the Slavic languages do not have the pronounced differences in the length of syllable. (95) This is equivalent to saying also that they are the languages in which there are no extreme differences in the stress of the syllables. The French also, along with the Spanish, modern Greek, and the Slavic languages, has a decided tendency to the open syllable, while the English and German have many closed syllables. (78)

In French the pattern of the alternating stressed and unstressed syllables may vary in the same breath group from speaker to speaker, and may vary from time to time with the same speaker; the variation depends on a difference of emphasis or on personal choice. As the syllables are not greatly varied in length, the rhythm is in the main trochaic and dactylic—the forms in which the length of the syllable is nearly the same. The frequent "mute *e*" and the occasional closed syllables make iambs possible; anapests are very rare. As it occurs in the breath group, the "word" stress of the French is not fixed. As a rule, the "mute *e*" does not have the stress, but it may on occasion; thus in a series of monosyllables with "mute *e*" there is a stress on the alternate syllables. The conventional stress of the isolated word is on the final syllable, of the word in context on the tonic syllable; but frequent "displacements" of this stress for emphasis and for rhythm are essential to a good French diction. Passy and Michaelis note the possibility of pronouncing "*impossible*" and "*excellent*" with a stress on any one of the three syllables. (61)

In English and German on the contrary, there are very pronounced differences in length of syllable and great differences in the force of the stresses. Sweet speaks of the possibility of distinguishing three different grades of length, and the customary notation of "primary, secondary and nul" distinguishes three grades of stress. With very rare exceptions the English contrasts with the French in having a fixed pattern of the word stresses. In French the stressing of the breath group determines the stress of the word; in English the stresses of the words determine the stress pattern of the breath group. The prevalence of syllables short in duration, and the extreme force of the word stress combine to give the English a prevailingly iambic rhythm. It is not unusual to find consecutive syllables stressed. Trochees and dactyls are common. While there is perhaps more variety of rhythmic pattern than in the French, the general character of the English is iambic. A. W. de Groot comments on the rhythmic difference between the English and German, and the French. (15)

This system of great difference of stress and of length of syllable gives important functions to the consonants which tend to maintain the difference of stress and length of syllable. The pronounced differences of lengths of syllables and the variety of rhythmic grouping make a place for the arresting consonants, whether followed by a vowel or a releasing consonant.

In French, on the other hand, the tendency is to evenness of stress on the syllables and to an even length of syllable. All consonants tend to become releasing in utterance at rapid rate, and all consonants in the arresting position tend to shift or drop; there are no heavy stresses and no great variations of length of syllable which would accommodate the arresting consonants and give them definite function.

The tremendous changes which have taken place in the "sounds" of the French as it developed from the vulgar Latin must have been due to something beside the ordinary changes to which a language is subjected. Side by side with the Latin, the Greek also has had a continuous history of development into a modern language; but the Greek presents no such extensive changes. There can be little question that a profound change in the rhythm underlies the extensive alterations during the transition from Latin to French. A new rhythm has produced a new language, reshaping the ancient words, eliminating syllables and shifting the stress to an alternation from syllable to syllable. Gradually the French tended to the open syllable, probably under the influence of a rhythm which prefers rapid and even syllables. The tendency to equalize the syllables, and the inevitable rate of utterance, resulted in the elimination of the arresting consonants (final and "appuyantes"). Other consonants brought into juxtaposition by the dropping of the syllables affected each other profoundly. Such a change of rhythm and of stress is apparent in the Hebrew over against the Arabic, and in the Czech over against the Lithuanian, and in the French over against the Italian.

A language mechanism is an interrelated set of movements in which the various traits have their function; they are not isolated. The habit of describing the "sounds" and the rhythms of a language as if they were collections of independent peculiarities overlooks the fact that they are part and parcel of each other. And changes which occur affect the entire language mechanism.

The changes occur at first as normal, synchronous changes which revert with the restoration of the rate and stress. Diachronous changes are such changes which have become irreversible because of perturbations in the language mechanism as a whole. (89, p. 46, 97)

APPENDIX I

A. Syllables Developed into Series with Doubles by Increasing the Speed of Utterance (Pronounced with English short vowels, if without indication)

Syllable	Number of series, '24	'26	Number of doubles measured, '24	'26
beb		8		1
bob	11	2	87	8
church	1		1	
dead		10		2
dud	11	8	78	17
fife		10		11
fuf	5	5	16	25
lul	11		78	
mom	2		10	
non	6		36	
peep		2		2
pep		3		1
pope		4		5
pup	13	10	85	33
shish	2		10	
sis	8	10	54	6
tet		5		5
tight		4		15
tut	9	4	56	6

B. Syllables Developed into Series with One-member Abutting Pairs by Increasing Speed

Syllable	Number of series, '24	'26	Number of pairs measured, '24	'26
bup	1		4	
pub	4		18	
fub	5		30	
buf	1		5	
beef	4			
fup	6		23	
puf	5		25	
lit	6		29	
til	2		9	
lun	2		6	
nul	5		18	
nit	5		21	
tin	6		23	
sat	6		27	
tas	5		30	
chide	4		13	
chin	5		22	
chit	4		18	
dish	4		13	
ditch	2		7	
nas	5		31	
nash	4		22	
natch	1		1	
shun	3		12	
shut	3		11	
thin	2		12	
tiz	3		15	

C. Syllables Developed into Series with Two-Member Abutting Pairs of Consonants by Increasing Speed

Syllable	Number of series, '24	'26	Number of pairs measured, '24	'26
bat	3		9	
bit	5		17	
tab	15		79	
bin	17		48	
bone	3		7	
nib	4		21	
nob	3		14	
boss	10		50	
sob	12		56	
dim	3		14	
dime	1		3	
tim	11		46	

Syllable	Number of series, '24	'26		Syllable	Number of pairs measured	'24	'26
time	1					3	
mad	8					31	
dip	3					18	
pod	5					29	
fan	10					35	
fine	1					3	
knife	10					33	
fuss	7					23	
safe	6					15	

Syllable	Number of series, '24	'26		Syllable	Number of pairs measured	'24	'26
mass	6					21	
Sam	17					69	
name	7					35	
nim	1					4	
man	6					12	
main	1					3	
nip	10					41	
pin	5					16	
pass		8					17
piece	7					19	
sap	2	6				4	9
sip	9					45	
pat	2	12				6	39
pit	11					37	
tap	3					6	
top	13					50	

Words			Words	
Ot' to	9		up' pup'	13
ought' to'	9		up' up	15
pup' py	12		up' spout	16
pup pie'	8		up' spring	59

Nonsense syllables			Nonsense syllables	
ma' mam	18		peb' pep	33
ma mam'	13		peb pep'	28
pa' pap	6		pe' pep	37
pa pap'	6		pe pep'	31
pa' pep	12		po' pep	9
pa pep'	9		po pep'	9
paw' pep	12		po' pep	12
paw pep'	8		po pep'	11
pay' pay	5		po' pop	12
pay pay'	5		po pop'	8
pop' up	16		ta' tat	17
pop up'	12		ta tat'	14
pu' pep	12		ted' tet	17
pu pep'	12		ted tet'	18
set' set	14		tep' tep	6
set set'	10		tep tep'	5
sit' sit	15		te' tet	33
sit sit'	12		te tet'	30
sot' sot	6		te' tet	12
sot sot'	5		te tet'	12
soots' tsoot	3		to' tot	6
soots tsoot'	6		to tot'	4
soot' soot	10			
soot soot'	10			

D. Abutting Pairs, and Arresting Consonants, "Constructive Doubles"

add A,	23		add T	12
a day	22		a tall D	47
add C	5		told E	39
add P,	5		at C,	24
add E	20		at E	24
a tea	32		pop up a	16
at E	24		pop up	12
at P,	35		Zeep Ope	68
at E	30		will be pope	59

E. Accented Groups of Two Syllables

Words			Words	
at' it	4		state'	6
a tit'	4		to state'	5
ba' by	16		test' it	21
ba boo'	13		test it'	20
de' bit	17		tes' tate	12
de bate'	18		es tate'	9
hit' him	8		test' S (ess)	20
hit' Tim'	8		test S' (ess)	16
in stall'	2		too' tight	13
			too tight'	8
in state'	42		up' late	18
			a plate	16

F. Accented Groups of Three Syllables

Words			Words	
in' stitute	50		up' pup' py	50
lob' Bob' by	25		up spring' ing	47
sed' ative	29		up spout' ing	14

Nonsense syllables			Nonsense syllables	
pat pat' pat	6		pup' up up	64
pet' pet pet	14		pup up' pup	40
pet pet' pet	9		pup up pup'	26
pet pet pet'	8		up' up pup'	18
			up' up up'	8

G. Accented Groups of Four Syllables

ba ba' ba bab	15		bub bub' bub bub	8
ba ba ba' bab	16		bub bub bub' bub	8
bay bay' bay bay	5		dot dot' dot dot	21
bay bay bay' bay	4		dot dot dot' dot	12
bō bō' bō bō	8		ma ma' ma mam	18
bō bō bō' bō	8		ma ma ma' mam	16
pa pa' pa pap	6		sap sap' sap sa	18
pa pa pa' pap	5		sap sap sap' sa	18
pas pa' pas pa	14		sep' sep sep se	58

APPENDIX I

Accented Groups of four Syllables:

pas pas pas' pa	10
pat pat' pat pat	47
pat pat pat' pat	32
pe pe pe' pep	61
pe pe pe' pep	55
pe' pe pe pe	40
pe' pe pe pep	29
pes pes' pes pes	5
pes pes pes' pes	6
pes' pes pes pes	53
po po' po pop	35
po po po' pop	44
po po' po pop	4
po po po' pop	4
pup pup' pup pup	9
pup pup pup' up	8

sep sep' sep sep	4
ta ta' ta tat	14
ta ta ta' tat	16
tay te' te tet	18
ted ted' ted ted	14
ted ted ted' ted	14
te te' tay tet	30
te te' tay to	17
te te tay' to	30
te te' te tet	15
te te te' tet	13
te te' te te	11
te te te' te	9
te te' te tet	4
te te te' tet	4
tō tō' to' tōt	4
tō tō tō' tōt	4

List of the words, phrases, and syllables discussed in the text: Words (dots following a word indicate that it is developed into a series.)

	Fig.	
apt...	74, 76	p. 108, 110
asp...	75	p. 109
bay...ac. group:	86, 87	p. 124
bee...	57	p. 96
beef...	57	p. 96
eat...	27	p. 66
fie...	49	p. 91
fife...	49	p. 91
halfpay	40	p. 86
hello		
instate	99	p. 136
institute	99	p. 136
pass...	63	p. 100
pat...	64	p. 101
Poe...	50	p. 92
pope...	50	p. 92
ac. group	112	p. 144
puff...	56	p. 96
pup...	43	p. 89
ac. group	83, 85, 98, 99	p. 122, 123, 135, 136
puppy ac. group	34	p. 77
Sam...	60, 61	p. 99
sap...	62	p. 99
sat...	58	p. 97
sedative, sed' tive	97, 98	p. 135
tea...	27	p. 66
tight	48	p. 91
Tim...	67	p. 104
top...	59	p. 98
up...	28	p. 67
phrase:	34	p. 77
ac. group	83, 84, 98, 99	p. 122, 123, 135, 136
upspring	78	p. 111
upspringing	78	p. 111

Phrases:

	Fig.	
a tall D told E	73	p. 108
at C, at E	68	p. 105
at P, at E	69	p. 105
an aim, a name		
Bobby don't boo at baby	22	p. 60
hit him, hit Tim		p. 84
I do, I'd do		p. 84
I'm Ike, I'm Mike		p. 84
I lie, I'll lie		p. 60
lob, Bob		p. 84
Lil' 'll lie low	88, 89	p. 125
Otto ought to	47	p. 90
pop up a pop up	113	p. 145
runnin' 'n' neighin'	111	p. 144
topic, top pick	39	p. 85
thus E, the C, thus C		p. 85
unknown		p. 84
up, Bob	46, 80	p. 90, 112
up up, up pup	35, 37	p. 77, 80
up, puppy	34	p. 77
whole ode		p. 85
hoe load		p. 85
whole load		p. 85
Z is Z	38	p. 80
Zeep Ope will be pope	112	p. 144

Nonsense syllables (dots following a syllable indicate that it is developed in series). (English short vowels, unless indicated)

	Fig.	
pup...	3, 4	p. 37, 38
pope...	10	p. 41
ispda...	77	p. 110
nas...	44	p. 89
ōp...	21, 36	p. 59, 78
pō...	26	p. 65
sis...	45	p. 90
sfa...	72	p. 107
tas...	71	p. 107
tee too tay		p. 66, 67
top...	59	p. 98

Nonsense syllables in groups:

a, a, a, a,	39	p. 85
ah ah ah ah	16	p. 57
ab-ba vak	36	p. 78
a la dad'	15, 17	p. 56, 57
ba, ba, ba, ba,	23	p. 60
bay bay bay bay	86, 87	p. 124
et es	31	p. 73
et ez	32	p. 74
pa ba ma	20	p. 59
pa pa ta	9	p. 40
pa pep	90, 91	p. 126, 128
pe pe pe pe	81, 103	p. 121, 139
pe pep	90	p. 126

Nonsense syllables in groups:

peb pep	93	p. 131
pe pe pe pep	100, 101	p. 137, 138
pes pes pes pes	82	p. 122
po pop, po pop, po pop	105	p. 140
pup pup pup pup	85	p. 123
pup pu pup	83, 84, 92, 94	p. 122, 123, 128, 132
pu pep	95	p. 132
ta tat, ta ta tat, ta ta tat	106	p. 141
ta tat, ta tat, ta tat	104	p. 140
te tet	96	p. 133
te te te te	102	p. 138
to to to tot	29	p. 67

APPENDIX II

SPEECH WITH ARTIFICIAL LARYNX

To be rid of misconceptions and to get a fresh view of phonetics, speaking with an artificial larynx is a process worth looking into. The artificial larynx is unfamiliar but its workings are simple and mechanical and will make some things clear.

When the larynx is removed, there is no longer a connection between the mouth and the lungs; the patient no longer breathes through the throat and mouth; instead, the patient breathes through the opening of the windpipe (trachea) just above the breastbone. As he recovers he can make articulatory movements but he can utter no slightest sound. The patient has all the coordinations of speech but they are disrupted by the removal of the larynx and the closure of the throat.

The artificial larynx restores the connection between the breathing apparatus and the mouth. A tube leads from the opening of the trachea to the cylinder containing the reed so that the patient can force air through the reed; from the cylinder the mouth tube leads air and voice into the corner of the mouth. The patient holds the cylinder as if he were to smoke a pipe connected with the trachea. He notes that he is breathing through the open vent in the cylinder below the reed; and he wonders how air and voice led into the front of the mouth can replace the air and voice which used to come through the missing larynx into the rear of the mouth.

The patient is asked to put the mouth in position for an O, to cover the vent and force air into the mouth; to his surprise the reed sounds and the result is a prolonged vowel "O". Then he is asked to make a series of quick pulses, "*Oh, Oh, Oh. . . .*" A series of quick pulses means that the abdomen-diaphragm muscles must be adjusted for the series while the quick pulses are made by the chest muscles (intercostals). Then a series "*E, E, E . . . .*" is produced. For "*I, I, I . . . .*" he finds that he must change the shape of the mouth during the pulse.

The patient is making his series of vowel syllables, starting the syllables with the chest muscles and stopping them with the chest muscles. There is nothing else to release the syllable and arrest the syllable pulse; the mouth is open and the mechanical reed is inert. The reed sounds when the pulse is released and the reed stops sounding when the pulse is arrested.

The series of "*Oh's*" or "*I's*" can be schematized OVO, OVO, OVO. . . . in which the -V- stands for the vowel shape, and -O- stands for the chest-muscle contraction which releases the air pulse.

Now the patient is asked to make the syllable "*a*" and close the lips at the end of the syllable, to say "*ape, ape, ape. . . .*". He has no trouble and presently he finds that he can manage the breath pressure above and below the reed so that he can distinguish "*ape*" with an unvoiced arrest from "*Abe*" with a voiced arrest. This consonant-arrested syllable may be schematized OVC to indicate that the syllable is arrested by a consonant.

Now it is easy for the patient to close the lips at the start of the syllable pulse and to release the lips to say "*pay, pay, pay....*" or "*bee, bee, bee....*"; a syllable consonant-released; CVO.

There remains one other type of syllable: the patient releases the chest pulse with a lip articulation and arrests the chest pulse with a lip articulation: "*peep, peep, peep....*", "*babe, babe, babe..*" "*mope, mope, mope....*" CVC.

Thus the patient without a larynx has mastered the four fundamental types of syllables: OVO, OVC, CVO, CVC. In a few hours practice he will have got back all the coordinations, handling speech by the manipulation of the chest pulses which are released or arrested either by the chest muscles or by the consonant articulations, or both. He depends on manipulating the air pressure above and below the inert reed to make the larynx voice the syllable factors properly, viz.: the vowel shape, and the releasing and arresting consonants. The ease with which the artificial larynx is mastered shows that the coordinations are very like the coordinations before the loss of the larynx. On the other hand, speaking with the esophagus, a somewhat novel process, is worth learning, but it takes a half year or more.

It is impossible of course to make a given vowel without releasing and arresting a pulse from the chest; shaping the vowel prepares for the syllable pulse of the vowel but the pulse must occur if there is to be a vowel. The lips or tongue may be in position to make the releasing or arresting stroke of a given consonant, but that does not constitute a consonant. The consonant is produced when the stroke releases or arrests the air pressure of the syllable pulse. The vowel is an articulation which has the function of shaping the vocal canal for the chest pulse; the consonant is an articulation which has the function of delimiting the chest pulse of the syllable. It is only in the coordination of the syllable pulse that they act as a vowel and consonant. They may be named as if separate, but that is merely a convenient abstraction. A vowel is a specific quality of a syllable when uttered through a specific vocal-canal shape; a consonant is a specific way of releasing or of arresting a syllable. Details of the process involved come later.

The syllable proves to have three invariable factors:

> The releasing factor: chest muscles or consonant movement; O- or C-; Oh OVO beau CVO.
> The vowel shaping factor: muscles of tongue, pharynx, jaw, lips; -V-; Oh OVO, pope CVC.
> The arresting factor: chest muscles or consonant movement; -O or -C; Oh OVO, ope OVC.

Any one of these syllable factors may be characterized by one or several significant aspects; these are the phonemes. A syllable may have no significant aspect, no phoneme, or it may have as many as seven significant aspects of the syllable factors, phonemes. There are compound consonants of two or three aspects, and there are compound vowels, diphthongs (and a few triphthongs). Details of the characteristics and processes involved in compound syllable factors come later.

APPENDIX III

THE HISTORICAL ASPECTS OF THE SYLLABLE, SYLLABARIES AND ALPHABETS

A system of writing may not be phonetic. The ancient Egyptians and the Chinese achieved a developed form of writing in which the words (and sometimes groups of words) came to be represented by single characters. In such systems the phonetic resemblance of words may occasionally figure in the symbolizing; words are often single syllables; and single "sounds" which play a part in the morphology may come to have specific characters. But neither a syllabary nor an alphabet appears. The writing may develop a semi-cursive form, but the signs run into the hundreds or even thousands and simplification does not take the form of phonetic representation.

The Sumerians were the first to develop a system of representing not the words or ideas, but the syllables. Based on ideograms, the construction of the language made it possible to find one-syllable words of all types, including released syllables of the form CVO, and arrested syllables of the form OVC and CVC. And finally, it is important that the Sumerian recognized the simple vowel as an independent syllable, e.g. *a*, "water", *e* "house", *e* demonstrative pronoun, *u* "ten", were among the common substantives, OVO. The form CVC, released and arrested by a consonant, is also common, so that the Sumerian had all the types of syllables, CVO, OVC, OVO, CVC.

The morphology of the language involves composite syllables:

za-ra "to thee"
za-a "upon thee"
za-ra-an-ze-en (za-ran-zen) "to you"
za-a-an-ze-en (zan - zen) "upon you"

The analysis and construction of Sumerian syllables compelled such fusions. There is definite orthographic evidence of the union of such elements in simple syllables.

The morphology led to recognizing the syllable as both released and arrested: me-es (mes), and za-an (zan). Thus the Sumerian came to notate three types of vocalization: 1) The common Semitic form, post-consonantal: za-a. 2) Pre-consonantal: a-an. 3) Inter-consonantal, za-a-an (zan).

The analysis and construction of such syllables evidently developed with the rise of the cuneiform syllabary and was perhaps furthered by foreign influence. A composite Sumerian syllable may appear orthographically as za-a-am, which may also be spelled with a single character in lieu of the three, zam. The same elaborate handling appears in Akkadian in sa-a-at (sat). (47)

Thus the structure of the Sumerian led to the recognition of the three factors in the syllable, each of which might on occasion be distinguished in notation.

1. Releasing factor, usually a consonant with an inherent vowel-suffix; za, ra.
2. Vowel shape giving the syllable a definite quality; -a-, -e-, -u-.
3. Arresting factor, usually a consonant with an inherent vowel prefix; -en, -at.

The treatment of the syllable in the Sumerian and derivative orthographies is remarkably consistent. The phonetic analysis is more acute and more consistent than that of some recent theorists. The derivative Sumerian orthographies, and notably the Hurrian and the Akkadian, show a practical mastery of the structure of the syllable as composed of the three essential syllable factors. In spite of the clumsiness of a syllabary, they handle the system so as to take account of the changes and shifts at the syllable frontier. The essential syllable factors, and the changes and shifts at the syllable frontier, which were treated later in the Greek and Sanskrit phonology and have been demonstrated in modern laboratories, were reckoned with in the second millenium B.C. (89, p. 60).

The Babylonian syllabaries (and derivatives) remained syllabaries however. Although the number of characters might be reduced, the method of marking each characteristic syllable factor, "sound", with a single specific sign was never adopted. The reading of the Bibylos inscriptions by Dhorme shows no more than 100 characters, and Dhorme has classified them by the releasing consonants of the Semitic alphabet; but the characters representing the same consonant with different vocalization have no resemblance. (17) It is called an "alphabet" but has none of the traits of the Semitic alphabet.

The first approach to a true alphabet is the systematic syllabary of the early Semitic. The Sinaitic "alphabet" followed the simple phonological structure of the Canaanite and represented each syllable by a releasing consonant vocalized. The importance and stability of the consonant "radical", and the morphological and inflectional changes, led to counting the vowel as a variable which was left without indication in the early orthography. The identification of the limited set of releasing consonants vocalized, which make up the corpus of the early Semitic syllables, and the adaptation of a simple series of acrophonic signs to represent these few releasing articulations, constitute the great phonological discovery and invention on which all the alphabets of both East and West have been based. The Semitic prototype, however, was not a true alphabet, but a very simple syllabary, in which twenty-odd characters each represented some four or five syllables determined by the inferred vocalizations. The early Semitic "alphabet" then was a corpus of perhaps 100 syllables. But there is this important difference from any other syllabary which has come to light: the releasing consonant is always indicated by a single specific sign; the releasing syllable factors have been isolated and notated. That is the beginning of the true alphabet.

Unlike the cuneiform syllabaries, the type of syllable represented in the early Semitic was limited to the one form CVO; the notation represented only the C-, assumed the -V-, and ignored the -O (chest arrest). A common form of double consonant did appear in various places in the inflection of the verb, but only in special positions, and was counted a 'sharpening'; it was never written with a repeated character which would have indicated a repeated syllable, but it was distinguished from a single consonant. With the decay of endings and extreme phonological change, closed syllables, CVC, were indicated very much later by the 'syllable divider'. The early notation involves the use of certain gutturals to indicate a vowel; the guttural selected gave some indication of the vowel to be assumed (scriptio plena), but there was never a full writing of the vowels, nor recognition of the function of the vowel in the syllable. The importance of the releasing consonant, the "radical", centered the interest on these consonants. In recognizing only one form of syllable (CVO) and marking it with the consonant sign, the Sinaitic and its derivatives differ radically from the cuneiform syllabaries which recognized the three syllable factors, including the vowel and deal with all four forms of syllable (CVO, OVC, CVC, OVO).

The Semitic "alphabet" and the neo-Sumerian syllabaries seem to have had no influence on each other. The Ras Shamra alphabet shows no indication of having been developed from an earlier syllabary; it is simply a Semitic "alphabet" written with cuneiform signs.

It remained to the Greeks to invent a true alphabet in which all three syllable factors are represented and all four types of syllables are written. Like the Sumerian, the Greek has all four varieties of syllables, often makes syllables by fusion, and recognizes the vowel as an independent syllable. And unlike the Semitic languages, in the Greek the vowel is quite as important and as stable a factor in the syllable as are the consonants. Therefore in adapting the Phoenician "alphabet", the Greeks faced a new problem. The structure of the Greek syllable was not limited to CVO; there are all four syllable types: CVO, OVC, CVC, OVO. It was not possible to make the opening consonant of the syllable the single character for the syllables having that opening consonant. There were not merely four-five CVO syllables; there were hundreds of syllables having a given opening consonant. Moreover, the Greek changes the vowel very little in inflection; the vowel of the stem is often quite as stable as the consonants.

The Greeks made the fundamental step of recognizing the vowel as the core of the syllable rather than the releasing consonant, and of defining the function of the consonant, simple or compound, as releasing when preceding the vowel, and as arresting when following the vowel in the syllable; therefore the vowel character was written on the line. The unity of the syllable and the division of the syllables are clearly indicated in the Greek morphology, accidence, and prosody. The consonant articulations were counted the same whether releasing or arresting, and the fundamental distinction between consonant and vowel was always clear. Vowels might combine with vowels to diphthongs, and consonants with consonants to compound consonants, but there was no fusion of vowel and consonant. The distinction between vowel and consonant was always clear; there were no indeterminate "clusters" in Greek phonology (palinskios, pa-tros and pat-ros, praksis). And always the vowel represented a syllable. Greek assimilation of abutting consonants made the double familiar and stressed the separate function in each syllable (en-leipo—el-leipo). The compound consonants are numerous and occur frequently, especially in the releasing position. The arresting compounds are rather few and rare. The convention which limits the ending consonant of a word to n, r, s, limits the arresting compounds to -nks, (sphinx) -ks (eks), -ls (hals), -ps (phleps). (30)

The Greek was the first language of the European type to be written, and its corpus of syllables runs into the thousands. Enumerating the syllables is not feasible. The description of the Greek consonants was unsatisfactory and was supplanted, but the Greek handling of the syllable factors was unerring. By indicating the syllable by a vowel, by indicating both releasing and arresting syllable factors as simple or compound consonants, by recognizing abutting consonants, including the double, the Greeks came to a perfected alphabetic orthography. The morphology and prosody favored such an achievement, but the adaptation of the Phoenician syllabary was a remarkable stroke. The Greeks preserved the simplicity of the "alphabet" and bent it to a much more difficult task. The Cypriotic syllabary shows another and inadequate solution. The Canaanites and the Greeks, favored by the structure of the language with which each worked, evinced the pioneering genius in phonetics.

APPENDIX IV

EARLIER STAGES OF MODERN PHONETICS

Alexander M. Bell had worked out "Visible Speech" to indicate the articulations for the deaf learning to speak. His pupil, Henry Sweet, turned to that system as best for a description of the historical and contemporary "sounds" of English. Meantime, F. de Saussure had undertaken to define the "sound" in question, since it was becoming evident that it was not invariable, as had been assumed, and that it was not a mere acoustic event. Saussure proposed the unit of the "phoneme".

Bell had defined the "sounds" as static positions; articulatory movements, "on- and off-glides" occurred between these positions. Sweet and Passy accepted this analysis and thought of speech as a series of fixed articulatory signs. Variations in the fixed signs were manifest, however. The obvious contrasts could not be ignored between whispering and speaking aloud, or between the speech of an orator and the speech of ordinary conversation. Saussure came to the rescue with the "phoneme". There is obviously an identity in this diversity. Although the actual acoustic patterns of whispered speech and of declaimed prose are unlike, there is certainly some characteristic for each "sound" which is in common and which hearers and speakers identify. That common characteristic Saussure called the "phoneme". Saussure had made his phoneme function in a syllable; but the I.P.A. group felt that they had no need of a syllable.

Although he had originally made the syllable a fundamental unit, Sweet, as well as Rousselot, and E. W. Scripture, all assume that there is no justification for the physiological subdivision of the breath group; they count words, syllables, and even "sounds" as fictitious divisions for grammatical convenience.

"The only division actually made in speech is that into breath groups due to the organic necessity of taking breath." (95, p. 14)

"Strictly speaking, the syllable has no physiological existence except in isolated monosyllables."

"The word like the syllable does not exist intact except in isolated.... The breath group has genuine individuality." (Rousselot, Principes de Phonétique Expérimentale, Welter, Paris, 1901–1908, p. 969, 972.)

"I do not believe, however, that a division of the flow of speech into separate blocks (termed syllables) has the slightest justification.... speech does not consist of any such blocks of sounds as the letters are supposed to indicate, or of any such large groups as syllables." (Scripture, E. W. Experimental Phonetics, Scribners, N.Y., 1902, p. 450.) Also: "Impossible to divide the verse, 'Somebody said it couldn't be done' into words, or syllables, or separate sounds." (Die Verskunst und die experimentelle Phonetik, Wiener Med. Wschr., 1922, 72, p. 1378.)

From the days of F. de Saussure, there have been two divergent trends: Saussure had defined the phoneme but had taught explicitly that the phoneme is always an aspect of the syllable and that the phoneme always has a part to play in the syllable.

Marichelle, a pioneer in teaching speech to the deaf, stressed the syllable and the role of the consonant and vowel in the syllable. (50, 51)

Herlin (Brussels), who developed a syllable method of teaching the deaf, Grammont, Sapir and his associates in the U. S., Sommerfelt (Oslo), Fouché (Paris), have all followed this trend. G. S. Haycock, a leader in the teaching of the deaf in England, like Marichelle and Herlin, knew the syllable and the syllable factors, and their importance in teaching speech.

Those who have recognized the syllable as basic have been ready to make use of experimental methods; although not all laboratory work has been done with the syllable in mind.

The other trend has been to make Saussure's "phoneme" the basic unit, while ignoring the syllable, or even denying the syllable as a phonetic event.

To isolate and classify the essential "sounds" (phonemes) of a language, i.e. to assemble the phonemic alphabet of a language, was an important project for Sweet and F. de Saussure, and a primary enterprise for Trubetzkoy. This was the impulse which lay behind the International Phonetic Alphabet, the first achievement of the phoneme doctrine.

Sweet noted that "sounds" differentiated words; at the hands of Saussure, Trubetzkoy and associates, the smallest phonic change in a word which shifts the meaning was made to indicate a new phoneme.

"Dans le 'projet de terminologie standardisée' soumis à la Réunion Phonologique Internationale de 1930, on trouve les définitions suivantes:

"Une *opposition phonologique* est une différence phonique susceptible de servir dans une langue donnée à la différenciation des significations intellectuelles; chaque terme d'une opposition phonologique quelconque est une unité phonologique; le phonème est une unité phonologique non susceptible d'être dissociée en unités phonologiques plus petites et plus simples." (Travaux du Cercle Linguistique de Prague, IV, p. 311.) (99, p. 232)

It is apparent that the method involves a resort to meanings and also to observations of articulations. Certainly, in one form or another, differentiating the significant articulations by differences of meaning will be important to any system. It is unfortunate that the scholars who have made the most of the method have not only ignored the syllable but have also insisted that the articulation occurs in the separate, concrete world of *la parole*, while the phoneme symbol occurs in the separate, ideal world of *la langue*; and so the phonemicists have made virtue of their ignorance of experimental methods of observation. There is no good reason for such deprivation.

The notion that each letter of the alphabet, and later each character modified from the International Phonetic Alphabet represents a separate event, has been strengthened by a logistic treatment of the phoneme initiated by Saussure, and developed by Trubetzkoy. The articulation and its physiological coordinations are counted a matter of *la parole*. In the world of *la langue* there are only symbols. Whether the syllable is an event in *la parole* need not matter if it is assumed that the syllable is superfluous in *la langue* which is composed of symbols independent of any physical correlates.

The assumption is false that the phonemes can be present as a row of symbols on a line. In articulate language the symbols are always phases of actual articulations; they are never disembodied and they never occur as a mere discrete row. Phonology is an objective science; the units must be studied in the one form in which experiments and observations can be made and repeated, and that is the form of actual speech; there is no "mental" world involved, no place for a series of disembodied symbols called "*la langue*". Jespersen was right in rejecting the postulated separation of *la langue* and *la parole*. Written characters are convenient as cues for the utterance of the syllables of an articulate language; but they are no more than cues; they are not entities in themselves.

Ignoring the syllable, it seemed possible to refer everything to the individual phonemes and their connections. Sievers believed that alongside Sweet's pressure pulse syllable (Drucksilbe) he detected another type of syllable in his own speech (without apparatus of course) due to differences of "sonority" (Schallfülle, Schallstärke). A "sound" of strong "sonority", contrasting with the neighboring sonorities, constituted a "sonority syllable" (Schallsilbe). Passy extended the sonority concept to cover *all* syllables. Actual sonority proved hard to demonstrate and so Passy added "apparent sonority" for good measure.

"Sonority" has not proved a legitimate concept in acoustics nor in audition, and the noncommital "prominence" is often substituted. (It is safe to say that a phoneme is prominent because of its prominence.) The sonority syllable was popular with the I.P.A. group, however, because sonority or prominence was considered a trait of the individual phoneme and thus the syllable was reduced to the relations of the phonemes. Stress and duration might be handled in the same fashion.

Saussure insisted that this series of stable phonemes in their syllables constituted the language proper, "la langue"; while the endless variations, omissions, and substitutions of phonemes in everyday usage were to be referred to speech, "la parole".

Thus "la langue", the series of stable phonemes, was caught up into a Platonic world quite apart from the changing and unstable articulations which imperfectly embody the phonemes in actual mundane speech, "la parole".

The I.P.A. of Bell-Sweet-Passy, the sonority (prominence) of Sievers-Passy, the phonemes of Saussure, and the separation of la langue and la parole of Saussure, all contributed to a system of signs which invited logical handling.

Saussure, Trubetzkoy, and le Cercle Linguistique de Prague, recognized the empirical nature of a science of linguistics including phonology. But in 1933 Trubetzkoy and Sapir turned to a mental world in which the observation and experimentation were to take place. For Trubetzkoy phonemes were distinguished by phonic differences in "what one imagines himself pronouncing"; Sapir asserted "the psychological reality of the phonemes". (99, p. 246) By 1939 the positivist position had prevailed and a mental world was no longer possible for observation and experiment. For an empirical science the material studied must be objective, i.e. accessible as it stands to any and all observers and investigators.

In what medium is articulate language to be presented for any and all investigators? It is impossible to appeal to a "linguistic consciousness" or to the imagination. If a phonemic or phonetic system is to be determined, a "phonemic transcription" or a "phonetic transcription", however meticulous, is subjective and begs the question. The slow, careful utterance of actual speech is the only objective material for the study of the units of an articulate language. Modern disks and films make it possible to play back for any investigator the actual utterance, i.e. the train of auditory signals; modern tracings from kymograph and oscillograph make the movements of articulation visible to any investigator. Phonemes and phoneme systems may be posited, but in an empirical science such hypotheses are subject to the test of the objective data of actual speech.

The series of characters which we read and write as representing an articulate language have given us a mistaken notion of the units which we utter and which we hear. The series of speech units cannot correspond to the series of "sounds" or "phonemes" set down on paper. Even "slow, careful utterance", let alone the rapid utterance of everyday, is much too fast for that. The maximum rate at which articulations can be uttered is 10–12 per sec.; and the maximum rate at which auditory signals can be identified is 14–16 per sec. A syllable of speech often indicates 2–7 phonemes; "do" has two, "tree" three, "quilt" five, "squelched" seven; the slow, careful rate of utterance is often 4–5 syllables per sec. Thus phonemes are often indicated 15–25 per sec. Obviously the phonemes are not uttered (or heard) one after the other; there must be extensive overlapping, as physiological tracings prove. The consonants do not prove to be separable units, they must have breath pressure behind them; the pressure is supplied by the pulses of the syllables in which they function. A consonant cannot be pronounced alone; it is always a characterized factor in some syllable. The supposed consonant "elements", which naive teachers assume that they are uttering, prove to be syllables with pulses from the chest, but often with the vowel shape unvocalized.

What is heard and said, therefore, is not a series of separate phonemes, but a series of syllables identified by overlapping articulations and grouped in breath groups. The series of separate phonemes is artificial, but it has proved a convenient way of representing a language on paper; although in some cases like the South Sea

Island group and the Japanese, a syllabary might be simpler. But the series of separate phonemes is misleading when it comes to the study of the articulations of speech, of the system of signals which are to convey meanings. The signals are not the separate phonemes, and the factors which the phonemes indicate do not occur as a simple series. Instead, the unitary signals of speech are the syllables, differentiated in various ways when made and heard. The syllable may be stressed, the syllable may have a different pitch (in 'tone' languages), the syllable may be started or stopped by a particular articulation, and the syllable may be emitted through a particular vocal-canal shape. What is identified is the syllable in its breath group, however its identifying factors may change, shift, appear and disappear, in the familiar modification which the play of articulations makes inevitable in varied utterance.

The schematized series of phonemes is not fitted to account for these connections and changes of the articulations which have their system and rationale in the speech apparatus and its movements. There has been an efflorescence of tonemes, prosodemes, neuremes, phones, allophones, phonemes segmental, phonemes supra-segmental, phonemes subdivided, posited, and multiplied, morpho-phonemes; positions (permissible sequence), phonemic phrases, junctures of sorts, boundary markers (Grenzsignale) etc.; and finally there has been this retreat into "description and classification only". All this serves to light the inadequacy of logistic manipulation of the phonemic signs. It is however becoming elaborate and confusing enough so that the next generation of phonologists may realize that learning the physiological mechanism of utterance and getting its bearing on the system, organization, and changes of the units of speech, is no more formidable and a great deal more rewarding.

Trubetzkoy's insight into the relative character of the limited number of significant articulations in a given language, and into the systematic relations of these articulations, and the substantial contributions of Trubetzkoy and his colleagues are not bound up with the arbitrary separation of *la langue* and *la parole*, and with the arbitrary definition of the phoneme as independent of the physiological movement of the syllable of which it is an aspect. The positive phases of Trubetzkoy's method will be considered in the proper place.

On the other hand, the positive contribution of Saussure-Trubetzkoy to phonology does not warrant the mistaken attempt to develop the Saussure-Trubetzkoy assumptions into a logistic phonemics in lieu of an empirical handling based on the physiological facts.

APPENDIX V

CONDITIONING AND THE UNITS OF SPEECH

How the Process of Conditioning Determines the Syllables and the Characterized Factors of Syllables

Bell, Sweet, Passy et al. undertook to define the "sounds" of language as auditory or articulatory patterns. It was soon apparent that while the words remained the same in varying conditions, the "sounds" changed.

F. de Saussure referred the constancy of the words to *la langue*, the conceptual language; and he referred the changing "sounds" to the varying physiological processes of *la parole*, the actual speech.

The constant words were assumed to be composed of stable "phonemes" which, as unchanging attributes, took the place of the former "sounds". And the phonologist faces the question of how all the variations of a "sound" of *la parole* come to be identified as the constant phoneme of *la langue*.

The fixation of the particular trait of the phoneme, and the way it functions as a differential in the syllable, depend on the process in psychology known as conditioning. The method by which an animal is conditioned and the method whereby the syllable is differentiated for the speaker of the articulate language are essentially the same.

Conditioning has been a fairly successful method of getting answers from the animal. The dog comes to respond to the signal which is parsed out and separated from the mass of noises round him. Sometimes the signal is a complex noise, a click, or hiss, or buzz; sometimes it is differential when the dog is expected, e.g., to learn the difference between the sound of a fork at 250 cycles per sec. and the sound of a fork at 260 cycles per sec., or to respond to the louder of two sounds, etc. So the members of the household come to distinguish the front doorbell, the rear doorbell, and the telephone; and to distinguish the high note of the whistle teakettle from the low hum of the electric fan.

Animals and human beings learn to respond to auditory signals in much the same way. The conditioning process is the same. Traits which are nearly alike but within the range of the human or the animal ear may be discriminated, or a group of obviously different traits may be counted as all-one. Thus similar traits may be sharply differentiated, or they may be 'generalized' and counted the same, depending on the circumstances and the resulting habit formation.

The differentiating trait is never presented as an isolated occurrence; it is always a phase, an aspect of a composite event. The experimenter may be interested in the pitch of the tuning fork which is sounded for the dog or child; but it is evident that the dog or child is reacting to a sound in context; and at first the context in which the sound occurs may be more important than its pitch. When the dog or child does not come to respond to the difference of pitch of the two forks, the pitch has not been discriminated as a separate factor, however apparent it may be to the experimenter. If instead of the usual tuning forks two pitch pipes are substituted, a new conditioning process is necessary. In time the dog or child may come to respond to a whole series of sound sources in which each pair differs primarily by this given pitch difference. One is not justified, however, in saying that the dog or child is listening for the pitch, although the pitch is the common factor in telling the occurrences apart. And if now you ask the dog or child to discriminate a tuning fork and a pitch pipe by this given pitch difference, you must undertake a new conditioning process. In fact, a skilled singer accustomed to a piano accompaniment may find it difficult to adjust to an organ or an orchestra.

All the traits of the sounds will figure, the quality, the loudness, the onset, the termination, the duration of the sound; and also the context of the sound in the course of the animal's actions, and of the series of stimuli to which he is responding. Though often overlooked, the context and the timing of the "sound" are part of the event to which the response is made.

Most recognition is based on the overall pattern of the event, not on the discrimination of a single trait. Only careful investigation will control or even reveal the "significant factor". That you may not demand of a witness the items on which his identification is based is an established principle in the law of evidence—since the days when the 'Law Lords' decided that a tailor might indeed know his own stitches but might not be asked how he knew them. The handwriting expert and the art specialist may study the details of strokes and brushwork, but the bank cashier or the art critic are not aware of unique details; they judge by the whole.

A notation convenient for the conditioning of animals is also available for the type of conditioning which stereotypes the articulations of a human language.

In a project of conditioning the dog, one may assume that there are to be these basic signal-events: a click, or a hiss, or a buzz, which have been conditioned so that they have definite meanings for the dog, i.e. to each of these signal-events the dog makes a definite conditioned response. These signal-events are always composite, and they occur in a specific context. The signal-events operate in the field of the dog's actual behavior. Such actual basic events can be notated: c = click, s = hiss, and z = buzz. They have an order in the dog's train of actions, and the order is very important in conditioning, but *order as such* does not figure as a signal or phase of a signal for the dog. (The dog can of course be conditioned to *order*, but that is another matter.) The signal is actually a process and may have an obvious duration, or may even involve a temporal pattern. The signals c, s, z, as events in the dog's behavior may occur again and again in a series of experiments, or in the course of a single experiment. They correspond to "*la parole*".

When the psychologists set up an experiment, they talk about these signals as items to handle in setting up experiments for the dog or other animal. And they want convenient signs for these signals, to refer to them in the experiment with the animal, to lay out the procedure in advance, and to make records of the experiment. It will be convenient to use C, click, S, hiss, Z, buzz, which will be distinct from c, s, z, which indicate the actual occurrences in the train of a given animal's reactions in actual life. C, S, Z refer to any possible occurrence of such signal to any animal producing a specific response, i.e. to any occurrence of c, s, z which has happened or will happen in context in the conditioned reactions of any animal in any laboratory. C, S, Z generalize c, s, z and refer to them regardless of any particular species, or any context, and as mere events, regardless of duration, they are "zeitlos". They correspond to *la langue*. Thus C, S, Z are the generalized events independent of any particular occurrence, c, s, z are the actual conditioned occurrences in a dog's behavior; these are "signal-events".

In the course of experimentation it may be interesting to see what the dog can make of signals in series; will he respond to a train of signals? The dog will learn a maze, which is an actual order in the train of the dog's behavior. If the maze is separated into "maze-segments", will the dog recognize the "segments" and respond to them in a new order, etc.? For this layout we will ask the psychologist to use a different sort of sign, with provision for order, and with means of separating groups of signs. C, S. Z as such will not do because they are generalized and refer to any occurrence of the basic events, c, s, z, without reference to order, repetition, duration, or grouping. The new signs are to be used when the click, hiss, buzz are items which occur for the dog in succession. Psychologists may not see the need of such special signs; left to themselves they would use the same old C, S, Z with some extra marks if necessary, and they would assume the C, S, Z to mean now the basic events c, s, z and now the c, s, z items as ordered and grouped when presented to the dog. We need some modification of C, S, Z which shows that we refer to the c, s, z as ordered items in the train of the dog's actions and we need certain extra marks to show the precise connections in the ordering and grouping. This corresponds to the transcription device used in phonetics.

Let these ordered items in a group be notated c s z s, e.g.; *that* c begins the group as *c-,* and that the second *s* ends the group as *-s*, and that the first *s* and the *z* are in the middle of the group as *-s-* and *-z-*. Let the fact that it is a group be indicated by the spacing, e.g., *c s z s s z c z c s.* In conditioning experiments it may prove that the distinction of *c-* and *-s* from *-s-* and *-z-* is important because the dog's response to a series when the *c-* is an initial item and to a series when *-c* is a terminal item may be unlike his response to a series when the *-c-* is a medial item. The trains may be as brief as two items. It is of interest to see how the dog responds with longer series when the same items occur again and again in the train.

Experiments may show that the response of the animal to a series *c s z s*, or *s z c* or *z c s* is not directly related to his response to c, s, and z. The group, the series, becomes a composite signal. The notation can be formulated as follows:

It seems so easy for the animal psychologist to keep track of 1) those different facts of the actual signals as they operate in the dog's behavior, and of 2) the different uses of the signs for animal signals in general, and also for the same items arranged in series, that he does not take the trouble to distinguish them. The fact is, however, that by inventing terminology, reidentifying the terms, mixing differential with concrete items, the psychologists have got conditioning into about as bad a snarl as is phonology.

It is taken for granted that the dog or other domestic animal will respond to speech signals quite as well as he does to the click, hiss, and buzz. The signal may be a single syllable, a whistle, or a group of syllables: "Come, Down, Gee, Haw; Here Jack, Lie down, Dead dog, Sic 'em; Sit up like a man, Go lie down." The dog's ear for the differences in phonemes could easily be tested by varying the phonemes of the command and making the differences significant.

The dog comes to respond to the specific command—a group of syllables—if it is properly introduced into the train of his actions. Some normal ('unconditioned') stimulus situation must lead to the response which is finally conditioned to the command. The dog responds only when the words occur in a definite situation. The dog does not hear (and respond) when the words occur in everyday speech even though they have the exact form of the command.

The dog—or cat—will "answer", i.e. bark, whine, miaow, in response to the speech signal "Speak" in the proper situation. The conditioning

1. Events in general as signals for animals.	C S Z __	A collection with the definite cardinal number 3; no determinate order.
2. Events in series as signals for animals.	*c s z* __	(Supplemented by additional marks, *c-, -c, -c-,* and by symbol of spacing). Linear series; an indeterminate number of events, since the same event may occur again and again. The order is determinate. Although not indicated, it is assumed to be uni-directional to match the temporal order of c, s, z, the basic events.
3. Basic events, signal-events for animals.	c s z __	Linear series of signals as they appear in a dog's actual train of behavior; the series has the definite uni-directional ordering in time (items may appear between the signals, but the signals retain the irreversible succession of the time line despite intercalations.)

depends on catching and stereotyping, and reinforcing the pattern with food or approval (which is the terminus of action and relaxes tension). When the dog is bent on winning through, when his whole musculature is straining toward a given response, his chance single bark, which may be counted "no", or a trochee bark, which may be counted "yes, yes", is fixed as the proper response in that situation. So the dog learns his answers to questions; so the dog learns to "ask" to be fed or let through a door.

The "talking dog" can imitate the rhythms and something of the general characteristics of the human syllable series, if the trainer starts with the dog's own barks and rhythms, and leads him on to learn a short, stereotyped train of "syllables". And the dog learns to respond to a stereotyped train of syllables with his own opposite train of syllables to get food or approval. But he gets mixed up with a repertory of more than four or five such "questions" and "answers". And if he gives the wrong answer, he may, in desperation, give you his whole box of syllable tricks, as if to say: "There they all are, take your pick."

Although dogs are far more intelligent than birds, a dog has rather little inclination to imitate. Food or approval give meaning to the signals for the dog or young child. But there are other animal "meanings". The parrot repeats all sorts of noises, and long trains of human signals; the mockingbird and the northern catbird are given to sitting on a branch at nightfall and rehearsing odds-and-ends of others' songs that they have picked up during the day. The odds-and-ends have some meaning to them, or they would not distinguish such items.

To a limited degree the parrot may make use of his remarkable repertory of human articulatory signals, e.g., "Polly wants a cracker"; and he may whistle a dog insistently, and when the dog comes up, puzzled, yell and shout "Get out", and the dog sneaks off. How near the parrot's animal signals come to human symbols—which he seems to use with a third species—and if the parrot and the dog "reason", and if not why not, can be left to the animal psychologist to explain to the owners of the pets.

Although the "talking dog" and the parrot imitate human syllables, they always handle the train of signals as a (composite) whole. The dog and the parrot distinguish "come" and "gun", but the series of consonant, vowel, consonant which the phonetician notes is not a 'series' to the animal. Every syllable has a release, a vowel shape, an arrest, and may be represented by RVA, rva. But for the animal, rva is a basic event; rva = c, or s, or z. So *rva rva* or *rva rva rva* are notated as serial items in the reactions of the talking dog and the parrot who make the responses in simple series.

The experimenter may speak of "speech signals" and record them as RVA_1, RVA_2, etc., but to the animal they are as unitary as the click, c; the hiss, s; or the buzz, z. If the experimenter is interested in the animal's ability to discriminate small phoneme changes in the "speech" signal—as he is interested in the animal's ability to discriminate small pitch changes in a signal—the following conventional notation will be convenient: "Ah, Go, Come, Down". The same notation may be used to indicate rhythmic speech signals, i.e. feet composed of these syllables.

The following table treats speech signals after the plan for signals of all sorts given on p. 164.

Groups 1 and 2 are types of notation used by the experimenter. While the items differentiate the overall character of the syllables, the items do not figure as such in the reactions of the animals.

1. Generalized signs for any occurrence of syllables (and syllable factors) with any animal (including man):

I.	Ah SYL_1	Go SYL_2	Up SYL_3	Come SYL_4	Down SYL_5	____ Conventional notation.
II.	RVA	RVA	RVA	RVA	RVA	____ Notation for syllables as units, indicating a factor for release, for vowel-shaping, and for arrest.
III.	OVO	CVO	OVC	CVC	CVC	____ Notation for syllables as units, indicating vowel and consonant; with chest release or/and chest arrest, indicated by O.

2. Schematized signs for any occurrence in group patterns of syllables and syllable factors with any animal (including man):

IV.	rva	rva	rva	rva	rva	____ Notation of syllable units in series, indicating the factors.
V.	OvO	cvO	Ovc	cvc	cvc	____ Notation of syllable units in series, indicating vowel and consonant, and chest release and arrest.
VI.	rva O O	rva goO	rva O p	rva k m	rva daun	____ Notation of syllable units in series, indicating the specific vowels and consonants.
VII.	Go rva goO ./...../	up, rva O p ....../.	up! rva O p ./	Ah, rva O O ./..	come rva k m /.........	down! rva daun ./.. ____ The underlining indicates the breath-pulse of which the releasing, vowel-shaping, and arresting movements are a part. The dotted lines indicate the breath groups of which the syllable pulses are a part.

3. Signs for actual signals as they occur in the train of actions of given animal (or human being):

VIII.	syl₂ rva goO /...../	syl₃ rva O p ...../	syl₃ rva O p	Dog climbs up	syl₁ rva O O /...	Dog stops	syl₄ rva k m /......	syl₅ rva daun ./..	Dog comes down	Syllables as actual units in course of dog's actions; syllables represent as pulses which compose breath groups.

Interpretation of the signs in the table above:
I. The conventional notation of the human speech signal "Go, come, etc.".
II. RVA, RVA indicates merely that they are "speech signals" and therefore have some type of release, arrest, and vowel shape; but there is no indication of the type.
III. OVO, CVO, etc., indicates the speech signals as syllables with the release and arrest by the chest (O-, O) or by a consonant (C-, -C); but no definite consonants (or vowels) are specified.
IV. rva, rva as in II, save that they are to occur in series.
V. OvO ovO as in III, save that they are to occur in series.

VI., VII., VIII.
rva
O O indicates chest release and chest arrest, and the specific vowel—
rva
goO indicates consonant g-releasing, chest arrest, and specific vowel—
rva
O p indicates chest release, consonant p arresting, and specific vowel—
rva
k m indicates consonant k releasing, consonant m arresting; specific vowel.
rva
daun indicates consonant d releasing, consonant n arresting, specific vowel -au-.

Group 3, syl₂, syl₃...., indicate the conditioned units in the behavior of the animal (or child). The analysis, goO, O p.. is the analysis of the experimenter but has no place in the animal's behavior. It is convenient for handling the specific differentials.

Conditioning of the Child to Speech Signals
(46, p. 21–38; 67; 102, p. 281)

At an early stage, three to nine months, the child often experiments, plays, with a variety of articulations without reference to the speech about him. It shows that the child's articulatory apparatus is as well fitted for any language as for any other. Anthropologists and psychologists are agreed that there is no specialization for language. In fact, any child learns any language with equal ease. It is uncertain if this early articulatory activity has any influence on the later speech of the child. Although a variety of articulations are practiced, the repertoire of the child's future language(s) may not be covered. This is the first appearance in the child's development of articulatory events suitable for articulate signals (cf. c, s, z and rva, rva, rva of the animal). It is to be noted that at this babbling stage, the articulations are always in the form of repeated syllables. Cf. Lewis and Velten, above.

Before he attempts to speak, the time comes when the child recognizes human articulate signals as does the dog. The child responds to his name, and looks for the dog or cat or toy when it is named, and comes to know the meaning of "no, no" with headshaking, and "yes" with nodding. He recognizes the signal "come" just as he does the gesture of beckoning; he knows the meaning of "go", "go outdoors", "buggy" just as he knows the meaning of bringing outdoor wraps, or the go-cart. He responds to the signal series "milk" just as he does to the preparation of his food. He may make random articulatory responses which are not words.

As with any other animal, the conditioning occurs because the train of articulations is presented with and before the act or object. The nurse calls his name as she enters the room, she says his name as she takes him up; she indicates by gestures with the proffered object that it is "for Bobby", etc. Getting his coat and hat occur before the walk outdoors, and "go", "go outdoors", "buggy" are repeated in the sequence of getting ready to go out. Reinforced by repeated outings the articulate signals come to mean going out. "Milk" is repeated as the bottle or the cup of milk is prepared and in turn comes to mean being fed. So the articulate signals become conditioned stimuli for the child's action or active expectation.

The gesture to 'come' may be the beginning of the act of being drawn to the mother and taken up, and both the gesture and the articulate signal become conditioned stimuli. Later, when the child is creeping toward the mother, "Come" is part of his reception. "No, no" and headshaking are followed by interference and possibly punishment and come to be inhibiting conditioned stimuli.

The rise of the child's own peculiar "words" is interesting. The child makes some chance vocal response to the coming food, and is immediately fed; the chance articulation if repeated is reinforced by more food, and presently the child "has a word" i.e. he has an articulate signal which will produce food (or pet or toy) which becomes "his word" for the object or act.

Still there is no articulate response to articulate signals and little that is reciprocal about these speech signals. They are still on the level of the dog's ways who responds to his name, performs tricks to articulate signals, and learns on his own to bark when he wants to get out or in, or to sit-up-and-beg when he wants food. To associate with human beings, to pick up their ways, and respond, marks the "domesticated" animal.

Then comes the time of reciprocal games and the child imitates what the other does. In peekaboo the adult hides and peeks, and the child imitates, and may reproduce the articulate signal "peek". The adult pats the child's palms together in "pattycake", then pats the child's palm against the adult palm and the child follows suit, and may repeat "pat, pat".

All along the child may be imitating articulations. When training the "talking dog", the trainer imitates the dog's chance barking; and so the adult imitates the child's chance articulation, then the child repeats, and makes a reciprocal game of the alternations of his own utterance. Presently he may try to imitate any repeated articulation of the adult. Words are pronounced which the child imitates, and which come in the course of the child's actions to have conditioned meanings, and the child comes to ask for things and to announce things.

It is natural enough to think of the syllables and breath groups which the child is to learn as a fixed pattern; we use such terms as fixing, stereotyping the consonants (the various ways of releasing or arresting the syllable) and the vowels (the various ways of shaping the vocal canal). We know that the pattern of the syllable and the breath group varies, but we are prone to think that the child first learns the slow, careful form which we count the true form; and then later, has to learn to recognize the variants from this standard form. But the fact is that the child catches and tries to reproduce the overall pattern of the breath group and is conditioned to the variation of the details from the beginning of the process of recognizing the breath group and of the process of learning to reproduce the breath group. So in other forms of conditioning the subject comes to identify as the same a wide range of signals; so in early language conditioning the child identifies as the same the range of the given breath group in which phonemes change and shift and syllables may disappear and reappear. And the child's reproduction often begins with a variation beyond the tolerance of the language; it is finally brought within the tolerated range of variation by the conditioning process of learning to speak to be understood. The child's efforts, however inadequate, always involve the whole pattern of a breath group. This is of primary importance in handling the changes, shifts, and restorations of phonemes and syllables.

It seems convenient to teach a foreign language, and to teach speech to the deaf, in terms of the slow, careful forms. The result is often a peculiar classroom dialect, badly infected with the native speech habits, which determines the silent pronunciation in reading and interferes in getting the colloquial language. The dialect can be understood only by the initiated. The war-time emphasis on colloquial practice from the start is an excellent corrective of American methods of language teaching. In some schools for the deaf curious travesties on the actual speech are taught and accepted as "correct" which no outsider finds intelligible.

From the first the articulations of the child are breath groups; they are usually of one syllable but they are uttered from the abdominal musculature, and often have considerable emphasis when uttered as a demand. The child's management of crying, and the small harangues, "jabbering", which some children indulge in long before they can talk, show that the mechanism of chest-pulse syllables in abdominal breath groups functions before speech appears. But at first the demands of the regulated utterance make one syllable enough to manage. Soon the child tries for two syllables, of his name or the name of some object. Sometimes the two syllables are the same syllable repeated, "mama, papa, babay, bub-bub". Presently a simple vowel variation may be achieved, "da-die, ba-bie, daw-die (doggie), Bobbie". Then come unlike syllables 'choc'et" (chocolate), " cwe²co" (ice-cream cone). Though the child may not be able to follow the detail of the pattern set, it is significant that the grouping and stress of the breath group, i.e. the rhythm of the breath group, is achieved: "Harriet" becomes "Ha-ha"; "water" becomes "wa-wa"; "Miss Cope" becomes "Ko-ko". This reduplication of a single syllable is common with children who learn normal speech very late. They get the rhythm of the breath group but often repeat a syllable to fill in where they cannot manage the articulations prescribed. "Persistent infantile speech" gives an excellent opportunity to observe the process of shaping up the phonemes and syllables within the breath group. However imperfect the child's speech, which only his associates can understand, he forms breath groups of the normal type and the rhythm within these breath groups is often the clue to his words and meaning. His sounds are often non-native; a glottal catch for an arresting consonant, especially k/g is common; and as he learns the correct articulation of r and l, e.g., his habitual substitutes of w lead him to labialize the l or r. But the character of the syllable as released or arrested is usually normal, and the grouping and stress of the breath group is attained. Unlike an adult learning a foreign language, he does not impose a false rhythm or intonation.

The fundamental movement of the breath group comes first with the child just as the main movements of skipping and dancing are learned first and the details of the steps come later. This ensures the basic train of syllables in the breath group, the grouping and stress, which constitute the basis for the traits of the rhythm and of the articulations. Children get the overall pattern of the breath group; they frequently omit syllables as well as articulations, but they seldom add anything. (67) The movements of speech constitute an organized system, not a collection of separate details of articulation. If the basic movements are right, many of the details of articulation and the combinations and modifications are mechanical and inevitable. The precise syllables and syllable factors and their wide variations are acquired *pari passu*, with the manipulation of the breath-group movements.

Traits like voicing, nasalization, vowel reduction, and aspiration come to the child in part by imitation when the syllable or phrase is repeated to him; and in part when he finds that his approximation is not understood and he tries for the conventional form which *works* and is thereby reinforced. The child and the adult who "picks up" a language, never undertake to separate articulations of the syllable nor even of the breath group. The repetition of the same syllable, preserving the rhythm of the breath group, the substitution of familiar articulation for the actual "sounds" in the course of the breath group, the folk etymologies (tu ora—trou aux rats;

asparagus—sparrow grass, etc.) show that such a learner is always handling the breath group of one or more syllables. For the child it is the syllable or group of syllables which is difficult to get, not some one articulation in the syllable. The sophisticated adult may practice some foreign articulation in a simple syllable, but it is hard to incorporate it into continuous speech; his native speech habits dominate.

Chance phonetic identities from language to language are unnoticed. The boy from the farm does not note that the calling of sheep (ü) and pigs ("pügg, pügg) introduces the umlaut; he struggles with the German "sounds" as something novel. The familiar affirmative-negative "grunts" (anh-hanh, unh-hunh) and the derisive "mp-yinh-yinh" are identical with the French nasals *an* (en) *un, in*. Only an acute observer notes the French *u* in the pronunciation of New York as "ny-york". -*Ng* is said to be arresting only, in English. But it must shift to releasing in "ring in. . . ." etc., which we realize when we hear the false, dialectic "ring-gin"—although in standard English the abutting group "*fing-ger, Eng-glish*", are common.

The precision of the child's conditioned articulations in the train of speech is no greater than the precision of the various expressive movements which make up the deportment of his particular nationality ("race"). The peculiar American swing of the shoulder and arms, the 'stealthy' tread of the American Indian, the palmsfront of the Javanese carriage of the arms, the "military" bearing of the school cadet, the soft, slow enunciation of the southerner, the high-pitched monotonous voice of the American in contrast with the low-pitched, throaty voice of the English woman, are all assumed in the course of the child's rearing. The bow, the lifting of the hat, the handshake are quite as specific and ingrained as is the national speech accent. Some of these actions are reciprocal and so subject to correction, "reinforcement", but some are primarily imitative and without direct reinforcement. The American in Japan or China is amazed to find that his whistle or call means nothing to the 'native' dog. Animals share to some extent in the national signals.

Meantime, at least by a year old, the child begins to reason, a stage to which the dog never comes, though he may be astute in other ways. The auditory signals to which the child responded at first became articulatory signals which the child employed. But now the articulatory signals, syllables in breath groups, have become articulatory symbols. (18) The child solves problems, forms concepts; and his ability to name objects, and actions, and to make verbal recipes, becomes important for this reasoning process. And thus language with its morphology and syntax gets under way. While the child is able to make all the syllables in breath groups with all their factors and aspects which his language involves, by two-and-a-half or three years of age, he will still be learning the morphological forms and fitting them into breath groups according to the basic syntax until perhaps ten years old; his vocabulary will grow rapidly to twenty-five, and more slowly thereafter. (105) Although it is not a problem in phonology, one may note that the child acquires the complex morphological-syntactic-semantic apparatus of any language by imitating, by making or failing to make people understand, and by problem-solving and invention and experiment of his own.

The early use of articulatory signals as symbols separates the child from the dog. The mockingbird imitates his fellows, and the parrot imitates the human species, and they rehearse what they have heard. But it is never the recital of past events; it is repertory, not narrative. On the other hand, the child of two years, just in from his walk, struggles to tell you what he has seen. He uses the simplest expression: "Wind b'ow", "Dog" "Chou-chou", " 'It' kitty", "Dow-down" (fall down), "Aw detty" (all dirty) etc. There are no connectives, only isolated substantives; but there are statements and there may be chronological or logical order.

In setting up a system of signals and symbols for human speech it is convenient to modify the table of:

1. General symbols for any occurrence of syllables and syllable factors, designated.
   Sign designs; which correspond to C S Z of animal psychology, p. 165. (There is seldom occasion to specify the sign designs for the articulatory signals used with animals). They constitute the (phoneme) alphabets, and the syllabaries.
2. Schematized symbols for any occurence in series of syllables and syllable factors, designated.

Sign events; which correspond to *c, s, z; c s z s s z c z c s* (p. 165); these are elaborate; constitute the written form of language; transcriptions.

3. The actual signals as they occur in the train of human speech activity. These are the phonetic events, sometimes composed of conditioned syllables with their specific characterized factors, which are mere trains of nonsense syllables. Sometimes composed of conditioned syllables (with their specific characterized factors) which have become symbols and carry linguistic meaning. They carry both the signal meaning to which the dog can respond, and the rational meanings which are always beyond him. The signal, which may be a symbol, or part of a symbol, is never less than the syllable; fact which Twaddell stresses in his version of phonemics.

The great bulk of non-literate language is embodied in 3, the actual signals, the phonetic events. The non-literate peoples find no occasion for the analysis of syllables into characterized factors, although they are familiar with rimes and varied word-plays depending on such items. It is the project of phonetic writing by alphabet or syllabary which forces such an analysis.

Long effort and experimentation in the course of history have produced the sign designs, and have made it possible to arrange sign events in the series of written language.

1. The Sign Designs: RVA, OVO, CVO, OVC, CVC, and the detailed, characterized factors of syllables, in which the releasing articulatory movements and the arresting movement proves to be the same movement with a different function in the syllable. Thus there are the occlusives; p/b, t/d, k/g, etc. A collection with a definite cardinal number; no determinate order, though an arbitrary one is common in alphabets and syllabaries.

    cf. 1. Generalized Signs for any occurrence of signals (p. 165)
    e.g. RVA   RVA
          p/b- -k/g
          t/d- -p/b
          k/g- -t/d

2. The Sign Events: Are a series of sign designs which constitute a linear series with an indeterminate number because of repetitions; the order is determinate; and although not symbolized, the order is assumed to be un-directional in order to refer to the temporal order of 3, actual articulatory signals.

    cf. 2. Schematized signs for group patterns of signals. (p. 166)

3. The Actual Articulatory Signals: Are the phonetic events which may be either signals or symbols for the human being.

    cf. 3. Signs for actual signals. (p. 166)

How the Child Learns to Read

By common consent, learning to read is postponed until the child has some command of the language in terms of the vernacular; and by common consent the vernacular is made the basis of the early instruction. The actual articulatory signals with their meanings are familiar to the child differentiated but unanalyzed of course.

The present method of teaching reading does not undertake even a rough analysis. The groups of signs, letters in series (sign events) are presented—but without reference to the individual sign events, the letters. There is no question that the child is not aware of a series of events in the "word"; he has no sense of "the factors of the syllable" nor of a series of separate signs on the page. The child associates the spoken word and the pictures of his primer with the (composite) symbol of each of the words. In the primer the "word method" with its pictures repeats each breath group again and again, and then repeats the breath group with a slight variation. This overall pattern of the word of one or more syllables is acquired rapidly by most children. There is no reference to "The Sign Designs", the collection of characters of the alphabet; the child is not sure of his separate letters and, to the horror of some of his elders, doesn't know the limited collection of letters in its (pointless) conventional order. "He doesn't know the alphabet and can't use a dictionary." He is in about the same case as those same elders when they try to read Black-letter capitals, or when they've come to the stage where they can pronounce a Greek or Hebrew text, but are not sure of the individual letters and have half-forgotten the alphabet in its order.

On the other hand, the printers and designers of type faces must handle the sign designs as clearly differentiated; and yet they may design the type, and they may set it, without knowing any of the "meanings". The type for many mathematical symbols must be so designed and many mathematical books so set. The printers and designers work entirely with the sign designs and the sign events. It is a matter of pattern, not of mathematical meaning; and they never consider the actual use of the signs in problem solving or in utterance.

The difficulties of an occasional child who is slow in learning to read by the "word method" throws light on the learning process. For a long time the child has no means of making out the word on the page for himself; the conditioned stimulus of the picture, or the unconditioned and reinforcing utterance of the teacher is necessary. If those fail the child is helpless. The likenesses and differences of the one-syllable words, and the division of words into syllables have not come to him yet. In time he will be conditioned to the various releasing, vocalic, and arresting factors of the syllables; he will react to the "-at family": "at, bat, cat, fat, gat, hat, gnat, pat, rat, sat, tat, vat"; to the "pi-family: pie, pike, pied, pile, pine, pyre, pies". And he will make an added -e mean a "long vowel"; "ate, hate, cate, fate, hate, pate, rate, sate; so pipe, pike, pile, pine, etc.". As an adult he will come to have a rough-and-ready system of "phonetic" pronunciation of English which the catalogs of phonographic records can depend on to help him ask for what he wants in the maze of foreign names and titles. The older teachers are probably right: the knack of picking the word off the page without outside help, which the adult finally gets, could be got much earlier and many children might be saved from balks in learning to read. But it is important to note that this does not involve taking the syllables of the words apart; but it does involve catching the resemblances of the syllables; using the phoneme to indicate a class of syllables, as Twaddell would insist. Effective reading in all its stages is to be taught without an attempt to break up the syllable and use the pieces; and this can be done by comparing the syllables and getting the child to see how the syllables are alike and unlike.

Interpretation and Evaluation of the Notation of Human and Animal Conditioning to Speech Signals

The notation of the signals for the talking dog and the parrot must be supplemented by a statement in detail of the situation in which the conditioning occurred. The list of speech signals of a convenient analysis (1, alphabet, syllabary, p. 165), and the experimenter's notated records, 2, p. 166, must be interpreted by the animal subject's way of dealing with the speech signals when perceived and reproduced. In animal psychology we resort at once to the actual signal events in the course of the subject's behavior.

1. The animal's physiological apparatus sets limitations in the case of the talking dog, which are less obvious in the case of the parrot.
2. The animal's capacity for reproducing the speech signals and for collating the signals with meanings differs; the dog will respond; he is far more capable of playing a social game of question and answer, and of collating the speech signals with meanings than is the parrot; but the dog does not have the parrot's remarkable ability to imitate the *sounds* of the signals.
3. There is no question that the dog and parrot deal with the speech signals in syllables and phrases, "words"; it is always syl_1, syl_2, syl_3 etc., and never OaO goO, O p, etc. The composition of the signals is written in the notation of 1 and 2, pp. 165–166, for the convenience of the experimenter; there is nothing corresponding in the course of the animal's behavior. The phonemic notation does not indicate the meaning which the signal has been conditioned for; for the meaning to the animal, we must consult the conditioning procedure.

The conditioning of the child to speech signals follows much the same pattern. He is in command of all the types of syllables of his language by the age of three, as already noted; which can be interpreted in terms of 2, p. 166, to mean that he "knows all the phonemes".

1. The human physiological apparatus for speech furnishes the human child with the range of articulatory movements.
2. The child's capacities for perceiving and reproducing speech signals will enable him to select from the range of articulatory movements the component, conditioned movements of the specific language mechanism. The controllable movements for the speech signals and the collated meanings are far more extensive than in

the case of the dog or the parrot.
3. Nevertheless, there is no question that the signal events, syl_1, syl_2, syl_3, etc., figure as units in the course of the child's behavior.

Reasoning will play its part in the development of the language system of the human being. The child and the adult will come to appreciate rime and the varied word plays, which an experimenter may analyze and notate in terms of the "phonemes" (i.e. the characterized factors of syllables), but the subject treats them always in terms of syllables in breath groups and phrases, "words", and knows nothing of the types of rime or of the composition of syllables.

Since the accurate determination of a phoneme alphabet must depend on physiological investigation, there is every reason to turn to the physiological process of utterance for a system which will account for these shifts, changes, lapses and restorations of the phoneme. Reversible change's, depending on variations of stress-and-grouping and on rate, are certainly systematic, and point to activities within the specific mechanism of the language in question.

And there is an interesting relation between the reversible changes of the contemporary language and the irreversible changes of historical phonology. At each stage of the historical change some generation or generations must have found the older form and the newer form of variation at that stage tolerable and intelligible, because the identity of the word or phrase has persisted through the most radical phonological changes. The study of the historical changes is an excellent clue to the physiological changes of a contemporary language.

The teaching of reading confirms the statements about the unit involved in speaking. The teaching of reading by the "word method" handles the language in syllable wholes. And it was true in the days when words were taught by their spelling, alphabetic or 'phonic', that learning by syllables occurred in spite of the tedious spelling.

APPENDIX VI

REDUCTION OF A LANGUAGE TO PHONEMES

If a language is literate, the orthography is bound to figure in the process of developing the scientific notation of the syllables. The orthography may be approximately phonetic, German, Italian, or it may be traditional and at variance with the present phonemes and syllables (English and French); or it may have been adapted from another language, with fairly adequate modification in case of the Russian orthography, or rather poor results in case of the Arabic characters used for Turkish and Malay.

If the language is non-literate, the natives know word plays, are aware of assonances, alliterations, and may use rime. If the verse of the language has a regular meter, this will help to determine the syllable and the permissible stress system.

For this essential phonetic analysis, Sweet, Saussure, Passy, Trubetzkoy and the phonemicists have depended on a traditional phonetics often inexact, employing now articulatory and now auditory criteria. Trubetzkoy (100, p. 17), "must be physiological"; Martinet (10, p. 273 f), "must have concrete individuality"; Pos (101, p. 78), Trager and Bloch propose a careful study of experimental data concerning segmental, prosodic, and rhythmic features, in the course of a discussion of "open juncture".

There is some general recognition of the physiological articulation as the fundamental event, but most linguists depend on what they assume to be an auditory impression. Experienced observation has been the principal resource; sometimes the investigator tries repeating the "sound" if it is in his own language, or tries to imitate the "sound" if it is foreign, to determine its characteristics, perhaps with the help of a "small mirror". Because of the practical difficulties there has been very little use made of such exact experimental methods as are now available.

An intelligent native of the non-literate language, with some practice in writing a culture language, is likely to do best in noting the essential articulations. In any case, only the phonetic distinctions which are significant for the meanings of the given language are to be noted.

The International Phonetic Alphabet as it stands is not available for the notation of a given language. Of necessity it does not fit the specific phonemic system of any language. Investigators modify the I.P.A. radically, introduce new characters, modify the stock characters, and set up various conventions as to breath-group, stress, and possibly 'tones'.

The analysis is of course to be in terms of the given language. For practical purposes 'phonemes' are always identified by reference to standard words of the given language. Phonetic treatises use a notation based on well-known languages; and the standard word lists for the "sounds" of pronouncing dictionaries identify the phonemes—at some risk—in terms of familiar words. It is the one way in experimental work to set patterns for a subject, and to indicate the actual syllables used, for other investigators. It is dependent on uniform habits of pronunciation.

In psychological terms it is dependent on stability of conditioning.

The number of syllables in the given language will vary from a minimum of 40 or 50 to as many as 5000 or more, depending on the permissible syllable patterns of the language. And variants of each syllable which involve traits which may be significant in the language in question must be noted. Vowels may diphthongize in stressed syllables, or reduce to schwa in unstressed syllables; an arresting consonant may change, shift to the next syllable, or drop; a releasing consonant may fuse with the preceding arresting consonant, or shift to arresting position in a preceding open syllable as its own syllable drops. In the final form of the corpus of the various syllables of the given language, there may be several variants of each basic syllable which are the various phonetic forms of the syllable. The basic syllables are determined by reference to meaning in morphone stems, affixes and infixes. If these syllable types are put on cards for machine sorting, a card will be punched for each variant of every syllable. (If new variants or new syllables are discovered in the course of the analysis, they are added, of course.)

Analysis of the Corpus of Syllables to Determine the Complete List of the Phonemes— the Phoneme Alphabet—not as "Elements, Segments" but as the Characterized Factors of the Syllables in the Breath Group

It is convenient to designate the phoneme by the form in which it appears in slow, careful utterance, and usually as it occurs in a single syllable in the breath group. The use of the syllables as conditioned signals with meaning has moulded the syllables to be analyzed; but in the process of analysis they are treated as nonsense syllables.

PHONETIC AND PHONEMIC ALPHABETS

Since the corpus of syllables is designated by phonetic signs for the specific articulations (characterized factors of the syllable) it would seem that the task of isolating the "sounds" is already accomplished. A phonetic alphabet has already been set up composed of such different articulations as are significant (conditioned to meanings) in the given language.

The phonetic alphabet, however, merely indicates the "sounds" as they occur in each syllable without reference to their relations, while the phoneme alphabet designates each type articulation and identifies its variants through all the changes, compounds, shifts, dropping and reappearances of the type articulation. The phoneme, then, designates the set of reversible forms which the type articulation assumes in the varying conditions of utterance of the syllable in the breath group. When the variant of the one phoneme comes to coincide phonetically with the variant of another phoneme, the phoneme sign designates which phoneme is actually represented by the ambiguous articulation. In such cases a change of rate and stress will cause the ambiguous articulation to revert to the type form of the phoneme. It is easy to apply the test: if the utterance keeps the same linguistic ("intellectual") meaning through the changes caused by rate and stress, the phoneme remains the same.

It is worth emphasizing how wide may be the "phonic difference" in certain conditions without changing the linguistic meaning of the utterance in which it occurs. The minimum "phonic difference" to produce a change in linguistic meaning is not a fixed difference, but varies radically with the conditions of utterance. In one situation the difference of voicing of a consonant (aspect of a syllable factor) may change the meaning; in another situation the change of voicing, or the dropping of the consonant articulation, or even of the entire syllable, may not change the meaning. The characteristics of the phoneme change with the changing situation (in which rate and stress are primary).

Analysis of the Relations of the Phonemes in this List Drawn from the Corpus of Syllables; Classifications, Differentiations, Various Relations and Groupings

The syllable is not a self-subsistent unit; it must be part of a foot and a breath group. The types of breath group and the position of the syllable in the breath group have a profound influence on the phoneme. Hence, for the phonemes of any language, 1) the types of breath group movement incorporating the syllables, and 2) the types of syllable movement (pulses) permissible in the given language, are of primary importance.

Certain traits of syllables and of breath groups are correlated. The breath group with light and heavy stresses and with varied feet, is the basic movement for a series of syllables with frequent arresting consonants, which drop, abut, and shift with the reducing of vowels and the dropping of syllables; such syllables are a part of such breath groups. Cf. English and German.

The breath group with light and rather variable "word" stress and with little variation in the grouping of the syllables into feet, is the basic movement for a series of syllables with few arresting consonants, slight differences in the syllable duration, relatively little variation in the quality of the individual vowel, and few or no repressed syllables. Such a series is essential to the dynamic structure of such a breath group. Cf. French.

PHONEMES FROM LANGUAGE TO LANGUAGE

1. Since the beginning of comparative linguistics it has been assumed that "sounds", later called "phonemes", are equivalent or identical from language to language. The types of breath group and the types of permissible syllables will seldom be the same in two languages. It can hardly happen, however, that the two languages have *no* syllable factors in common (enphonic phonemes). A number of syllable factors will be somewhat alike. Nevertheless, the syllable types and the breath-group types of the respective languages make the like syllable factors unlike members of a phonetic system. If the essence of the phoneme is in its specific unlikeness to the other phonemes of the system peculiar to the one language, the handling of the 'phoneme' common to two or more phonemic systems, each in a different language, needs to be considered. Saussure insists: "Ce qui importe dans lemot, ce n'est pas le son luimême, mais les différences phoniques qui permettent de distinguer le mot de tout les autres." (75, p. 163)

"The phonic difference capable of differentiating intellectual meanings in a given language" (98; 99, p. 232) cannot be applied when there are no common meanings. Apart from meanings and in terms of nonsense syllables, it is certain that the phonemes of one language, i.e. the characterized syllable factors, cannot be equivalent to the phonemes of another language however closely alike the articulations may be. The English "do", and the German "du", and the French "doux", are all represented by the I.P.A. /du/. But the English series, "How de ye do, how de' do, how d'-do", shows possibilities quite foreign to the French. The French "doux" has a consonant form for the d- unlike the German and English releasing consonant, due to the difference in breath pressure. (89, p. 83; 61, p. 115)

The unit of utterance in which the phoneme of two languages is handled cannot be a "free form", for it is seldom that the same 'form' will occur in the two (or more) languages. The like syllables of the two languages, independent of morphology and of any form of meaning, must be the unit of utterance for the enphonic phoneme. In some sense such an enphonic phoneme is only a potential phoneme; the I.P.A. is a set of possible phonemes. When incorporated into specific syllables in breath groups, the enphonic phonemes become phonemes in the specific system of a language.

2. The development of the I.P.A. and of various notations for different language groups has been in response of the need of enphonic units. The processes of comparing and identifying the 'sounds' of the different living languages which have yielded the enphonic articulations for languages, both ancient and modern, has been carried on by bi-lingual speakers (or multi-lingual speakers). In the case of non-literate languages, members of the culture language have learned the non-literate language, often as children and without an accent; and members of the non-literate people often acquire the culture language in childhood. The practical business of devising an alphabet to write and print the non-literate language forces the consideration of the 'sounds' in terms of the stereotyped orthography of the literate language.

Where two peoples of different culture languages are in contact there must be bi-lingual speakers. Common religious-, business-, government, craft-, and art- terms are bound to interpenetrate and to be notated in the characters of both languages. Approximate and actual equivalents are found, and the unique 'sounds' noted. The brogue of the neighbors becomes familiar to each people, and picks out the minor differences of the 'sounds', if not the more fundamental differences of the breath-group and syllable-organization. There is the famous bit of practical phonetics in the "shibboleth" incident of the Old Testament when a phonetic variant meant life or death (Judges 12:6).

The recovery of the approximate values of the early characters is one of the amazing achievements. The Sanskrit grammarians undertook phonetic descriptions of the 'sounds'; the Greeks made a less successful analysis. Since the early descriptions and classifications of the 'sounds' could not be exact, the value of the ancient sign has ultimately to be worked down to the living language.

The ancient physiological descriptions must be verified by present-day manipulations of the speech apparatus. The ancient character may be traced down to living languages in various ways. There are many lines of evidence: a single alphabet has often been adapted to various unlike languages, hence many writing systems stem from the primitive Semitic alphabet. The cuneiform syllabary was extensively employed for languages of all sorts. On occasion words occur written in two or more notations. Hurrian and Akkadian are written in derivatives of the Sumerian syllabary, and also in the Ras-Shamra alphabet. Greek words are written in the Greek alphabet and in the Cypriote syllabary.

The various living Semitic languages furnish the clues for the values of the early signs. The vocalizing of the Late Egyptians has been established in some degree by a study of the Old Coptic 'sounds' determined in turn by reference to the phonological history of Coptic. The continuous history of Greek as a living language down to the present day—with all its recorded changes—and the comparative study of the Romance languages, have yielded a fair idea of the earlier values of the Greek and Latin at various epochs. And the two languages have furnished the alphabets for the notation of the European languages and have been adapted for the speech of many non-literate peoples. The Slavic languages are written in some cases in an alphabet derived from the Greek; and in some cases in an alphabet derived from the Latin. Arabic has been used for many unrelated tongues: Turkish, Persian, Urdu, Bantu, Malay. In general, the notation of a common culture language is likely to spread through its entire territory and may persist through all changes for centuries.

Words persist through the vicissitudes of phonological and lexical changes, and furnish the continuous chain by which phonological states are held together and the changes can be traced and defined. The method of comparison of modern forms in different languages and dialects has been made to yield remarkable results as to ancient values.

RELATIONS AMONG THE PHONEMES OF DIFFERENT LANGUAGES

Affiliation

The history of a given language and of its collaterals, all derived from a common source, demands an identification of common sounds' and a study of their changes. This is the basis of the historical phonology of the comparative philologists.

The relations of the phonemes and of the syllable and breath-group units of languages which are actually connected are due to conditioning to meanings from generation to generation. The word or locution proves to be more stable than either the lexical meaning or the phonetic factors of the syllable. The word or locution survives, though the breath-group and syllable organization may change radically—as in the case of French from Vulgar Latin. This makes it possible to trace the change or persistence of the phonemes. However marked the transformation in the course of centuries, even in times of rapid change the users of the language in each generation have found the variants equivalent.

Where the derivative languages have been isolated, their parallel histories may be very unlike. But all these changes have the common chain of utterances conditioned to meanings; the phonemes have been modified as they passed down, but the locutions have kept the continuity.

Such relation of phonemes have had a large share of the attention of linguists and may be called affiliated.

Association

Contemporary languages are to be compared and grouped according to their phonogical relations, whatever their connections may have been.

The relations of phonemes from language to language may be due to regional diffusion among languages which have few or no other connections. Regional diffusion or morphological and lexical influences may or may not occur where enphonic diffusion is striking, as in the case of American Indian languages, or the occurrence of the Hottentot (and Bushman) 'clicks' in the Bantu Zulu. The process of such peculiar transfers is uncertain and may vary from case to case. Such cross influences due to propinquity may be termed associated.

Parallelism

Independent groups of languages which can never have had common influences nevertheless present striking likenesses. Cf. Speiser (80, 81) and Z. S. Harris' comparison of American Indian Yokuts and Semitic (23, p. 210). The possible types of breath groups and of correlated syllable organization are limited; the possible types of syllables are limited; and the characterized syllable factors which the race finds available are limited. Therefore such (apparent) relation is due to parallel developments.

The (special) mechanism of each language must be a specialized version of the general phonology which can be stated in physiological terms, independent of meanings. It is not surprising that there are striking chance resemblances. A general phonology was the hope of Trubetzkoy. Such chance likeness may be called parallel.

Groups of languages may be set up in reference to the phonological types. The correlations between types of breath groups and types of syllables, and the influence on the characterized syllable factors have been noted. German, English, Scandinavian and Dutch languages belong to a group with heavy, fixed stresses in the breath group and frequent closed syllables and varied feet. French, Japanese, and the South Sea languages tend to the open-syllable type which is correlated with a lighter and often variable stress in the breath group while the duration of the syllable is less varied.

Although the morphological units have had extensive consideration, we have had, as yet, rather little study of the breath-group types, and of the correlated syllable types. E. Hermann (30) made some interesting observations:

1. He established the status of the syllable in the history of Greek phonology.
2. He adopted the sonority concept, but his careful findings are in line. His use of "sonority" and of the "mora"—postulated unit of length within the syllable—does not vitiate his findings.
3. He recognized the simple or compound releasing consonant in a train of syllables.
4. He recognized the abutting group of arresting and releasing consonant as basic for the prosodic "length by position" of Greek grammarians.
5. He recognized the simple and compound consonants, and the abutting pair.
6. He recognized the singling of the double consonant.
7. He compared the Greek alphabetic notation with that of the Cypriote syllabary which confirmed his findings.
8. He followed the study down through the Latin and the derivative Romance languages, and noted the general tendency to make the consonants releasing, which reaches its ultimate form in modern French.

No study is available of the Greek Septuagint form of the Hebrew proper names and technical terms, nor of the Greek transliteration of cuneiform words. There is a mass of evidence to be mustered on the points which Hermann stresses.

Metrical formulations often illuminate the breath-group organization. If the discussion of "juncture" in the form of "Grenzsignale" had reached the stage of considering the reciprocal relations of the types of "juncture" and the corresponding modifications of the syllable frontier, it would have opened the problem of types of breath-group organization. But the "juncture" method deals with the apparent boundaries and not with the organized movements.

APPENDIX VII

SEGMENTATION

Phonemicists assume a phonemic series and a parallel articulatory series. Pike finds articulations are to be defined by a physiological system which he sketches; but he assumes a linear series of articulations parallel to the series of phonemes. (63)

Bloch assumes a simple, single movement which is to be unchanging in direction and speed. Either the member remains in one position, or it moves without perceptible change of acceleration or direction (or it is set into vibration). This simple, single movement is identified by the perception of articulatory movements (5, p. 12). Thus the criterion is essentially subjective, mentalistic, and incapable of experimental verification.

Joos has a series of neurological waves which overlap but seem to be essentially in a single linear series. This series derives from cerebral engrams (39, p. 111) and is organized in lower brain centers into the consecutive series (39, p. 109). Joos objects to ballistic movements and syllable factors on the score of the form of the actual movements of speech; but muscular contractions and mass-velocity factors are inevitable, however the neutral impulses are ordered (39, pp. 106–107).

None of these segmentation schemes takes into account the inclusive function of the phonetic units:

The syllable includes the syllable factor, with accessory movements.
The foot includes the syllables.
The breath group includes the feet.

Thus the syllable factor, the syllable, the foot,

a. A vowel alone
b. A consonant and vowel
c. Compound consonant and vowel
d. Consonant, vowel, and consonant
e. Compound consonant, vowel and compound consonant

and the breath group are all present in any simplest articulation. The simplest possible utterance will be a breath group of a single one-syllable foot.

The phonetic units are of course movements which include each other. In all skilled movements the elements of the movements are included in larger units. A movement must be started and a movement must be stopped. In piano playing a series of small movements, the finger strokes, are united and included in the arm movement for the figure and phrase, and the arm is supported by the trunk posture.

When the articulatory movements are reduced to the logistic symbols of a phonemic alphabet, the notation cannot ever be that of a simple series of signs, they must include each other. This will be true whatever aspect or layer the signs are made to represent; the phonemic unit will be "bound". To Trubetzkoy's opposition, conjunctive, and disjunctive must be added: included, and including. Failure to note the inclusive character of articulatory movements and the bound character of the phonemic signs is one of the fundamental difficulties of the segmentation of the phonemicists.

Joos has a type of indeterminancy which limits the number per second possible of the elements of speech; .05—.06 sec. is the duration of a "smear" which limits the linear series to ca. 18–20 per second. This is roughly correct for one-member repetition, and articulation is a one-member coordination. The limiting rate is actually 8–10 syllables per second. It is not a rate of phonemes per second. The rate of the phonemes depends on the number of phonemes per syllable, and the type of syllable:

10 per sec.	ah, ah, ah....
10 per sec. 20	be, be, be....
10 per sec. 30	tree, tree, tree....
3.5 per sec. 10.5; ca. the rate of (a) above	
3.5 per sec. 17.5; ca. the rate of (b) above	

But if the movement coordinated is of two members, as in piano playing, the values are different. The notes, which are equivalent to the syllables, can be struck at the rate of 16–18 per sec. Each note has at least pitch and stress, so that at a minimum, there are 32–36 tonemes per sec. If tone quality (timbre) and dynamic level (loud-soft) are added, the number of musical tonemes per sec. rises to 64–72 per sec.

It is to be noted that the limits of toleration in making and hearing syllables and notes depend on the rates of movements possible, not on some inherent acoustic or auditory property.

Joos' interpretation of speech coordinations depends on outdated neurological notions: A cerebral engram is a single static neural pattern in storage; at some lower level these static patterns are combined into the forms of speech. Such neural speculation has been given up: there is no experimental warrant for such assumptions and the concepts raise far more problems than they solve.

Chapter V of Joos' monograph is a medley because of various speculations at odds with the fundamental facts of included and including movements. There is a tangle of accessory hypotheses:

a. Segmentation—assuming consecutive segments (p. 98).
b. Decomposition (cutting) simultaneous components "in layers" (p. 98–99).
c. Phonetic congruence (p. 98, 112).
d. Aspects (98–99):
   1. brain selectivity and innervations
   2. articulation including labial, lingual, glottal, "pulmonary"
   3. acoustic aspect
   4. hearing (audition), ear and lower levels, not exclusively speech
   5. speech perception
   6. language, neural patterns in speech center—engrams.
e. Slur: simple (p. 104), mixed (115–116); linguistic layers have interpenetrated.
f. Neureme—engram (d, 6 above) (p. 112).
g. Juncture, consonant (p. 113, 118).
h. Vowel-allophone (p. 113).
i. Layers, e.g. labial, lingual, glottal, simultaneous and overlapping; compounding supposedly in cerebellum to produce slur (e above) (p. 114).
j. Re-cutting (p. 116).
k. Multiple cutting (p. 118).

The layers which interpenetrate, the segmentation with the various neural assumptions, the cutting (decomposition) with re-cutting and multiple cutting, the various "aspects" will straighten out if speech movements are subjected to the same treatment as any system of skilled movements. Piano playing or violin playing might also be reduced to a similiar tangle of segmentation, decomposition, cutting, re-cutting, and multiple cutting, of "aspects" to which some new musical concepts would be added. Singing would then be analyzed into a complex more complicated when all the segmentation and decomposition demanded by musical pitches and by musical rhythm, with its figures and phrases, are fused with the segmentation and decomposition already demanded for speech. Singing as a musical performance and as a speaking performance uses the one and the same neuromuscular mechanism; it is quite possible to handle the movements involved as a neuromuscular coordination. But there is little hope of an analysis which proceeds in terms of segmentation, decomposition, aspects and various other logistic concepts. As they stand they cannot be translated into movements.

APPENDIX VIII

REDUCTIONS OF TRUBETZKOY'S PHONEMICS TO MOTOR TERMS

1. Trubetzkoy has carried on Ferdinand de Saussure's tradition of the "phoneme" as a symbol, and therefore a member of the system of *la langue*; the symbol is opposed to the signal, the articulation, which belongs to the system of *la parole*. This is Trubetzkoy's fundamental division between phonemics and phonetics.

2. Trubetzkoy supplements F. de Saussure's treatment of the phoneme by insisting that the individual phoneme is always to be defined in terms of the system of phonemes of the particular language. Trubetzkoy's basic phoneme is an articulation; he is aware that the acoustic traits are scant, variable and at present difficult to define. But Trubetzkoy did not carry his study of the physiological basis of the phoneme, the articulation, into the specific apparatus of speech on which the system of a language must depend. (100)

3. For both phonetics and for phonemics the main types of phonological language systems are important. The word stress in the breath groups gives two obvious types; 1) the light, variable stress and the resulting variable grouping within the breath group of the language; 2) the heavy, fixed stress with well-defined feet within the breath group of the language.

4. Further, the nature of the syllable gives two language types: 1) a system with nearly all syllables open, i.e. without arresting consonant (chest-arrested, but this is not noted as a specific mark); 2) a system with many syllables closed; an open (chest-arrested) syllable becomes notable.

5. These two classifications are related and the most obvious main phonological types appear to be:

a. Breath groups with light, variable stress, and varying rhythmic grouping into feet. Nearly all syllables are open (without consonant arrest) and there is rather little change at the syllable frontier, owing to the absence of arresting consonants.

b. Breath groups with heavy, fixed word stress and well defined feet, with many syllables closed upon which the stress may fall. All the phenomena of abutting, doubling and dropping (singling) consonants appear at the syllable frontier, in the form of "assimilation, sandhi, visarga".

6. It is in those terms that Trubetzkoy must carry out his system of "oppositions". An opposition consists of a contrast of differentiation between two "words" (in its lowest terms between two syllables) due to a simple change of articulation; such an opposition distinguishes two phonemes.

7. There are four movement units involved:

a. Breathing cycle; respiratory act modified for speech: sentence, period, stanza.

b. Breath group; subdivision of the breath cycle: phrase, verse line; due to the

abdominal movements, with or without intake of air.
c. Foot; rhytmic grouping of the syllables about a single syllable due to the individual movements of the abdominal muscles (vs. diaphragm) for the stress and the grouping of the syllables. It is usual for a language to distinguish three grades of stress. Trubetzkoy recognizes this as the function of producing culminations, (p. 29, Gründzuge)—feet of verse and of prose.
d. Syllable; a chest pulse released by the chest muscles (intercostals) or by a consonant; and arrested by the chest muscles (intercostals) or by a consonant. This syllable proves to be the movement peculiar to speech, as the note is peculiar to singing.

8. Definition of the articulation:
Whether a distinction can be drawn between the articulatory signal and the phoneme as a signal according to Trubetzkoy, is left to later discussion.
For the discussions of phonetics at least, speech consists of a series of articulatory signals. The articulation, i.e. the phoneme, is to be the simplest unit, the element of this train of articulatory signals.

9. The basis for Trubetzkoy's differentiation of the phonemes is the change of meaning. If an articulatory change affects the meaning of the "word" (strictly it should be the meaning of the simplest utterance possible, which is the syllable) then it constitutes a "phoneme". Trubetzkoy is clear that this is to be a movement. He comments on the fact that often the auditory signal varies, and that the auditory description of the phonemes is scant and unsatisfactory.

10. We may say that the oscillograph records show acoustic fusion and continuity. The extent to which the sounds interpenetrate becomes apparent. But the study of oscillographic records shows that the interpretation must be in terms of articulatory movements.

11. Thus Trubetzkoy's definition of the phoneme becomes: "A controllable movement which changes the meaning of the syllable." This he recognizes as a phonetic definition of the phoneme (100, 17 and 20), and he makes haste to add that the higher stages of phonological description are free from phonetics.

12. This fundamental "opposition", contrast, differentiation, is the basis of the system: if it is due to the presence or absence of a controllable movement, it is counted a "correlation" e.g. correlations of voicing, correlations of nasality. If it is due to two different main movements (by different members) it is counted a "disjunction" (98; 99, p. 235).

13. In actual speech the simplest utterance, the smallest actual unit proves to be the syllable which Trubetzkoy, following De Groot, characterizes as the prosodic unit and which is comparable to the note in music. (100, pp. 17, 83, 84, 85, 166). He cites Motor Phonetics as to the handling of the syllable. Variants of a syllable can be distinguished, but nothing less than a syllable can be uttered. In the same fashion, variants of a note are possible, but nothing less than a note can be sung. The phoneme is the symbol designed to represent this speech signal. The phoneme represents a speech signal which has no independent existence but must occur in a syllable. It can be put on paper but it remains an articulatory symbol whose meaning is the speech signal.

14. Phonetics deals with the apparatus of the articulations and their relations. In this system of movements the breath group proves to be the simplest movement which cannot become implicit in a rate-modified pattern; the characterized factors of the syllable, (i.e. vowel and consonant) may "drop" to reappear at the proper rate; but the breath does not drop.
The breath group, however, is not bounded by syllables as auxiliary movements; syllables do not stop and start the breath group; the order of syllables and nature of the syllables is incidental.

15. The syllable, however, the peculiar movement of speech, is a pulse which is released and arrested in specific fashion (by chest muscles or by consonant articulation) and the pulse is emitted through a vocal canal which has a specific shape which is termed the vowel.

16. The fundamental distinction, opposition, then, is between the shaping vowel movement which opens the vocal canal, and the releasing or arresting consonant movement, which constricts the vocal canal. Both the acoustic analysis from Stumpf's time, and also the study of the articulations has led to a division of the vowels, the shape qualities, into two series, with three

cardinal positions or main vowels. The starting point of both series may be made the most open position of the vocal canal for the syllable pulse. This gives the vowel *ah*, [a]. The extreme narrowing of the front orifice at the lips gives *oo*, *ou* [u]. The extreme narrowing of the rear orifice, tongue to palate, gives *ee* [i]. The series *a–u* has a single main resonance, zone (formant) indicating that the mouth cavity is acting as a single resonator with orifice. The series *a–i* has two resonance zones (formants) indicating that the mouth cavity is acting as a pair of coupled resonators with an orifice between.

17. Between these three cardinal vowels there are two graduated vowel series. In English the vowels *a–i* are *a, æ, ε, e, I*. And between *a–u* are *u, u, o, U*. This gives an English vowel system of perhaps 12 vowels, without including diphthongs, and the various reductions toward shwa produced by the heavy English word stress.

18. Many languages have combinations of the two basic positions, in which both the front orifice and the rear orifice are narrowed. Shwa (dark-e, French e muet) is the most common; it can be looked on as the 'neutral vowel', i.e. the vowel produced by the least possible movement of the vocal apparatus for the emission of the syllable pulse. The series of German umlauts and the French *u* belong to this combined series and account for an additional four or five vowels in these European languages. In English most of these can be looked on as the result of reduction of a simple vowel toward shwa. Thus the English vowel system could be reduced to perhaps 13 vowels. But usually some 15 to 18 are recognized and notated. This variation shows that they are not due to presence-absence conditions of shape, but to a graduated series of positions. This is common to many phonetic "disjunctions" (to use Trubetzkoy's term.)

The Consonants

19. The consonants are auxiliary movements which release and arrest the syllable pulse, in lieu of a release or arrest by the intercostal muscles. Sometimes the auxiliary movement merely assists the chest release and arrest. Thus the consonant always has a mechanical function; it is part of the mechanism of the syllable pulse and therefore subject to the conditions which vary the syllable mechanism and which are apparent at the syllable frontier. The basic disjunction of Phonologie (Phonemics) is that of *vowel-consonant*.

20. While the consonants present many types of specific presence-and-absence of a given movement and therefore group in correlations, there are also a large number of disjunctive relations. There are several organs which give the main stroke of the consonant articulation: the lips (and jaw), lips and teeth, tongue tip, tongue blade, tongue rear, glottis and adjacent structures. In the case of the tongue, the bearings of the stroke to the palate may vary in position, making a graduated series of positions which may include and group together rear, blade, and tip. Such a graduated series, involving all the tongue, is sometimes convenient in explaining certain diachronous phonetic changes (cf. French development Caesar to César.)

21. It is convenient to treat Trubetzkoy's elaborate classification of the phonemes by proceeding from the largest classified groups to the smallest. This follows Trubetzkoy's own basic distinctions.

22. The fundamental distinction is between the vowel and the consonant. The movement differentiation depends on the fact that the vowel represents the shaping of the vocal canal for the emission of the syllable pulse, and the consonant releases or arrests the syllable pulse. As Trubetzkoy puts it, the vowel opens the vocal canal and the consonant constricts it; and he cites Menzerath's discussion (100, p. 83–84).

23. In English, as an example, this fundamental distinction makes two classes:

The vowels, some 15 perhaps; and the Consonants, some 24.

The movements involved are functional in relation to the syllable pulse.

24. The next largest division is between the releasing and the arresting consonants. This is not often cited in English and in German because, with few exceptions, the consonants function as both releasing and arresting.

The releasing consonants include *w, wh, y*, and *h* which function only as releasing (23 in English). The arresting consonants include -ng, which functions only as arresting (21 in English). This is true also of the glottal stop (') which does not occur in normal English. The movements involved function in the syllable pulse.

25. The distinction between the voiced and unvoiced consonants, on the other hand, is nearly always recognized.

The number of voiced consonants exceeds that of the unvoiced:

Voiced consonants: b, v, y, m, w, d, th, z, j, dj, l, r, n, ng—14 in English.
Unvoiced consonants: p, f, wh, t, s, th, sh, ch, k, h—10 in English.

This is not a functional movement; it is not essential to the function of the syllable pulse; it is a controllable movement which may be added or subtracted from the consonant complex; an accessory movement which is an aspect of the syllable factor. It is not, however, simple; it is the pressure-differential complex with the apposition of the vocal folds.

26. The distinction between the occlusive (stop) and the continuant is generally recognized and is often important.

There are the occlusives: p/b t/d, k/g, ch/dj—8 in English.

There are the continuants: f/v, w/wh, m, s/z, sh/zh, n, l, r, ng, h—14 in English.

The distinction is not functional and it is not due to the presence or absence of a single movement. It describes the closure of the consonant as tight, or leaky; the muscles involved are as various as the members involved. It is an accessory movement.

27. Still smaller classes are determined by the member involved e.g.:

Labials: p, b, f, v, wh, w, m—7 in English.
These may be sub-divided into stops and continuants:
labial stops: p–b
continuants: f–v, wh–w, m
or into voiced and unvoiced labials:
voiced: b, v, w, m
unvoiced: p, f, wh.

In such groups appear the unidimensional pairs which Trubetzkoy emphasizes: p–b, f–v, wh–w. In German, Trubetzkoy cites 13 of 190 contrasts (100, p. 62) which are counted the simplest "oppositions" (contrasts, differentiations). Though the simplest, they are not to be counted especially significant. The pluri-dimensional groups are much more common, since they involve contrasts between articulations of different members.

28. There are various cross-classifications sometimes cited, e.g.:

The sonants, including the vowels and the voiced consonants—28 in English.
The continuants, including the vowels and the continuant consonants—29 in English.

A graded series of constrictions might be made from the most open vowel, ah, through the "liquids" (n, l, r, ng), to sibilants, and finally to occlusives; but it has no significance. The one relation between the vowels and consonants which is important is in the case of the cardinal vowel u and the consonant w; and the cardinal vowel i and the consonant y. If the constriction of the u is forced to closure, and suddenly released, the result is the consonant w. If the construction of the i is forced to closure, and suddenly released, the result is the consonant y. This interplay appears in some phonetic changes.

29. It is easy to see, when the movements of Trubetzkoy's classifications are analyzed, that the bases for phonemic classification are varied:

a. Essential functional movements: vowel shaping, consonant arresting and releasing.
b. Presence or absence of a movement factor in a complex: voicing, or nasalization.
c. Articulatory member concerned in the particular consonant: labials, linguals, etc.

It is apparent that many classifications are possible. Most commentators on Trubetzkoy's elaborate system make haste to add that other schemes are possible. But it is clear that his network of contrasts proves to be a system of related movements whose control leads to the significant shifts which change the meaning and are therefore significant phonetic signals.

30. On occasion these differentiations appear in graduated series, as in the vowel series from *ah* to *i* and from *ah* to *u*. The choice made from language to language is arbitrary, as to the steps chosen and stereotyped. For instance, the series of positions on the palate, bearings for the tongue strokes, which again form a series, is significant, for example, in the shift of the Latin gutturals to the modern Romance sibilants.

31. It is obvious that a reference to the speech apparatus organizes and explains the elaborations

of Trubetzkoy's system, and at the same time makes it apparent that other schemes are quite as feasible. The final elements for Trubetzkoy are these contrasts due to controlled movements. He does not always think in terms of syllables, or of breath groups, and he loses sight of the fact that the basic utterance is never less than a syllable. Strictly speaking it is never less than a breath group composed of a single syllable. Within the syllable, and within the breath group, the individual signals may or may not appear in the familiar pattern; they may shift position and they may disappear to reappear. This is true of individual contrasts, of individual phonemes, and even of individual syllables. This confronted Trubetzkoy in the guise of "neutralization". The contrasts which he counted essential to a system of phonemes was lost.

32. The problem of "neutralization", and Trubetzkoy's proposal of an "archiphoneme", clear up if one refers to the movements underlying the speech process. An examination of the conditions will show that rate or stress has changed and has affected the movements involved, but that the complex pattern of signals of the syllable as a whole, or breath group as a whole, carries the meaning; and that a change of rate or stress will lead to the reappearance of the lost contrast within the pattern. This is a commonplace in any system of phonetics and will be found in any and all rapid movement patterns: in writing, in the playing of musical instruments. The same processes which appear in speaking appear also in singing.

The pressure on the arresting consonant in a language like German forces it to become surd when the rate is rapid or the stress is heavy.

The closure of a stop may become imperfect and a leaky variant appears; so the Greek thala*tt*a becomes thala*ss*a.

With a heavy word stress, the vowels of the unstressed syllables are neutralized, i.e. they are reduced toward shwa, and it is impossible to distinguish the original vowel, although a shift of stress brings back the original shape and quality.

The arresting function of a consonant is often neutralized; the consonant arrest is replaced by the chest arrest, and the consonant either shifts to the releasing function in the next syllable or drops.

33. Another phase of the speech movements which Trubetzkoy does not provide for in his logistic classification, but which can be handled by a direct reference to movement, is the connection between these "phonemes". The release of the syllable is unlike the arrest of the syllable. The feet and the breath groups and the breathing cycle are articulated as all movements must be. The connections and the stops and starts of movements are parts of the pattern to be perceived and produced.

34. "Junctures" are a part of the coordination of movements, and must present various phases in the system of movements which constitutes speech. Speech is a modification of the breathing cycle. The largest movement complex to be organized and articulated will be that of the breathing cycle, the differentiation of sentence, period, or stanza. The opening of the sentence will be marked by the rapid intake of air through the mouth. The expiration will be slow, consisting of a series of stages, marked by the action of the abdominal muscles giving stresses (Trubetzkoy's culminations), and sometimes marked by pauses and sometimes by brief intakes of breath. At the close of the expiration, the vocalization ceases; there is a pause and the rapid intake for a new clause. The fundamental boundary indicator (Grenzsignal) is the pause and the abrupt intake of breath for the next clause.

35. The breath group is set off by its pause or brief intake, and is marked by the stress or stresses of the abdominal muscles which give the "culmination" to the breath group. Within this breath group the syllables are joined. Between little clusters of syllables, the feet, there may appear abutting or double consonants which link the syllables, or rather, link the closing and opening syllables of the feet composed of syllables. Assimilation and sandhi occur at the syllable frontier. This is a specific type of "juncture" in that the constriction for the arrest of the last syllable of the foot fuses with the constriction for the release of the first syllable of the next foot. The movement form involved is characteristic and is considered in detail in the text. In languages with heavy "word stress", as in English and German, the syllables are affected by the stress. The syllable on which the heavy stress falls tends to lengthen (either in the vowel, or the arresting process). Meanwhile the unstressed syllables are

reduced; the vowels approach shwa or may disappear. On occasion the syllable itself disappears (Aladad and Aragon become "Al-dad and Ar-gon", e.g.).

36. The more detailed questions of "juncture" concern the movements of the syllable. The opening of the syllable is marked by a releasing movement, which may be of the chest in an "open syllable", or may be of a consonant acting with the chest. The function of the consonant is specific and there may be differences; *w, wh, h* function only as releasing consonants; they are always boundary indicators. Continental phonologists are accustomed to distinguishing two types of English "l". The bright *l* is always releasing and is therefore an indication of the release of a syllable.

37. In a rapid train of syllables, the arresting consonant of the preceding syllable appears in the releasing position of the following syllable. This shift marks the opening of a new but closely connected syllable, i.e. one within the foot. One may generalize and say that the presence of an arresting consonant, either alone or in an abutting (doubling) pair, marks the foot division within the breath group.

38. The "junctures" within the syllable are coordinations of the auxiliary movements of the syllable pulse; they are often overlapping or concurrent: the releasing consonant's back stroke overlaps the vowel; the arresting consonant's beat stroke overlaps the vowel. Continuants of all sorts fuse with the adjacent vowel because of the common movement; liquids and sibilants may be concurrent with, or may replace the vowel.

39. The constituents of the compound consonants fuse as far as possible. Rousselot notes that the beat strokes of the constituents are as near simultaneous as possible. A special "juncture" is often formed when the arresting consonant fuses with the releasing consonant of the next syllable. Vice versa, at the close of a foot the compound arresting consonant may divide into an abutting consonant marking the "juncture" with the following foot.

40. The junctures of vowels and consonants are indicated by the fact that the vowel is the shaping movement for the syllable pulse, and the consonants may be the releasing or the arresting movements for the syllable pulse; the "junctures" are of delimiting, auxiliary movements for the main movement.

41. The series of junctures and the related units of utterance may be summarized:

Inter-clause (breathing cycle): the rapid intake indicates the sentence or stanza.

Intra-clause, inter-phrase: the pause and intake mark the frontier between phrases.

Intra-phrase, inter-breath group: the pause and possible intake mark the frontier between breath groups.

Intra-breath-group, inter-foot: the culminating stresses and the arresting consonant (abutting, double also) division of compound consonants mark the frontier between the feet.

Intra-foot, inter-syllabic: shifts from arresting to releasing, fusion of consonants to compound consonants, various sandhi changes, mark the frontier between syllables.

Intra-syllabic, inter-phonemic: shaping, releasing and arresting (delimiting) functions, movement fusions of compound consonants mark connections within the syllable.

42. Music furnishes an analogy to the units of utterance and the so-called junctures:

Inter-period: Pauses, final cadences, mark the periods.

Intra-period: inter-phrase: pauses, rhythm, harmony, mark the phrases.

Intra-phrase, inter-figure: grouping accents, harmonic progressions, voice leadings, mark the figures.

Intra-figure, inter-note: specific beats mark the notes; staccato, legato, portamento mark the note connections.

Intra-note: attack and termination (staccato, legato) swell of long note.

43. We may note that the coordinations of the movements of speech are of various types. Aside from the simple controllable movement which may be present or absent in a movement complex (as in nasalization, aspiration), we may also consider:

44. Movements may be bound. The process in hand is due not to a single member, or muscle group, but to a complex process. The following movements are common:

a. Voicing is due not only to the apposition of the vocal folds, but also to the contraction of the chest muscles producing pressure from beneath and the lowering of the larynx-mass, which reduces the pressure above. It is properly called the "differential-pressure complex."
b. The lips do not function alone but are always bound to the movements of the jaw.
c. The tongue, front and back, the larynx-mass, and the jaw-and-lips, all figure in the formation of the cavity or cavities and orifices of the vowels.
d. The abdominal-diaphragm contraction reinforces and groups the chest pulses forming the stresses and the foot-and breath-groups.
e. The manipulation of the vocal folds is reinforced by variations in the shape of the vowel cavities in the production of musical pitch in singing, and of intonation in speech.

45. Movements may be mutually exclusive:

a. The movement of a consonant excludes the movement of a vowel, and vice versa. A semivowel is a consonant closely related to the extreme position of the vowel orifices but it is in no wise partly a vowel.
b. The shaping of each vowel excludes the shaping of other vowels; there is a definite limit to the number of combinations, "Umlauts", of the front and back positions.
c. Many movements like the up and down movement of the jaw, and the forward and backward movement of the tongue, are the same movement in reverse and of course mutually exclusive.

46. Movement processes may be considered as conditioned by other movements:

a. Aspiration and the emphatics are due to a combination of movement factors.
b. Long and short syllables and vowels are due to several processes, in which both the force of the chest movement and the resistance of the articulations have a part.
c. Rate changes condition a variety of articulatory movements at the syllable frontier.
d. Stress and rhythmic phrasing prolong and diphtongize the vowels of the stressed syllables, and reduce the vowels of the unstressed syllables, and may eliminate syllables.

47. Position Analysis:

Sometimes it is proposed to recast Trubetzkoy's system of "oppositions", contrasts, and differentiations, in terms of the positional distribution of the phonemes. What phoneme may come before, between or after given phonemes is made the basis for a definition of the specific function of the phoneme. The sign designs, the list of phonemes, are to be defined by the occurrence of the sign events as they actually appear in language.

48. It is easy to see that the phonemes cannot take position until they have been isolated, differentiated, and designated by some process. Trubetzkoy's basic "contrasts" are essential to determining the phoneme alphabet before anything can be said of the preferred and tolerated positions of various phonemes in reference to each other. There can be no "privileges of position" until there are entities to assign the privilege.

49. In addition, the function of the factors in the syllable, of the syllable in the breath group, of the breath group in the clause, cannot be determined by mere observation of the possible distribution of the phonemes. Some of the changes with rate and stress of syllable, foot, breath group and clause will be left quite unexplained.

50. Position, both with and without the substitution of other phonemes, is an important factor in the analysis of the phonemes, *once the phonemes are known*. But of course it is useless until the phonemes have been determined by some independent method.

51. Position, as indicated by phonologists, I always in reference to a functional element in the syllable, as the terms 'post-vocalic' and 'pre-vocalic', 'syllable-initial' and 'syllable-final' illustrate. The basic distinction recognized by everyone, though sometimes minimized, of vowel and consonant, is actually a reference to a difference in function of the vowel core and the accompanying articulation.

52. The effect of varying rates shows the

functional difference. As far as mere position is concerned, there should be no difference between CVO and OVC; both merely represent a vowel adjacent to a consonant. But the series CVC CVO.... may run to 8–10 per sec., while the series OVC, OVC.... cannot exceed 3.5–4 per sec. When consonants are adjacent, much depends on whether they are compound consonants or abutting consonants. If compound, their rate may be very rapid; tree, tree.... may be uttered at 8 per sec. The vowel occupies about half the interval, so that the rate of the t, r may be as high as 30 per sec. If the consonants are abutting, as in tha*t r*eel, the arresting t must drop as the rate increases to 4 per sec. Position within the syllable and position between syllables proves to be very different for the same sequences.

54. Thus a characterization of articulations by mere position is unsatisfactory. Position with reference to the units, syllable factors, syllables, breath groups, is fundamentally important. The connection, the stress, and the rate of the articulatory movements determine the nature of a "position".

55. The positional analysis does not take into account the difference between coordinations which are determined by the movement apparatus of all speech, and the preferences of a given language. Languages may exclude all arresting consonants, as do the South Sea Island languages, and Japanese in the main. A language may not tolerate a syllable opening with a vowel which is true in general of the Semitic group. A language may avoid compound consonants, as is the case with most of those just mentioned, or it may be very rich in compound consonants, as are the Russian, German and English.

56. In addition to these matters of structure, most languages show preferences and aversions for particular combinations which might not seem out of place in their systems. It is arbitrary that w, y, and h in English are always releasing, and the -ng is always arresting. Tl- and dl- do not appear in English, although pl-, bl-, and kl- and gl- are common. Sb-, sd-, sg-, zl-, etc. are not tolerated; ts-, ps, ks- occur only in foreign words, although they are common in the arresting position. Although the contrast between delta and theta is preserved in the present Greek, the sonants b, d, g must be represented by mp, nt, nk (or gamma-kappa).

57. Greek and Spanish have the theta-delta sibilants so familiar in English, but most of the European languages are without them, though they once had them. English has lost the *ch* so prominent in German. English cultivates a variety of lingual sibilants, while the Semitic tongues specialize in gutturals unfamiliar to Europeans. The presence or absence of particular articulations, and the choice of the vowel system of a language, seem rather arbitrary and accidental.

58. Such traits are subject to rapid change; neighboring, unrelated languages borrow phonemes. The Zulu "clicks", borrowed from the Hottentots and Bushmen, are a striking illustration. It is hard to say whether the glottal stop appearing in the Midlands and the south of England is a survival from the Danes or a thing sporadic. Such traits can be noted, but they are evidently matters of habit formation and not the result of a language mechanism and its various coordinations.

APPENDIX IX

AMERICAN VERSION OF PHONEMICS (PHONOLOGIE)

Phoneme

There is no clear statement of the articulatory nature of the phoneme. The definition is allowed to stand in the logistic terms of Sweet-Saussure-Trubetzkoy: a phonic difference which distinguishes one word from another constitutes a phonemic difference. Often the phoneme is treated as a differential; and often it is counted a *class* of articulations, or of articulatory attributes. The phonic difference must be due to a controlled movement (muscular contraction) which modifies the articulation. It is a class of articulations in that a series of articulations may be modified by this same muscular contraction. The nature of the "opposition", whether a group of related shapes, as with the vowels, or as the presence and absence of a particular attribute,

---

The following may be cited as representative of the American version of Trubetzkoy's Phonologie:

Trager, G. L., & Bloch, B. Syllabic phonemes of English.
   Lang., 1941, 17.   TB, (97)
Bloch, B., & Trager, G. L. Outline of linguistic analysis.
   Ling. Soc. Am. 1942.   BT, (6)
Hockett, C. F. System of descriptive phonology.
   Lang., 1942, 18.   HS, (31)
Harris, Z. S. Phonemicist version of Yokuts.
   IJAL, 1944, 10.   HY, (24)
——————Phonemicist version of Navaho.
   IJAL, 1945, 11.   HN, (25)
——————Phonemicist version of Kota.
   IJAL, 1945, 21.   HK, (26)

---

is determined by the apparatus in terms of which the phonic differences and therefore the definition of the phoneme must be formulated.

In motor phonetic terms the phoneme is a characterized factor of a syllable. The factors of the syllable are the canal shape (the vowel through which the syllable pulse is emitted), and the release of the pulse by the chest muscles or by consonant, and the arrest of the pulse by the chest muscles or by consonant. Various aspects of the syllable factor characterize the syllable: vocalization, nasalization, constriction, etc. The phoneme always involves a syllable factor. The classes to which the phonemes are reduced are classes of syllables produced by these characterized syllable factors. The simplest "word" to be differentiated by a phoneme is a syllable. The phoneme can appear only in a syllable.

Formation of Speech Sounds: BT (6, p. 12)

The statements made as to the production of human speech are quite wrong, as experimental study of the speech apparatus shows. A free flow of a column of air under steady pressure through an enclosed passage is postulated, and the mechanism is compared to a clarinet or flute. It is "a kind of 'playing' on the column of air" which is said to produce the sounds of human speech. The notion of a free, steady flow, is false; the air is emitted in pulses, and the chest pressure between syllables is often neutral. The clarinet and flute are not analogous to speech; the comparison should be with the brass of the orchestra, the notes of which are made by pulses of air from the chest, precisely as the syllables are made by the speech apparatus. The study of speech with an artificial larynx reveals the function of the chest in making the individual syllable pulses. The reed of the artificial larynx is always ready to sound; the stopping and starting of the syllables must be done by the chest muscles. The function of the releasing and of the arresting consonants and the whole structure of the syllable cannot be properly understood unless the fundamental movement of the syllable pulse is clearly conceived (87; 91; 64, p. 319).

Simultaneous Components of the Phoneme: HN (25, p. 243).

On logistic grounds, Harris proposes to break up the phonemes into simultaneous components. No articulatory mechanism is proposed, and the analyses are not consistent. *T* and ' are assumed to give a single phoneme *t'*; a glottalized *t* is quite possible; but *h* and *l* are assumed to give *l̥*, in which the aspiration of the *h* cannot coexist with the voiced *l* in *l̥*.

In motor phonetic terms, such a simultaneous component will be defined as a significant accessory movement concurrent with the syllable factor: i.e. glottalization, vocalization, nasalization, etc.

Sound Types: TB (97, p. 223, 223 n)

"The sound-types constituting a phoneme must be phonetically similar, complementarily distributed, and congruently patterned; and the class thus composed must be in contrast with and mutually exclusive of every other such class in the language. Sound-types, as members of a phonemic class, are called allophones. The sound-type is a class of phonetic events called sounds; each sound is a sum of sound-features (as voicing, aspiration, occlusion, labial position, etc.) which may occur in various combinations. The repetition of what is perceptually the same combination constitutes the sound-type, which is thus an abstraction from a series of utterances clustering about a norm."

In motor phonetic terms, "perceptually the same combination" means conditioned to meaning as the same articulation, in the context in which it occurs.... in which it has been conditioned. Therefore the phoneme is *not* "a series of utterances clustering about a norm" because the conditioning does not concern a series of minor variations but concerns an articulation with variants so different that they may coincide with the variants of other phonemes; and may be reduced to zero. The context is all important in determining the conditioned response. The users of the language have come to recognize the variant of the phoneme in that context. The use of the term "type" is good; the conditioned articulation is the "type" with an indefinite number of variants in the varying stimulus pattern to which the movement is conditioned. In cases where there is overlapping of the variants of different phonemes, it is easy to identify the phoneme by changing the rate and stress.

Phoneme as Segmental: BT (6, p. 41)

"May be regarded as segments of utterances." Such a definition of "segment" is quite inadequate. They are said to follow each other in the stream of speech, but the syllable factors are not merely sequential; they inevitably overlap (64). The fundamental representation of "sounds following each other" and therefore of "segments" corresponding to the "sounds", is at fault. The notion of playing sounds like the notes on a flute or clarinet was mistaken to start with.

Allophones: HS (31, p. 9)

Variants of a given "sound" are obvious. The context determines the variants. The varying function of the consonants in the syllable, the compounding of consonants, and the influence of stress and grouping on the vowels all modify the type movement of the syllable factor. To account for these variants within the phoneme, the term "allophone" has been devised.

In motor phonetic terms such variants are referred to the varying functions of the syllable factors, and the reciprocal influence of the movements.

Morphophonemes: HN (25, p. 243, 245), HK (26, p. 285)

In discussing Emeneau's treatment of Kota, Z. S. Harris speaks of the reasons for assuming morphophonemes. "For every morphoneme he assumes a base form, which is composed not of phonemes but of morphophonemes. When the morphophonemes occur in words (i.e. in speech), the morphophonemes of their base forms are replaced by the corresponding phonemes: morphoneme k by phoneme /k/, and so on. In some cases the replacement is not by the corresponding phoneme but by some other; e.g. morphoneme n, when it is due to follow a morphophoneme l, is replaced by phoneme /n/. This occasional non-corresponding replacement is, of course, the only reason for the setting up of base forms and morphophonemes." This is the clumsy result of setting up logistic units, instead of dealing with movements which inevitably influence each other. But the Kota system has to be carried out with further complications, and there prove to be "two levels of replacement", etc. The morphophoneme is a device for logistic classification of phonemic variants directly due to context. The logistic method does not provide for a changing articulation in context, but names each stage of the change as a separate entity, the "morphophoneme", and then collates them with the appropriate phonemes.

Instead of such cumbersome morphophonemes replaced by phonemes, etc., motor phonetics deals with the changes in the type form n when it follows l; experimental observation will show that the change is due to the influence of one movement on another and this makes all the logistic paraphernalia superfluous.

Prosodic Features: Quantity, Accent, Rime, etc.:
TB (97, p. 238), BT (6, p. 34)

Suprasegmental Features: TB (97, p. 224),
BT (6, p. 41, 49–50), HS (31, p. 8),
HY (24, p. 205)

These various terms are applied to the traits of the syllables in feet and in breath groups. The term "suprasegmental" is general, and might apply to any and all of the "prosodic features". The prosodic features refer to the rhythmic organization of the feet and breath groups. But in all cases the analysis is based on a string of phonemes to which these features are added; there is no means of organizing the prosodic features and the phonemes into a common movement, and yet the practical handling of such features always involves the unit of the syllable. The logistic scheme adds terms but provides no organzation.

In motor phonetic terms the syllable proves the fundamental pulse in which the phonemes have their function as syllable factors, and the syllable pulses are organized by larger inclusive movements into the feet, and the breath groups. It is a matter of the coordination of movements; the syllable pulses are produced by the chest muscles; they become a part of the coordinating inclusive movements of the feet and breath groups produced by the abdominal movements involving muscles of abdomen-diaphragm.

The Vowel—Consonant Contrast:
BT (6, p. 18)

This is a fundamental contrast, and appears in all phonological treatments. The contrast depends on the radically different functions of the consonants, which delimit the syllable pulse, and the vowel, which shapes the canal to emit the pulse. But the logistic handling does not recognize the syllable in which the consonants and vowels function, but deals in "position" of phonemes in reference to each other and in "oppositions" of phonemes. So the distinction, though recognized, is said to be "blurred" (6).

In motor phonetic terms the syllable is the pulse in which the consonants and vowels are factors; the function of the consonant and of the vowel in the syllable is always distinct; and there is no chance of "blurring" the distinction.

Clusters, Doubles: TB (97, p. 229),
NH (25, p. 240–242), HS (31, p. 10)

Since the logistic system does not specify a function for the consonants and vowels, the "cluster" remains an arbitrary sequence of two or more consonants, or of two vowels. The phonemicists are consistent in making clusters of vowels as well as of consonants, although the combination is quite different.

Motor phonetics deals with the clusters of consonants as compound consonants and abutting consonants; and with clusters of vowels as diphthongs. The releasing or arresting compound results from a fusion of the movement of two or three consonants into a single consonant stroke; and it can be shown that there are conditions in which the compound consonants will become abutting consonants, and vice versa. The diphthongs result from the fusion of two vowel shapes; but unlike the consonants, the movements are consecutive—the shape changes during the syllable; it is usually possible to show how the diphthong developed.

Distribution, Structure: BT (6, p. 45 f.)

Distribution of phonemes is the logistic equivalent of the system of habits which make up the language mechanism conditioning the occurrence of the phonemes. The logistic analysis undertakes to handle the structure by noting the permissible sequence and contrasts. The classification of the phonemes results.

This amounts to the classification of the motorphonetic syllable and of its factors; and the classification of the function of the syllable in the foot and breath group.

Syllable Appears Unannounced:
TB (97, p. 224), HY (24, p. 206), BT (6, p. 22)

Since the phoneme is the primary unit, and is defined without reference to the syllable, the syllable is treated as 'suprasegmental', as something added to the phoneme series. No provision is made for the syllable in the original specifications. Hence it appears as an arbitrary addition to the phoneme series.

In some cases the syllable is avoided, as in Z. S. Harris' version of Yokuts. As it is not counted essential, a formula which ignores the syllable seems more general.

The definition of the syllable reverts to "sonority" (or "prominence") although the concept has no place in acoustics, and is meaningless. The syllable is obvious, as they all agree, and it is natural to use a paraphrase of that fact, and count the distinguishing trait "prominence".

The motor phonetic definition of the syllable makes it the basic chest pulse; the phonemes have their occurrence in the syllable only; it is an inclusive movement in which the syllable factors function not a "suprasegmental" unit added to the phoneme series.

Vowels Nuclear, Consonants Marginal—
TB (97, p. 224)

*Syllable Implied—*HS (31, p. 10, 14)

*Base Forms—*HK (26, p. 284–285), HN (25, p. 245)

*Syllabic Consonants—*BT (6, p. 28)

*Coarticulation—*BT (6, p. 29)

Syllabic Division; ambisyllabic Consonants—
TB (97, p. 234)

*Onset of Stress—*TB (97, p. 234)

All these terms fall into line when the syllable is made fundamental; they consist of various generalized observations of the phases of the syllable.

Phonemic Phrases—Stress Culmination—
TB (97, p. 226), HS (31, p. 6)

*Contour of Stress—*BT (6, p. 41)

*Intonation—*BT (6, p. 42)

This is the term of the phonemicists for the breath group. In one form or another, the breath group is recognized, since stress and grouping play an important part in morphology and syntax.

In motor phonetics the breath group appears as the inclusive movement for the syllables and feet; it is an inevitable coordination of the breathing movements in speech.

Junctures and Boundary Markers:
TB (97, p. 225)

Pause as a unit: TB (97, p. 225)

Juncture as a gap or as an entity:
HN (25, p. 240, 243, 244)

The joining of larger units of speech forces attention because the phonemes are modified at the joining of these larger units. Although the phonemicists ignore the inclusive movements, they are aware that the boundary markers at the ends of the larger units are like the boundary markers between subordinate units, and therefore generalize the concept of juncture to cover all boundary phenomena. It would be better to count a juncture the case where two termini come together, where two ends abut. This would have eliminated the inconsistency of an "external open juncture" which does not join anything.

In motor phonetic terms, the beginning and the end of the inclusive movements are naturally marked, and the syllables and syllable factors which come together between movements are modified by the juxtaposition, which can be studied in its detail in the laboratory.

External Open Juncture: HK (26, p. 283 f.)

Internal Open Juncture:

Close Juncture:

These junctures are actually terminal phenomena. They become "junctures" only in the case of "internal open juncture" and "close juncture" between breath groups, feet, and syllables. Within the syllable, conditions are entirely different, although the phonemicists have not taken the difference into account. The logistic handling is such that internal open juncture and close juncture may alternate, depending on the rate and stress. The observations are not consistent, and there is no consideration of the variations with changes of rate and of stress.

The boundary markers (Grenzsignale) define the inclusive movements. They assume importance in a logistic system because they are the only recognition of the coordination of the movements which underlies the process of speech.

In a motor phonetics the boundary marks have their natural place as the indications of the limits of the movements which folow each other, but which are knit together by the underlying movement.

APPENDIX X

THE DEMARCATION OF THE SYLLABLE

The question of the syllable as an individual unit, and the question of the demarcation of the syllable, "the division of the syllable", are essentially the same problem. But they may be discussed separately. If the syllable is made an individual unit, it must be one indissoluble movement. It should be possible to define this one movement so as to show how it is delimited.

In all languages it is possible to make the syllables stressed or unstressed beats in a metrical pattern without doing violence to the nature of the syllable. Whatever the supposed character of the syllables so arranged, whether syllables by breath pressure or by "sonority", whether divided by "implosion-explosion" or by "discontinuity of intensity", they can all be represented by a rhythmic series composed of simple nonsense syllables. The rhythmical scheme of any actual verse or prose group can be adequately set out with "ta, ta . . .". Cf. De Groot (15). Instead of saying that "the syllabic sonant has sonority, real or apparent", which produces a subjective beat, it is simpler to say that the sound of the syllable, whether prominent or not, naturally occasions in the hearer just that ballistic pulse which makes the syllable for the speaker. "Sonority" is not recognized as a property in acoustics or audition; the attributes which occasion a "subjective" beat are duration and intensity, the attributes of a movement.

The observation of Rousselot, already cited, that in subcortical aphasia the syllable is preserved, bears on the same point. There are as many expiratory pulses as there are syllables in the phrase which the patient attempts to say.

The problem of *one* movement as applied to the syllable may be generalized: it is the problem of defining one movement in any series of rapid, skilled movements. How are we to define a single movement?

The syllable belongs to the type of movement characterized by a beat or pulse. Occasionally the movement may be prolonged when the ballistic pulse is continued into a prolonged, controlled (tense) movement. Speech may be very "slow" just as piano playing may be very slow; but in either case the pulse of the chest stroke and the pulse of the finger stroke is quick, ballistic, though the syllable or note continues.

The syllable is one in the sense that it consists essentially of a single chest pulse, usually made audible by the vocal folds, which may be started or stopped by a chest movement or by a consonant movement. These auxiliary articulatory movements cannot be considered independent because their essential function is to delimit the chest pulse, and their characteristics depend on that function.

This reduction of the movement of the syllable to a ballistic chest movement eliminates Sievers' distinction between "pressure" syllables (Drucksilben) and "sonority" syllables (Schallsilben). All syllables become pressure syllables in that the pressure is due to a sudden breath pulse. The concepts of the "variation of sonority", or of "relative prominence" are unsatisfactory. As W. Perret points out, it is possible to run through the whole gamut of vowels in a single syllable. (62, p. 25, 67)

And it may be added that the order of vowels may be varied, and slow consonant movements introduced; the one thing essential to a long continuous syllable is simply that no second ballistic movement occur; it is not a matter of variations in sonority nor of any other quality. To make a new syllable, the change in the velocity of utterance must be rapid enough for a ballistic pulse, but not too rapid. The *a-i* of the English "long i" shows a striking change in quality, but no second syllable develops because the change occurs during the one ballistic chest movement. Sievers' "*a-la*" does not prove to be pronounced as two syllables with only one breath pressure. Laboratory recording (Fig. 15, 17, *a la dad*) shows the two chest pulses. In the breathless mouthing of syllables with the glottis closed, the movements of lips, jaw and tongue coordinate with functionless chest pulses. Cf. the buccal whisper of the laryngectomized. The same thing is to be said of the pronunciation of the first two syllables of the word "Aragón" suggested by Navarro Thomás.

In this connection Navarro Thomás makes an interesting suggestion as to the nature of the syllable; after speaking of it as separated acoustically by the diminution of sonority, he continues: "Considered from the physiological point of view, it is an articulatory nucleus contained between two successive diminutions of the muscular activity." (57, p. 28)

Certain traits of the syllable division which have been noted on occasion are to be explained in terms of the consecutive ballistic chest pulses. It often happens that there is a "reduction in the force of utterance" at the syllable frontier. The "s" is continuous in the double sibilant of "*this sigh*" (cf. "*this eye*"), and there is a reduction in the intensity at the syllable frontier when the new chest pulse occurs. Diminution of intensity cannot be made, however, the general principle of syllable division. Passy states: "The separation of the syllable is marked by the point where the intensity is at its minimum" (60, p. 45).

There are cases in which the new chest pulse occurs without "diminution of intensity". Instead, a sudden rise in intensity marks the entrance of the new chest pulse. Rousselot has published records of a series "à, à.....". in which the laryngeal tone is continuous from à to à but there is a sudden rise in the intensity as a result of a change in the breath regulation (régime du souffle), i.e. a new chest pulse occurs for the new syllable. (70, p. 349)

F. de Saussure's division between the syllables was made to depend on an implosion-explosion juxtaposition; this means the arrest of the chest pulse followed by the release of the following chest pulse. And it is to be remembered that syllables without consonants on either side of the syllable division present just this same arrest-release phenomenon. Saussure's observation of the implosion-explosion as a sign of vowel demarcation is good; but to assign a series of "explosions" to a sequence of consonants and vowel, as in "t r y a" (in which *t*, *r*, *y* are all counted as explosions), is a mistake; there can be but one release of the syllable movement. The same objection is to be made to a series of "implosions" like "a r s t" (a, r, s, t, implosive); a syllabic movement can have but one arrest. It is also a mistake to assume that a given "sound" can have but one phase in a given syllable. In any syllable there is a release and an arrest of the pulse, so that a syllable consisting of a single vowel like the English word "a" or the French word "y" has both the release and the arrest, and would present, in Saussure's nomenclature, "explosion-implosion", "explosion" at the release of the vowel and "implosion" at the arrest of the vowel in the syllable.

F. de Saussure's description of the syllable division as a shift from one syllabic process to another recognized the syllable as a unit, and assigned functions to his phonemes. Ne was not aware of the chest pulse of the syllable, and phrased the delimitation of the syllable in terms of a process first of opening the articulatory apparatus, which continued to the mid-point of the syllable, and second of closing the articulatory apparatus from the midpoint to the end of the syllable. His formulation was far better than that of Rousselot who condensed the opening and closing of Saussure's syllable into the tension-tenue-détente of a single "sound".

The "pressure syllable" (Drucksilbe) describes the new chest pulse which makes the new syllable. In some cases this new pulse was not apparent to theorists working without experimental means of observation, and the "sonority syllable" (Schallsilbe) was added. The demonstration of the chest pulse for all syllables eliminates the "sonority syllable". The part played by the releasing and arresting factors of the syllable accounts for "diminution of intensity" if it occurs between syllables and for the equivocal prominence. There are various indications of the end of one chest pulse and the beginning of the new chest pulse.

The relation of the syllable division to the double consonant, and of the other forms of abutting consonants at the syllable frontier, will be considered later.

Prominence

Since the concept of "sonority" has no standing in acoustics, and the practical measurement of some such quality in the form of the carrying power of the "sound" proved impossible, sonority has been given up and non-committal "prominence" is used as the criterion of syllable demarcation. Speech is thought of as a series of peaks and valleys. They are, however, matters of process; they are not static. The syllables have prominence as they pass by, whether due to stress, or loudness, or any other quality. And the peaks and valleys are not fixed; there are constant shifts across the valley, both forward and backward. On occasion the peaks fuse in utterance.

In the process of utterance the syllables must be essential; peaks and valleys are not optional; there is nothing to correspond to the variegated plain; the foothills do not give way to rolling prairie. Utterance progresses peak by peak, however flexible the process; and the shifts of peaksides across valleys follows regular laws and can be explained in terms of the process of utterance. Prominence explains nothing and is not even a good description, since it does not provide for the factors of the syllable and their relations from syllable to syllable. There is nothing in prominence, in peaks and valleys to explain sandhi.

The close relation of juncture of the syllable train, whereby syllables are always separated by juncture, and the syllable factors are supposed to be connected by juncture, and the breath groups are set off by juncture, is not incorporated into the prominence conception; the junctures have nothing to do with the peaks and valleys.

Juncture

The term is used in phonemics to describe two very different and opposite functions.

1. Juncture is a separation, gap, pause, which may be of indefinite duration. "Open juncture" may be open for all time.
2. Juncture also means a seam or joint where things are connected, brought together.

Since the phonemicists deal in isolated symbols and have no provision for organizing these units, it is natural to assume that juxtaposition means union of some sort; that a slit is a seam, a gap is a joint, a split is a splice. When syllables fuse, when articulations and syllables are elided and reappear, "juncture" must come and go, and becomes another element. If an initial or final element disappears in the "open juncture" on either side of the breath group or phrase, it somehow makes its way back as a "close juncture". Since the consonants often move "across the juncture", i.e. from syllable to syllable, it seems possible to cross the gap; although sometimes the juncture is thought of as an element inserted between two other elements.

When it comes to a consideration of connections of the intra-syllabic factors, it is apparent that the 'juncture' is of a different order. "Close" and "open" juncture are not enough; there is an extensive overlapping of the factors; in fact, in the case of consonants of two different members abutting between syllables, the arresting and the releasing factor may come to coincide. Cf. in the series "pat pat . . . ." at rapid rate. Fig. 63. The notion of "juncture" to cover such a connection is inadequate.

If a basic process is provided for, of which the factors are a part in the syllable, and of which the syllables are a part in the breath group, the notion of joints between elements becomes intelligible, and their closure or overlapping is normal. The connection between members of the group need not be lumped with the silence which occurs before and after the group, and which may be indefinite, as in the case of any other movement complex.

If the terms prominence and juncture are defended as merely descriptive, then description is not enough. The important phenomena need far more than mere description to account for the evident laws of behavior of the syllables and their factors. Phonology has passed the stage of mere description; phonetics must be motor phonetics: the mere shuffling of symbols on a line is not enough.

APPENDIX XI

TABLE 1
Various phrases recorded to show the contrast between the double and the single consonant

Subject	Phrase			No. of phrases meas.d	Extremes of length single conson.s	Extremes of length double conson.s	Air-pres. curves of double	Conson. curves of double
C.	Otto ought to	A	43 e	5	.06–.13	.23–.33	bmr	bm
			42 d	9	.12–.19	.26–.31	bm bmr	bmr(af)
			42 e	4	.12–.14	.31–.38	bml	af(bm)
			38 d	6	.10–.13	.25–.45	bmcc	bma(a)
			38 e	5	.11–.20	.27–.40	cc	bma(a)
			39 b	7	.08–.10	.24–.33	bm cc	bm(a)
			39 c	8	.09–.13	.24–.47	cc(bm)	bm, (bml)
			70 f	11	.08–.12	.19–.34	bmr, bm	af(bmaf)
E.			53 a	5	.12–.16	.33–.45	bmr	bmal
			53 b	5	.18–.22	.34–.40	bmr	bma, bmal
			53 c	5	.16–.18	.33–.39	bma(a)	bmaf
			53 d	4	.12–.17	.25–.31	ai, cci	bma
			53 e	4	.14–.18	.23–.32	a(bm)	bma(af)
S.			47 d	11	.06–.12	.17–.34	icc	ai, a
			47 e	5	.07–.11	.18–.22	acc	a
			40 c	6	.06–.08	.16–.20	abm(al)	a
			40 d	5	.10–.18	.18–.23	abm	a
			40 e	5	.14–.16	.20–.24	abm, bm	a
C.	Hit him, hit Tim		41 a	5	.07–.10	.19–.28	bmr, bm	af(bmaf)
			41 c	6	.06–.11	.22–.28	bm(bmcc)	bml(af)
S.	I do, I'd do		40 a	3	.12–.17	.21–.28	bm	bm
			40 b	3	.13–.20	.28–.32	bm	bm
C.	I'm Ike, I'm Mike		71 d	3	.32–.50	.45–.48	bm	bma(af)
			68 a	5	.08–.14	.10–.24	bm	al, bml
			69 a	6	.10–.13	.20–.30	bm, bma	afl(bm)
			69 b	5	.10–.15	.22–.26	bma	bma(a)
			69 c	6	.09–.12	.20–.28	bm	a(bm)
			69 d	9	.07–.10	.16–.21	bm	bma, a
			69 e	8	.08–.12	.20–.27	bm	bmal, a

APPENDIX XI

Subject	Phrase		No. of phrases meas.d	Extremes of length single conson.s	Extremes of length double conson.s	Air-pres. curves of double	Conson. curves of double
C.	Whole ode, whole load	48 e	3	.06–.16	.22–.26	—	bm
		48 f	3	.12–.18	.23–.33	—	bm
		48 g	5	.08–.10	.12–.20	—	bm
		70 d	6	.12–.16	.26–.32	—	bm
E.		56 a	3	.19–.25	.33–.34	—	bmr, ar
		56 b	2	.25–.25	.32–.34	—	bmr
E.	I lie, I'll lie	59 c	3	.13–.28	.31–.35	—	bmr
		59 d	4	.18–.22	.32–.38	—	bmr(bmf)
		59 e	3	.17–.18	.25–.35	—	bm(a)
H.		66 d	5	.06–.13	.22–.32	—	al
		66 e	6	.09–.13	.20–.22	—	bml(al)
C.	Hello	70 a	6	—	.43–.61	—	bm
		70 b	7	—	.35–.45	—	bm
C.	Unknown	70 e	12	.10–.18	.30–.39	—	bm(al)
		70 g	3	.19–.34	.30–.40	—	bml, al
E.		54 a	6	—	.29–.36	—	bm, al
		54 b	5	.20–.25	.32–.39	—	bm, bmf
		52 a	3	.13–.21	.21–.22	bmr, bmf	a
		52 a	6	.17–.30	.23–.36	bm, a	al
		50 b	6	.18–.24	.20–.22	bm, n	a
		50 c	3	.24–.26	.22–.23	bmr	af
		55 a	4	.22–.24	.18–.25	bm, a	al
		55 b	3	.20–.26	.20–.25	bm	al
		55 c	5	.20–.26	.19–.22	bm, a	al
		55 d	4	.20–.27	.18–.25	bm(a)	al
		50 b	6	.19–.24	.20–.22	bmn, n	a
	Unknown, unown	50 c	3	.18–.20	.21–.36	bm, a	bm, a
		50 d	4	.15–.22	.25–.28	bm	bm
S.	Unknown	62 a	2	.19–.20	.46–.54	—	bm, bmr
		62 b	6	.10–.13	.26–.30	bm	bm(al)
		62 c	7	.14–.16	.26–.33	bm, cc	abm, (a)
		62 d	7	.14–.18	.20–.27	(bm)	a(bm)
H.		66 a	6	.16–.22	.19–.30	—	bml, al
		66 b	9	.12–.20	.18–.23	—	al(bml)
		66 c	7	.15–.17	.18–.26	bm	al
E.	This eye, this sigh	2 a	3	.16–.20	.25–.34	af	af
		2 b	3	.18–.23	.29–.37	af	af
		2 c	3	.16–.18	.29–.31	bm	bm
		2 d	3	.17–.24	.23–.37	a, ar	bm, af
S.		1 a	7	.18–.24	.29–.50	a, bm	a(bm)
		1 b	7	.14–.24	.27–.29	af(bm)	bm, af
E.	Z is Z	60 a	6	.22–.32	.32–.43	bm	bm
		61 a	5	.26–.42	.33–.42	bm	bmf
		61 b	4	.26–.33	.38–.57	bmr	bmf(af)
		61 c	4	.28–.35	.36–.41	bml	bmf
		61 d	5	.30–.38	.44–.57	bma(bmr)	bmf
S.	Z is Zinc	45 b	6	.22–.30	.48–.66	bml, a	bml
		45 b	6	.21–.28	.22–.40	—, ai	bmr

(*continued*)

Subject	Phrase		No. of phrases meas.d	Extremes of length single conson.s	Extremes of length double conson.s	Air-pres. curves of double	Conson. curves of double
C.	Up puppy	6 a	13	.06–.08	.14–.36	ncc(bm)	a(bm)
		6 b	10	.11–.22	.22–.32	cc(bmcc)	a(bmal)
		6 c	10	.15–.22	.25–.32	ccl(bmcc)	bma, al
		7 a	10	.06–.10	.24–.32	bm(cca)	bml
		5 d	11	.08–.08	.19–.27	bmcc(cc	abm
C.	Top pole	86 a	8	—	.25–.34	cc	bml, al
E.	Up puppy	3 a	8	.08–.10	.22–.36	bml, bmr	bm, bmaf
		3 c	9	.08–.14	.25–.36	bm, cc	bm(al)
	Topic, top pick	58 a	5	.09–.10	.33–.36	bmr	bm
		58 b	4	.06–.10	.30–.37	bml	bm
	Top egg, top peg	57 a	3	.11–.12	.36–.38	bm, bmcc	bm
		57 b	3	.14–.17	.32–.36	bm	bm
		57 c	3	.16–.26	.40–.52	bmr	bm, bmf
		57 d	3	.17–.18	.39–.40	bm, bmr	bm
		57 e	3	.17–.19	.36–.38	bmr	bm
S.		65 a	4	—	.20–.23	bmrf	a
		65 b	5	—	.18–.27	bmf	a, bmal
		65 d	8	—	.16–.25	bmf	a
		65 e	6	—	.20–.30	ccf	bm, al
		63 a	4	.10–.14	.14–.18	—	a
		63 b	4	.10–.13	.14–.17	—	a
	Topic, top pick	64 b	1	.07	.17	c	a
		64 d	4	.06–.10	.20–.22	cc	a
		64 e	2	.06–.06	.17–.20	cc	a
	Up puppy	9 f	13	.06–.11	.14–.33	bm	a, bm
		9 e	12	.10–.17	.18–.31	bm	a, bm
		9 a	9	—	—	bm	a
		46 a	8	.06–.12	.21–.30	bmr, bml	bm, a
		46 c	10	.06–.09	.18–.33	bmn	a, bm
		44 b	8	.06–.08	.17–.24	bman, bmcc	a
H.		4 e	8	.06–.14	.27–.42	bm	bml
		4 f	8	.09–.13	.33–.40	bm	bml
		44 a	9	.07–.10	.19–.31	bm	bml
		44 b	7	.08–.10	.18–.32	bmr, bml	bml
	Topic, top pick	67 c	6	.08–.11	.21–.40	bm(a)	bml
	Top egg, top peg	67 b	7	.10–.16	.42–.48	bm, a	bml
C.	Lob Bob	55 b	9	.11–.14	.19–.30	bml	al(bm)

The following abutting consonants, quite like the "doubles", are added for comparison:

C.	Hell no	70 c	8	—	.27–.34	—	bma(a)
E.	Unlike	53 c	6	—	.23–.31	a(bm)	bml(a)
		53 d	3	—	.27–.36	—, bm	bm
H.		66 f	7	—	.18–.31	—	al
		66 g	6	—	.16–.30	—	al
C.	Up Bob	5 a	10	.11–.16	.22–.32	bml	a, al
	Humbug	86 a	8	—	.19–.29	bmr	al, bm
	Half pay	86 c	9	—	.36–.41	cc(bmcc)	bmar(a)

APPENDIX XI

Subject	Phrase		No. of phrases meas.d	Extremes of length single conson.s	Extremes of length double conson.s	Air-pres. curves of double	Conson. curves of double
E.		58 c	6	—	.35–.43	nbm(cc)	bmr, bmf
		58 d	7	—	.32–.36	bmr	bmr, bmf
		58 e	5	—	.31–.38	bmr	bmf
S.	Up Bob	9 c	8	.08–.14	.18–.23	bml	a (bml)
		9 d	11	.09–.14	.20–.32	bm, bml	a
		46 d	10	.07–.18	.17–.26	bmr, bml	a (abm)
		46 e	12	.06–.15	.19–.23	bm	a (abm)

Key to abbreviations for air pressure- and consonant-curves:

bm – bi-maximal
  f — flat; affixed to abbreviation for curve form
  r — stress on right doublet; affixed to abbreviation
  l — stress on left doublet; affixed to abbreviation

a — rounded ("*arch*")
cc — "convex-concave"
i — pointed
n — "inflected curve"

Abbreviations in parentheses indicate a curve form which appears but once.

APPENDIX XII

Check List of English Compound Consonants

Releasing Consonants		Arresting Consonants		Releasing Consonants (con.)		Arresting Consonants (con.)			
bl	blow	bd	rubbed	sp	spa	lmz	elms	rths	girths
br	brave	bz	dubs	spl	split	lp	help	rv	starve
bry	brew	cht	pitched	spr	spray	lps	helps	rvz	starves
by	beauty	dz	adds	spy	spew	ls	pulse	rz	scars
chy	chew	fs	puffs	st	stay	lsh	Welsh	sht	pushed
dr	chew	fth	fifth	str	strike	lt	cult	sk	ask
dr	dry	fths	fifths	sty	stew	lth	health	sks	asks
dry	drew	gd	rigged	sw	swing	lths	healths	md	hummed
dy	dew	gz	bugs	sy	sue	lts	wilts	mp	lump
dw	dwell	jd	judged	thr	through	lv	shelve	mps	lumps
fl	fly	nt	tent	thw	thwart	lvs	shelves	mt	tempt
fr	fry	nts	tents	thy	thew	lz	bills	mts	tempts
fry	fruit	nth	tenth	tr	try	rb	herb	mz	hums
fy	few	nths	tenths	tw	twist	rbz	herbs	nch	lunch
gl	glow	nz	ones	ty	tune	rch	scorch	nd	burned
gr	grow	ngd	hanged	vy	view	rd	hard	nds	ends
gw	Gwenn	ngk	ink	zhy	azure	rdz	herds	nf	Banff
gy	gewgaw	ngks	inks	zy	presume	rf	scarf	nfs	Banff's
jy	Jew	ngkt	inked			rfs	scarf's	nj	plunge
kl	cloth	ngz	sings			rg	erg	njd	plunged
kly	clew	ps	maps			rgs	ergs	ns	once
kr	crawl	pt	mapped			rj	barge	sp	clasp
kw	quick	ks	ax			rk	bark	sps	clasps
ky	cue	ksth	sixth			rks	barks	st	list
ly	Lew	ksths	sixths			rm	arm	sts	lists
my	mew	kt	act			rms	arms	thd	lathed
ny	new	kts	acts			rn	burn	ths	smiths
pl	play	lb	bulb			rns	burns	tth	eighth
pr	pray	lbz	bulbs			rp	harp	tths	eighths
py	pew	lch	milch			rps	harps	thz	paths
shr	shrink	ld	pulled			rs	scarce	ts	hits
shy	sure	ldz	holds			rsh	harsh	vz	doves
sk	scold	lf	shelf			rt	part	zd	raised

APPENDIX XII

Releasing Consonants		Arresting Consonants		Releasing Consonants (con.)	Arresting Consonants (con.)			
skl	sclerotic	lfs	golfs		rts	parts	zm	spasm
skr	scrap	lfth	twelfth		rth	girth	zmz	spasms
skw	squeal	lfths	twelfths					
sky	skew	lj	bulge					
sl	slow	ljd	bulged	Releasing and Arresting Consonants:				
sly	slew	lk	bulk		sk			
sm	smell	lks	bulks		sp			
sn	snow	lm	helm		st			

APPENDIX XIII

COLLATION OF VISIBLE SPEECH PATTERNS WITH KYMOGRAMS OF MOTOR PHONETICS

R. H. Stetson and C. V. Hudgins

It is quite possible to make simultaneous recordings of the "patterns of visible speech" by means of the sound spectrograph developed by the engineers of the Bell Laboratories[1], and of the movements and air pressures of motor phonetics.

For this purpose the Kay engineers designed an independent circuit to indicate the overall acoustic intensity and so make the syllables apparent. (The apparatus used was built by the Kay Electric Company, Pine Brook, New Jersey, under license.)

Thus we recorded simultaneously:

1. The visible speech patterns
2. The acoustic intensities
3. The tracings of motor phonetics which give:
   a. Movements of lips, tongue, and jaw.
   b. Movements of chest and abdomen.
   c. Air pressure in mouth.

The motor phonetic tracing Chest Pulse for the syllables parallels the acoustic intensity line. This marks the identity of the syllable as it appears in the acoustic patterns and as it appears in the motor phonetic tracings.

In the visible speech patterns the vowels are marked by the modulation bars. The influence of the consonants on the vowel is seen in the warping of the bars in the same syllable.

In kymograms of motor phonetics the detail of the consonant movements which is not apparent in the visible speech patterns, is given by the tracings of lip- and tongue- contacts and the tracings of air pressure in the mouth.

The two types of recording confirm and supplement each other.

---

[1]Visible Speech. New York: D. Van Nostrand Co., Potter, Kopp and Green, 1947.

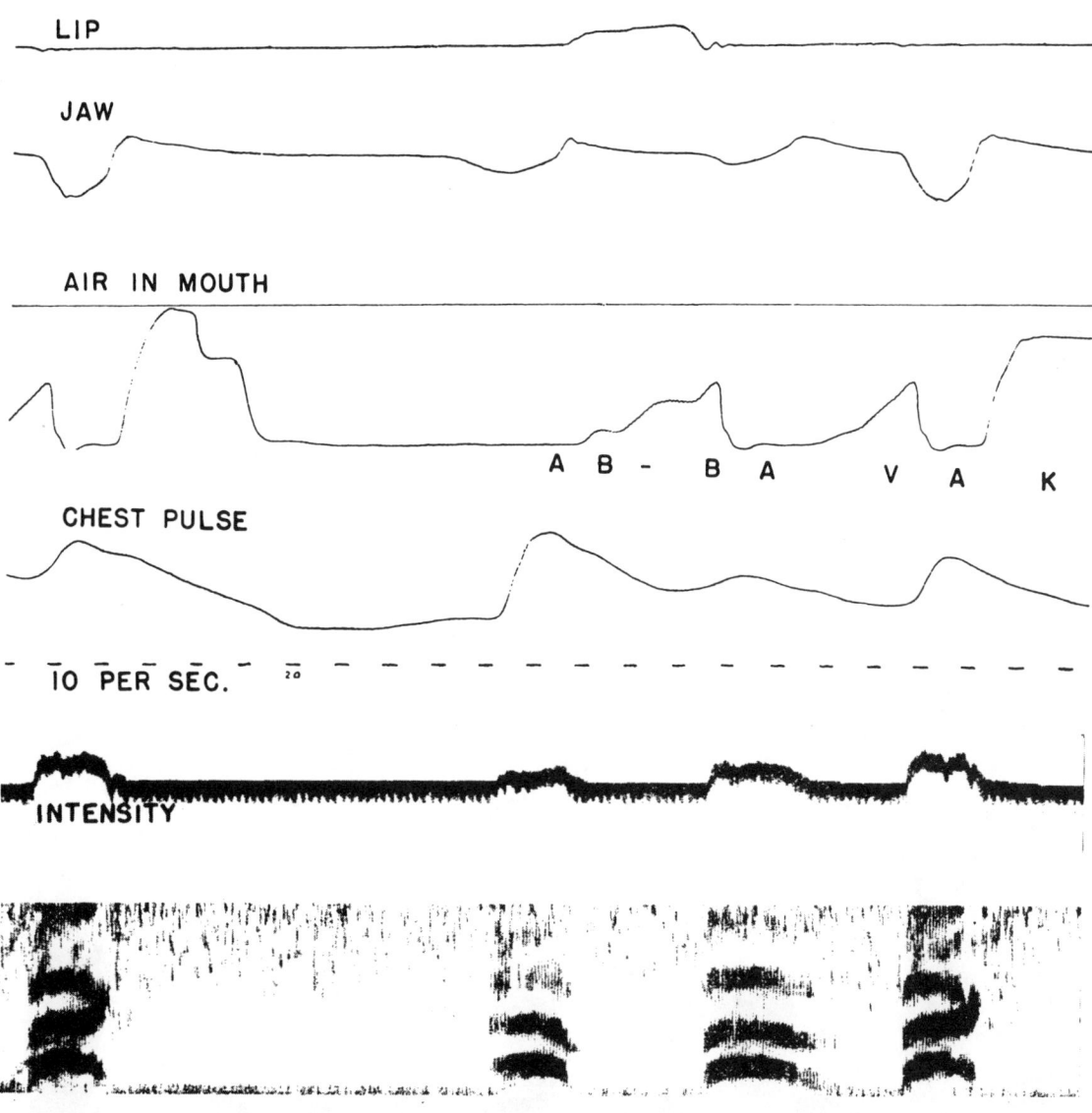

FIGURE 114

Syllables: Ab-ba vak.

The syllable pulses are indicated by:

1. The intensity line of the acoustic recording.
2. The chest pulses of the kymograph tracing.

The syllable factors are indicated by:

1. The vowel patterns of the visible speech modulation bars.
2. The delimiting syllable factors are not indicated by the acoustic record, but appear in the consonant movements of the tracings, *ab-ba*, and *vak*. The doubling (abutting) form appear between the syllables of *ab-ba*.

The feet appear in:

1. The stress and durations of the visible speech recording.
2. The overall grouping of the chest movements.

The breath group is indicated by the entire expression. (If a tracing of the abdominal movements had been added it would confirm this.)

This recording of actual speech should be compared in detail with the diagrammatic drawing, Fig. 36. (The intensity line is not shown in this diagram; the intensity line had not been developed when the drawing was made.)

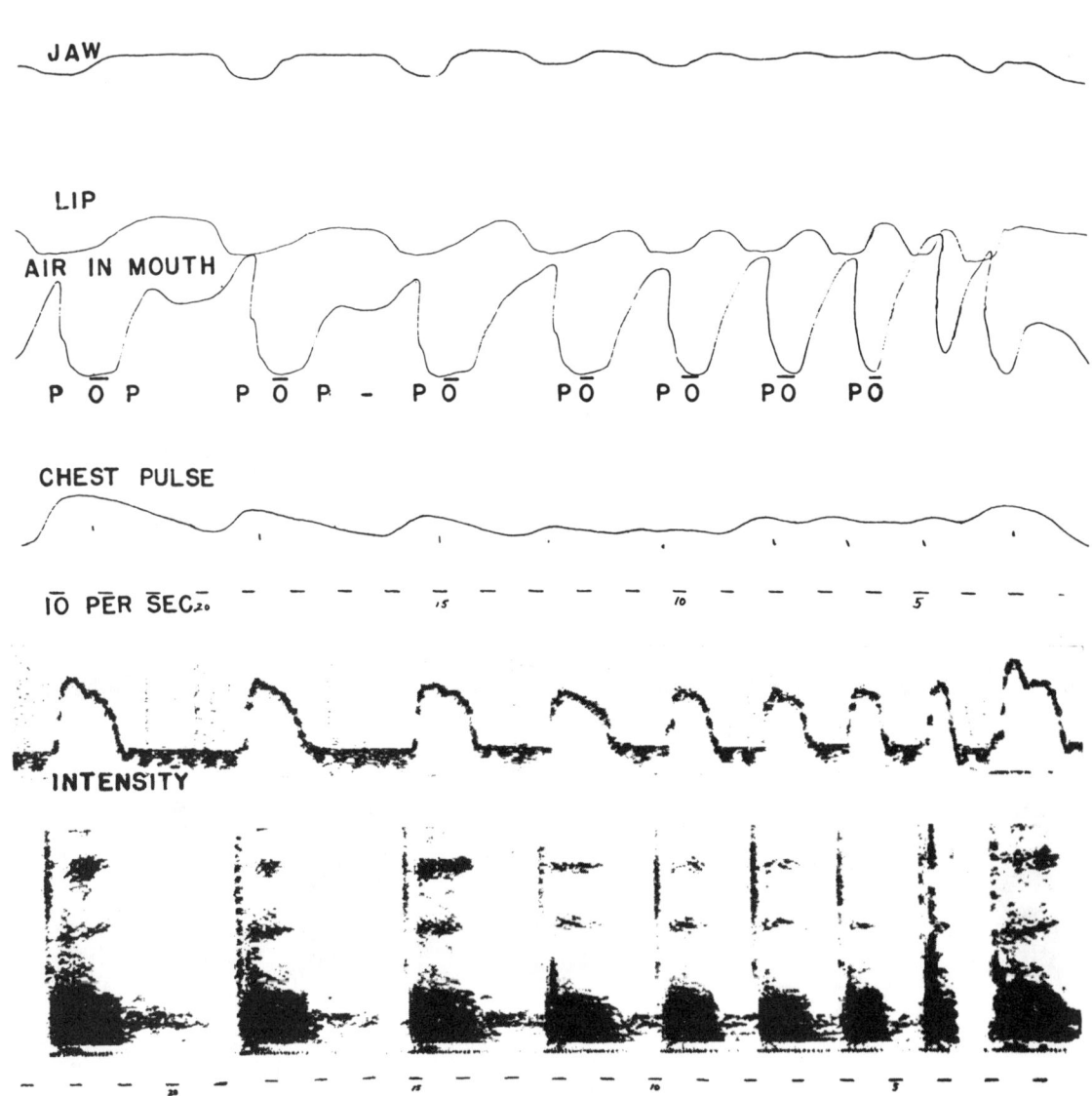

FIGURE 115. A Carrier Train of Syllables with Gradually Increasing Rate

Visible speech patterns show syllables clearly in the intensity line. The modulation bars of the vowel are warped downward at both ends by the adjacent p- and p- in the early syllables; when the arresting -p drops with the increasing rate, only the beginning of the vowel bars is affected.

Kymograph tracings show what is happening to the consonant where the acoustic recordings tell nothing.

Kymograph tracings of the chest pulses show the syllables, and the grouping of the syllables.

Air pressure in the mouth shows the releasing and arresting forms of the consonants, and the doubling (abutting) forms between syllables.

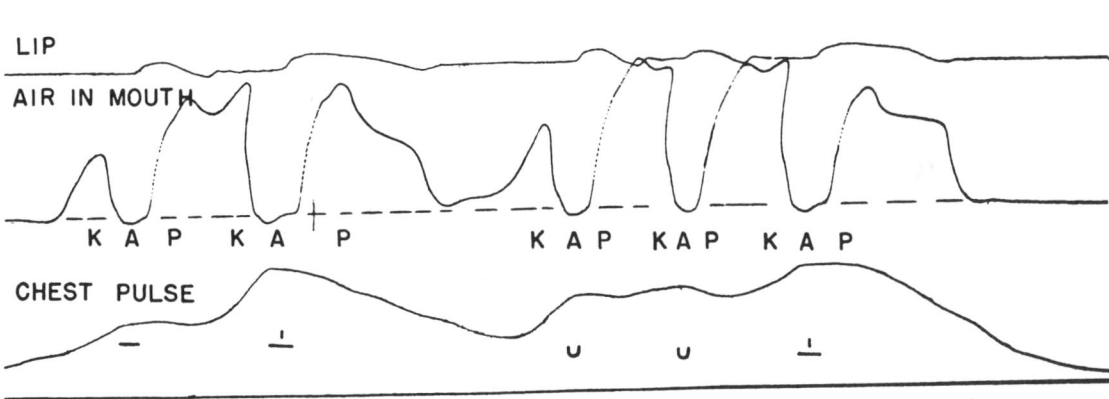

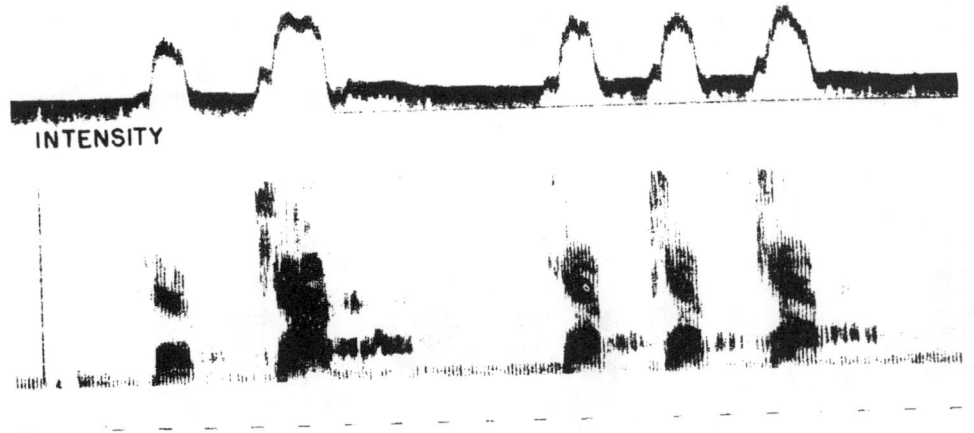

FIGURE 116

Syllables: *Kap kap' kap kap kap'*.
  Visible speech patterns:
  Intensity line marks the syllables and indicates stress and syllable duration.
  Modulation bars are warped upward by the *k*- and downward by the -*p*.
  This phenomenon is marked in: *kap kap kap'*.

Kymograph tracings show:
  Lip marker, indicating the consonant contacts for P. K is not shown.
  Air pressure in mouth which delineates the functions of the consonants; first the abutting K–P, then the fused forms.
  Chest pulses showing the feet and the subordination of the pulses to the main stresses.

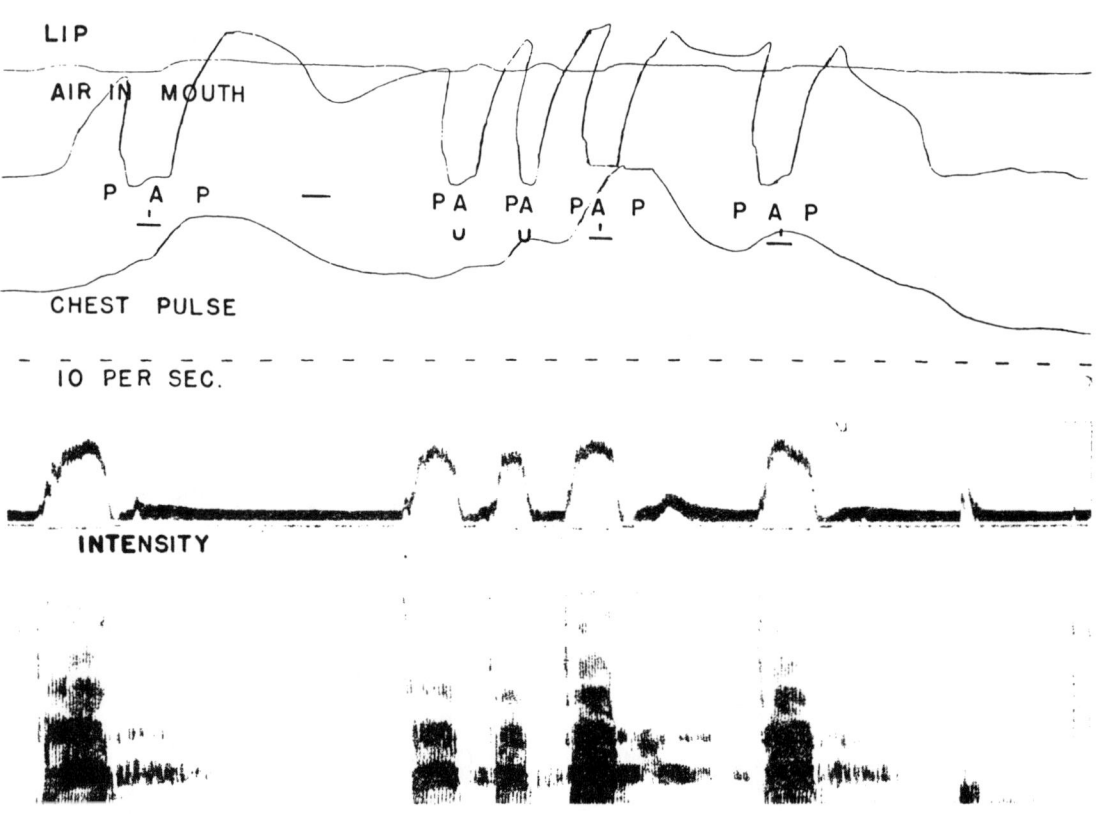

FIGURE 117

Syllables: *pap' pa' pa' pap' pap'*.
  Visible speech patterns:
  Modulation bars show the warping down at both ends for the accented syllables.
  Kymograph tracings:
  Chest pulses show:
  Preparation for the breath group (tracing of the abdominal movement would have been more pronounced).
  Air pressure in mouth shows releasing and arresting forms.
  Doubling is apparent in the air pressure in the mouth.
  Lips show the doubling forms.

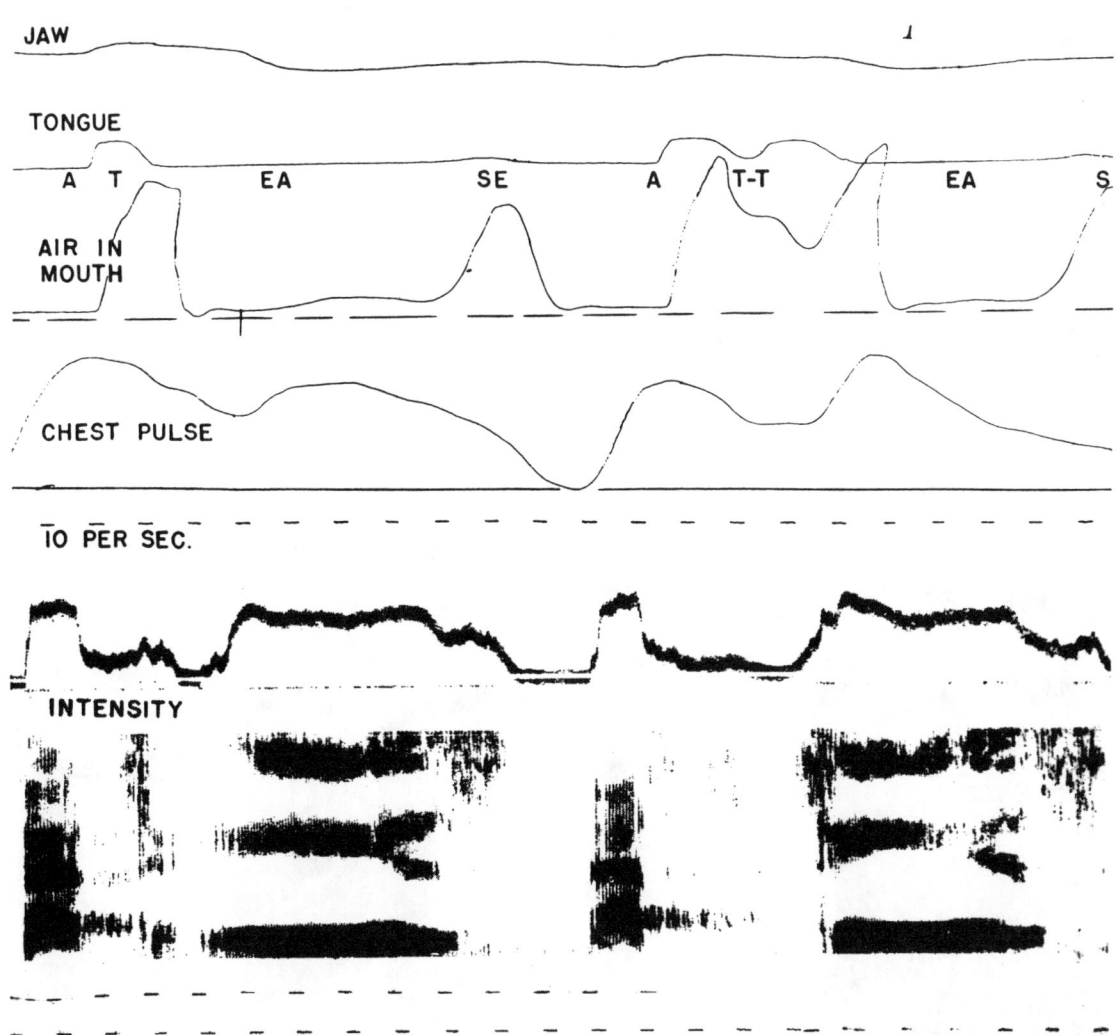

FIGURE 118

Syllables: *At ease, at teas*.

Visible speech patterns:

The warping of the modulation bars is not present in *ease*, because the arresting *-t* belongs to the preceding syllable.

The warping of the modulation bars shows both for the arresting *t* of *at*—and for the releasing *t-* of *teas*.

The kymograph tracing shows the releasing and arresting forms, and the double in "*at- teas*" clearly in the air pressure in mouth.

The tongue marker shows the double form in *at- teas*.

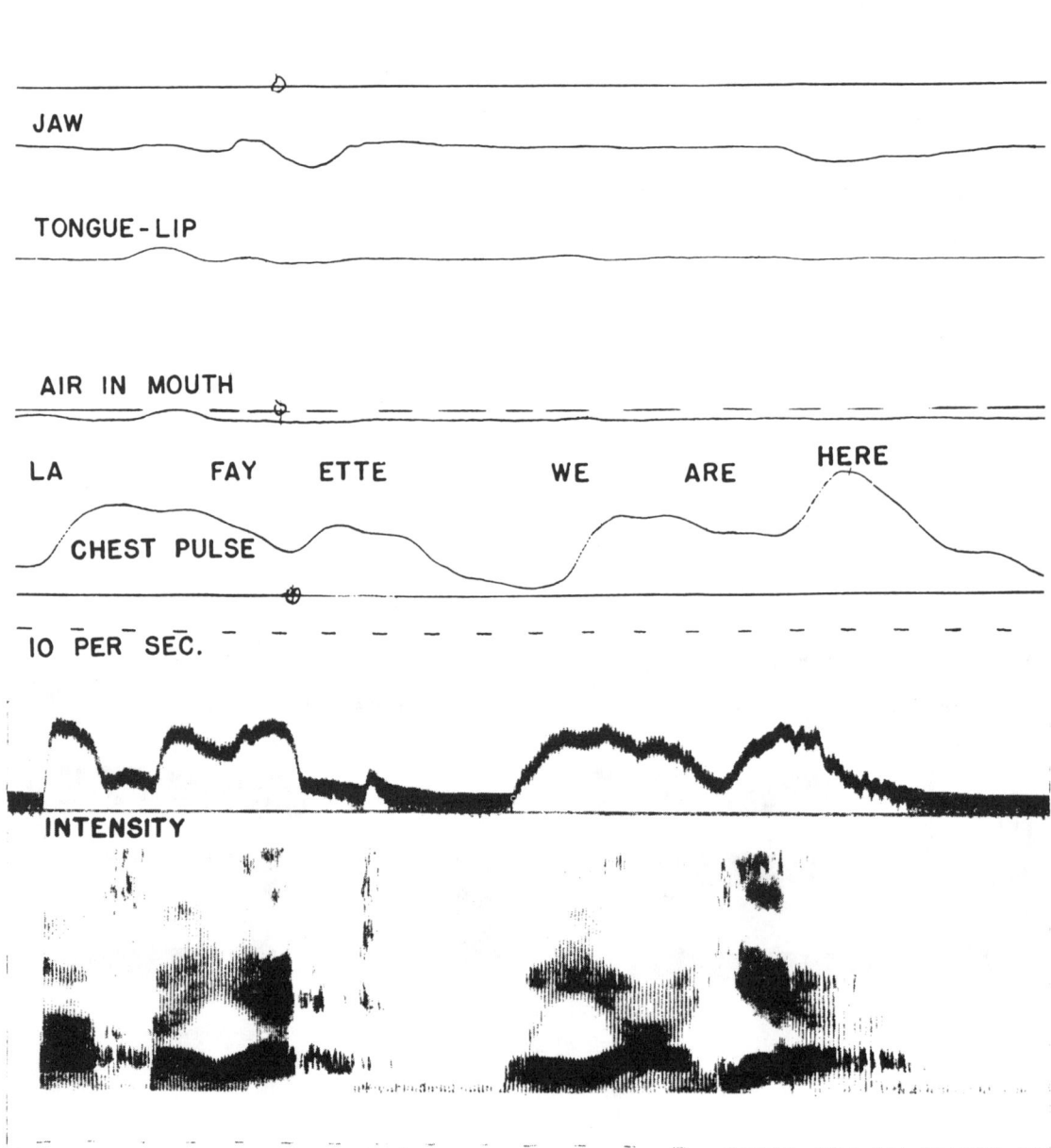

FIGURE 119

Syllables: *Lafayette we are here.*
Intensity line of the acoustic patterns, and the chest pulses of the kymograph tracings are parallel. Modulation bars of the acoustic recording give much more detail of the vowel shaping movements.

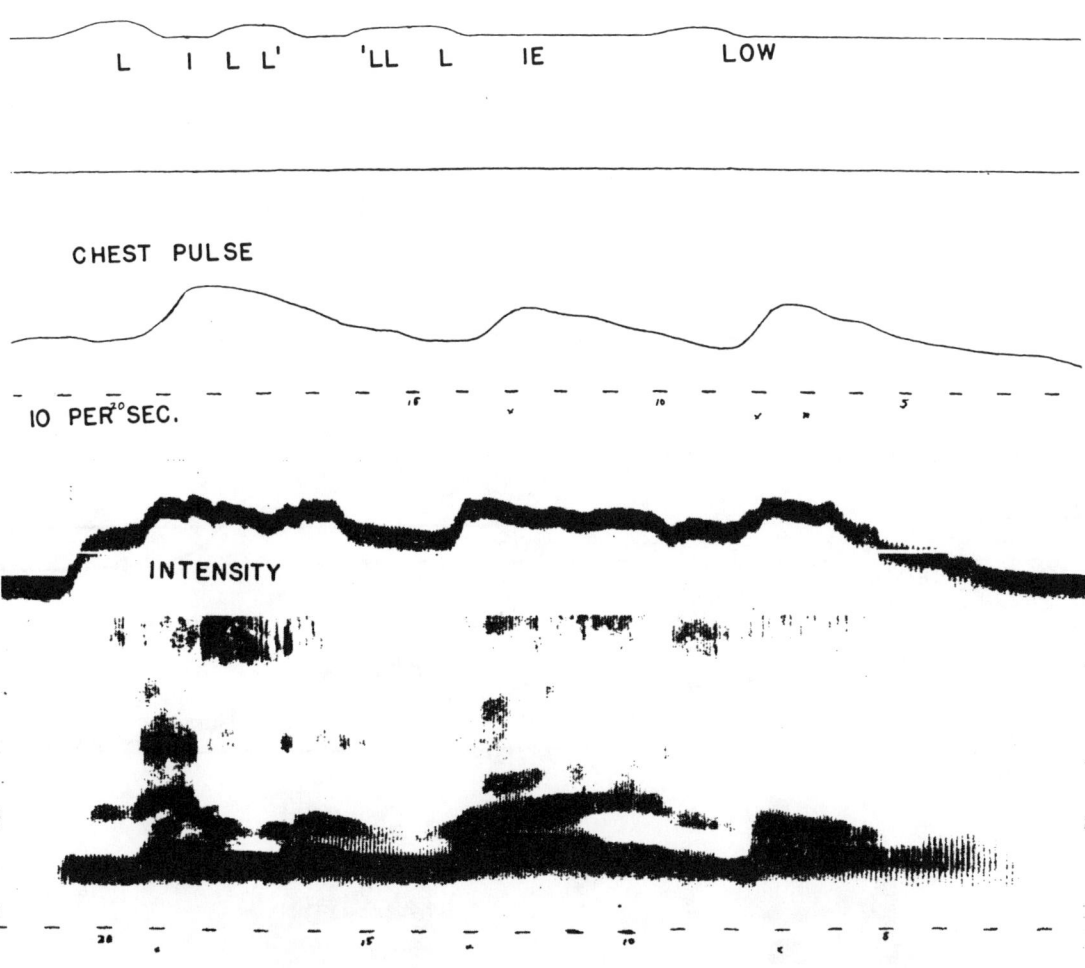

FIGURE 120

Syllables: *Lill' 'll lie low.*

The intensity line and the chest pulse tracing are parallel in showing the syllables. The intensity line gives rather more detail. (See also Figs. 88 and 89, p. 125.)

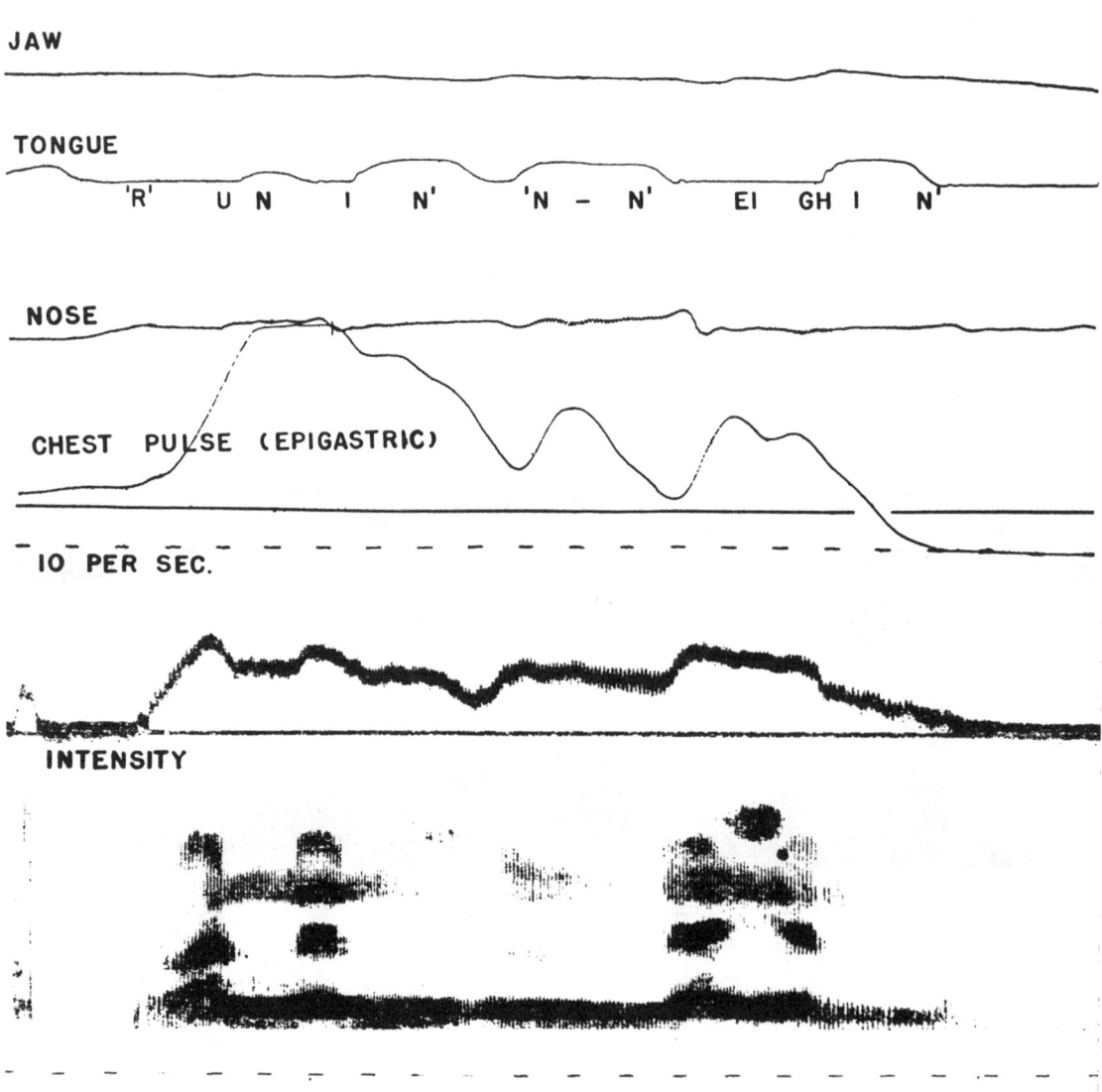

FIGURE 121

Syllables: *Runnin' 'n' neighin'*.
Intensity line and the chest pulse tracing show the same syllables. (See also Fig. 111, p. 144.)

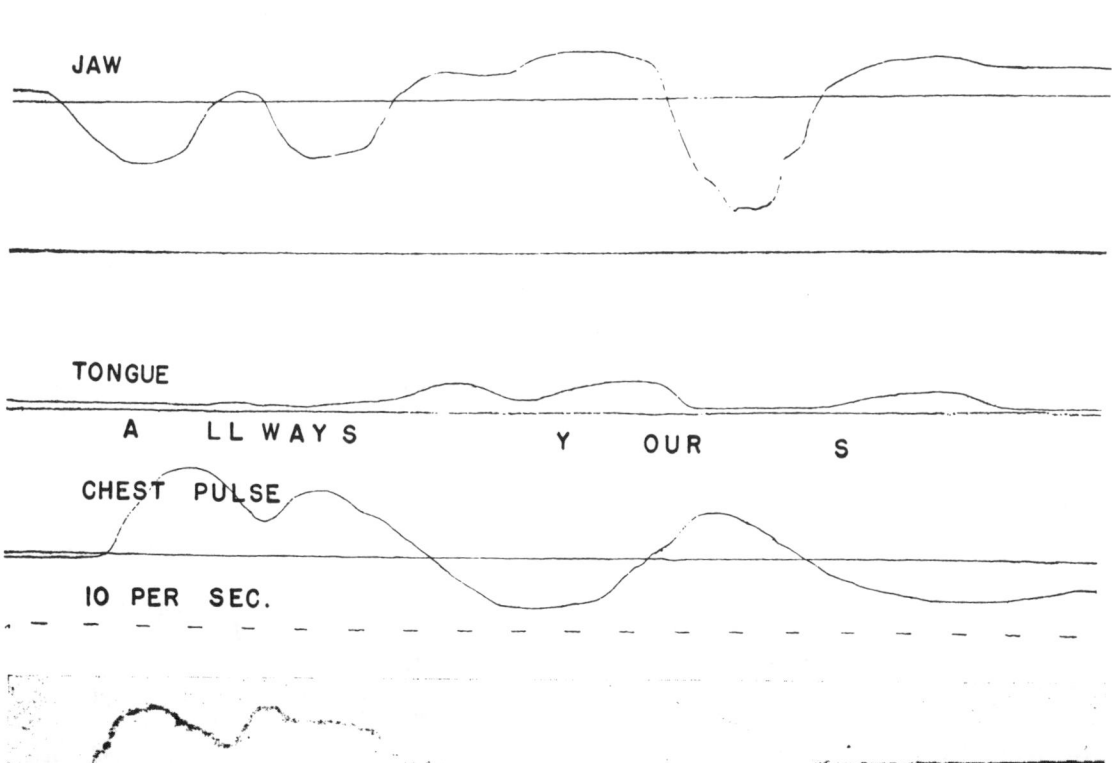

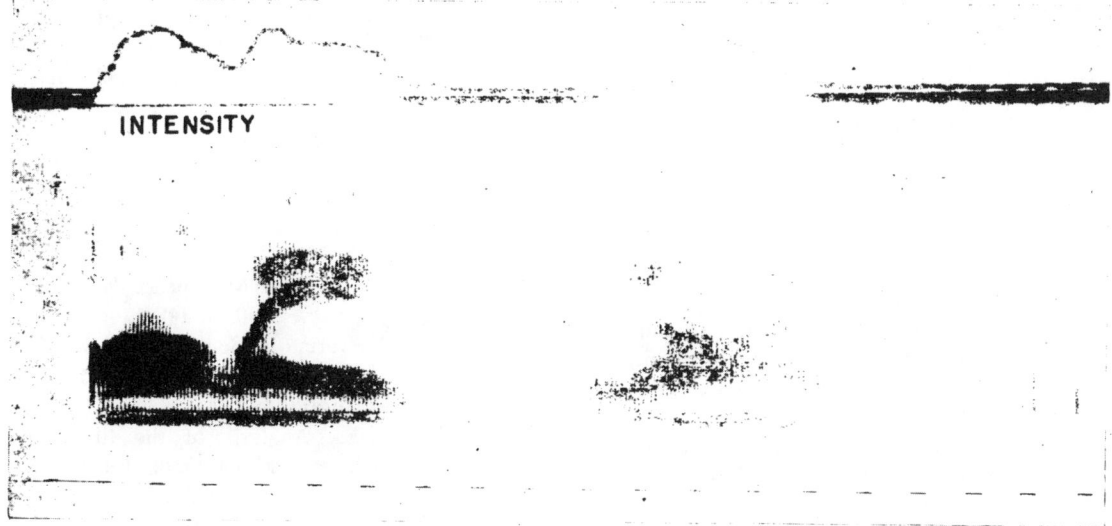

FIGURE 122

Syllables: *Always yours*.

Visible speech pattern:

Intensity line shows the syllables, and the grouping of the feet.

Modulation bars show the rapid shift for the *w* and the *y*.

Motor phonetic tracings:

The chest pulses show the syllables clearly, and the grouping into feet.

The tongue tracing shows the abutting consonants *s-y* and the composite group *-rz* of *yours*.

The jaw tracing shows the dip for each syllable clearly; the dipthong of *-ways* is suggested by the slight shift in the jaw movement.

REFERENCES

1. Abas, A., L'Accentuation syllabique en néerlandais. *Arch. néerl. Physiol.*, 1925, 10, 82–154.
2. Bell, A.G., The mechanism of speech. New York: Funk and Wagnalls, 1907, p. 80.
3. Bell Telephone Systems Monograph B. 1415. Reprint of articles. *Acoust. Soc. Amer. J.*, 1946, 17, 1–89.
4. Binet, A. & V. Henri, Les actions d'arrêt dans les phénomènes de la parole. *L'Année psychologique*, 1894, 5, 446–448.
5. Bloch, B., Set of postulates for phonemic analysis. *Lang.*, 1948, 24, 3–46.
6. Bloch, B. & G. L. Trager, Outline of linguistic analysis. Baltimore: Linguistic Society of America at the Waverly Press, Inc. 1942.
7. Bloomer, H. & H. H. Shohara, The study of respiratory movements by roentgen kymography. *Speech Monogr.*, 1941, 8, 91–101.
8. Brown, P. F., Characteristics of pneumatic recording systems. *J. gen. Psychol.*, 1939, 20, 505.
9. ———, Action current recording. *J. gen. Psychol.*, 1939, 20, 511.
10. Clédat, L., Manuel de phonétique. Paris: Librairie Hachette, 1917.
11. Coleman, H. C., Intonation and Emphasis, Miscellanea phonetica, International Phonetic Association, 1914.
12. Crandall, I. B., The sounds of speech. *Bell System Tech. J.*, 1925, 4, 586–626.
13. Curry, R., Speech recording and analysis with the cathode ray oscillograph. *Arch. néerl. Phon. Expér.*, 1935, 11, 107–118.
14. ———, The mechanism of the human voice. New York: Longmans, Green & Co., 1940.
15. De Groot, A. W., Le syllabe. *Bull. de soc. linguistique*, Paris, 1926, 27, 1–42.
16. Devaux-Charbonnel, La photographie de la parole. *C. r. acad. d. sci.*, 1908, 146, 1258–1260.
17. Dhorme, E., Déchiffrement des inscriptions de Bibylos. *Syria*, 25, 1946–1948.
18. Forbes, J., Development of speech in children. Master's Thesis, Oberlin College Library, Unpublished, 1931.
19. Gemelli, A. & G. Pastori, L'analisi elettroacoustica del linguaggio. Milan: Universita Cattolica del Sacro Cuore, 1934.
20. Grandgent, C. H., Vowel Movements. *Pub. Mod. Lang. Assoc.*, 1890, 5, 148–174.
21. Grégoire, A., Variations de duree de la syllabe française. *La Parole*, 1899, 9, 161–176; 263–280; 418–433.
22. Groff, M. L., Analysis of the first-year vocabularies of schools for the deaf. *Amer. Annals of the Deaf*, 1934, 77, 78, 79.
23. Harris, Z. S., Yokutz structure and Newman's Grammar. *I.J.A.L.*, 1944, 10, 210.
24. ———, Yokutz structure and Newman's Grammar. *I.J.A.L.*, 1944, 10, 196–211.
25. ———, Navaho Phonology and Hoijer's Analysis. *I.J.A.L.*, 1945, 11, 239–246.
26. ———, Phonemicist version of Kota. *Lang.*, 1945, 11, 283.
27. Heffner, R. M. S., Notes on the length of vowels. *Amer. Speech*, 1937, 12, 128–134 1940, 15, 74–79, 377–380; 1941, 16, 204–207; 1942, 17, 42–48; 1943, 18, 208–215.
28. ———, A note on vowel length in American speech. *Lang.*, 1940, 16, 33–47.

29. Helmholtz, H. L. F., (Tr. A. J. Ellis) On the sensations of tone. (rd ed.) New York: Longmans, Green, & Co., 1895.
30. Hermann, E., Silbenbildung im griechischen und in den andern indogermanischen Sprachen. Göttingen: Vandenhoeck & Ruprecht, 1923.
31. Hockett, C. F., A system of descriptive phonology. *Lang.*, 1942, 18, 3–21.
32. Hofbauer, L., Ueber Interferenz zwischen verschiedenen Impulsen im Centralnervensystem. *Arch. ges. Physiol.* (Pflüger's), 1897, 68, 546–595.
33. Hudgins, C. V. & L. M. DiCarlo, An experimental study of assimilation between abutting consonants. *J. gen. Psychol.*, 1939, 20, 449–469.
34. Hudgins, C. V. & R. H. Stetson, A unit for kymograph recording. *Science,* 1932, 76, 59–60.
35. ———, Voicing of consonants by depression of the larynx. *Arch. néerl. Phon. Expér.*, 1935, 11, 1–28.
36. Hudgins, C. V. & R. H. Stetson, Relative speed of articulatory movements. *Arch. néerl. Phon. Expér.*, 1937, 13, 85–94.
37. Jones, D., Analysis of the mechanism of speech. *Nature,* 1917, 99, 285–287.
38. ———, An outline of English phonetics. (4th ed.) New York: E. P. Dutton & Co. Inc., 1934.
39. Joos, M., Acoustic phonetics. *Lang. Monogr.*, 1948, 23, 1–136.
40. Josselyn, F., Etudes expérimentales de la phonétique italienne. *La Parole,* 1901, 11, 227–252.
41. Klestadt, Zur qualitätiven Analyse der Sprechatmung. *Zschr. Hals-Hasen.- u. Ohrenh.*, 1925, 12, 257–277.
42. König, W., H. K. Duin & L. Y. Lacy, The sound spectrograph. *Acous. Soc. Amer. J.*, 1946, 18, 19–49.
43. Kopp, G. A. & H. C. Green, Basic phonetic principles of visible speech. *Acous. Soc. Amer. J.*, 1946, 18, 74–89.
44. Lewy, F. H., Die Grundlagen des Koordinations mechanismus einfacher Willkürbewegungen. *Z. ges. Neurol. Psychiat.*, 1920, 58, 310–326.
45. ———, Tonusprobleme in der Neurologie: Untersuchungen zur Bewegungskoordination. *Z. ges. Neurol. Psychiat.*, 1921, 63, 256–270.
46. Lewis, M. M., Infant speech. London: K. Paul Trench, Trubner & Co. Ltd., 1936, pp. 21–38.
47. Lutz, H.F., Selected Sumerian and Babylonian Texts. Philadelphia: The University Museum, 1919.
48. Marage, M., Contribution á l'étude des consonnes. *C. r. acad. d. sci.,* 1911, 152, 1265–1267.
49. Marey, E. -J., In H. Marichelle's *La Parole.* Préface. Paris: Delagrave, 1897.
50. Marichelle, H., La Parole. Paris: Delagrave, 1897.
51. ———, La chronophotographie de la parole, Avec 79 figures d'aprés des Photographies de M. Marey. Paris: Institution Nationale des Sourds-Muets, 1902.
52. Meyer, E. A., Englische Lautdauer. Uppsala: Akademisha bokhandeln, 1903.
53. Miller, D. C., The science of musical sounds. New York: Macmillan, 1916.
54. Millet, A., Précis d'Expérimentation phonétique. Paris: Didier, 1925, pp. 108–115.
55. Morris, A. R., The orchestration of the metrical line. Boston: Badger, 1925, p. 16 and f.
56. Musehold, A., Akustik und Mechanik dei menschlichen Stimmorgane. Berlin: Springer, 1913, p. 51.
57. Navarro Tomás, T., Manual de Pronunciación Española. (4th ed.) Madrid: Hernando, 1932, p. 28.
58. Oakley-Coles., In Marichelle, H. *La Parole.* Paris: Delagrave, 1897.
59. Parmenter, C. E. & S. N. Treviño, Length of the sounds of a Middle Westerner. *Amer. Speech,* 1935, 10, 129–333.
60. Passy, P. & H. Michaélis, Dictionnaire phonétique. (2nd ed.) Paris: Soudier, 1914, p. 23.
61. Passy, P., Petite phonétique comparée. (3rd ed.) Leipsig: Teubner, 1922.
62. Perrett, W., Some questions of phonetic theory. The perception of sound. Cambridge: Heffer & Sons, 1919.
63. Pike, K. L., Phonetics. Ann Arbor: Univ. Michigan Press, 1943.
64. Potter, R. K., G. A. Kopp & H. C. Green, Visible speech. New York: D. Van Nostrand Co. 1947.
65. Riemann, H., Musikalische dynamik und agogik. Hamburg: D. Rahter, 1884.
66. Rosapelly, M., Apparatus for larynx movements. *In* Rousselot, P. -J. *Principe de phonétique expérimentale.* Vol. 1. Paris: H. Welter, 1897–1901, p. 98.
67. Röttger, F., Phonetische Gestaltbildung bei Jungen Kindern. München: Beck, 1931.
68. Rousselot, P. J., Les modifications phonétiques du langage. Paris: Charente, 1891.

69. ———, La parole avec un larynx artificiel. *La Parole*, 1902, 12, 65.
70. ———, Principes de phonétique expérimentale. Paris: H. Welter, Vol. 1, 1897–1901; Vol. 2 1901–1908.
71. ———, Principes de phonétique expérimentale. Paris: H. Welter, Vol. 1, 1897–1901, p. 49
72. Rousselot, P. J. & F. Laclotte, Précis de la prononciation française. (2nd ed.) Paris: H. Welter, 1913.
73. Russell, G. O., The vowel. Columbus: Ohio State University Press, 1928.
74. ———, Speech and voice. New York: Macmillan, 1931.
75. Saussure, F. de, Cours de linguistique Générale. (2nd ed.) Paris: Payot, 1922.
76. Scripture, E. W., Experimental phonetics. New York: Scribners, 1902.
77. Sen, A. C., Proceedings, 2nd International Congress of Phonetics, London, 1935.
78. Sievers, G. E., Grundzüge der Phonetik. (4th ed.) Leipzig: Breitkopf & Härtel, 1893.
79. Snodgrass, J. M., Simplified tracings of muscle action currents. *J. gen. Psychol.*, 1939, 20, 503–504.
80. Speiser, E. A., Phonetic method in Hurrian Orthography. *Lang.*, 1940, 16, 319–340.
81. ———, Introduction to Hurrian. New Haven: Amer. Schools of Oriental Research, 1941.
82. Steinberg, J. C. & N. R. French, The portrayal of visible speech. *Acous. Soc. Amer. J.*, 1946, 18, 4–18.
83. Stetson, R. H., Rhythm and rhyme. *Psychol. Rev. Monogr.*, 1903, 4, 413–466.
84. ———, A motor theory of rhythm and discrete succession. *Psychol. Rev.*, 1905, 12, 346–347.
85. ———, Speech movements in action. *Trans. Amer. Laryngol. Assoc.*, 1933, 55, 29–41.
86. Stetson, R. H. & J. A. McDill, Mechanism of the different types of movement. *Psychol. Monogr.*, 1923, 32, 18–40.
87. ———, Motor phonetics. *Arch. néerl. Phon. Expér.*, 1928, 3, 1–216.
88. ———, The breathing movements in singing. *Arch. néerl. Phon. Expér.*, 1931, 6, 155.
89. ———, Bases of phonology. Oberlin: Oberlin College, 1945.
90. Stetson, R. H. & H. D. Bouman, The coordination of simple skilled movements. *Arch. néerl. Physiol.*, 1935, 20, 177–254.
91. Stetson, R. H. & C. V. Hudgins, Functions of the breathing movements in the mechanism of speech. *Arch. néerl. Phon. Expér.*, 1930, 5, 1–30.
92. Stetson, R. H., C. V. Hudgins & E. R. Moses Jr, Palatograms change with rates of articulation. *Arch. Néerl. Phon. Expér.*, 1940, 16, 52–61.
93. Stumpf, C., Tonpsychologie. Vol. 1. Leipzig: Hertzel 1883.
94. Swadesh, M., The phonemic interpretation of long consonants. *Lang.*, 1937, 13, 1–10.
95. Sweet, H., History of English sounds from the earliest period, with full word lists. Oxford: Clarendon Press, 1888.
96. Thorndike, E. L., A teacher's word book of the twenty thousand words found most frequently and widely in general reading for children and young people. New York: Teachers' College. Columbia Univ. Press. 1931.
97. Trager, G. L. & B. Bloch, The syllabic phonemes of English. *Lang.*, 1941, 17, 223–246.
98. Trubetzkoy, N. S., Anleitung zu phonologischen Beschreibungen. Brno: Cercle linguistique de Prague, 1935.
99. ———, La phonologie actuelle. Psy. du lang. Paris, 1933.
100. ———Grundzüge der phonologie. Prague: Cercle linguistique de Copenhague, 1939.
101. Trubetzkoy, N. S., Wie soll das Lautsystem einer künstlichen internationalen Hilfssprache beschaffen sein, Études phonologiques dédiées à la mémoire de Prince, N. S. T. Travaux du cercle linguistique de Prague, 1939.
102. Velten, H. V., The growth of phonemic and lexical patterns in infant language. *Lang.*, 1943, 19, 281–292.
103. Viëtor, W., Elemente der Phonetik des deutschen, englischen und französischen. (7th ed.) Leipzig: O. R. Reisland, 1923, p. 357
104. Wachholder, K., Willkürliche Haltung und Bewegung insbesondere im Lichte elektrophysiologischer Untersuchungen, *Ergebn. d. Psysiol.*, 1928, 26, 568–775.
105. Wooton, M. H., The phrasing of children's speech. Master's Thesis, Oberlin College Library, Unpublished, 1939.
106. Wundt, W., Volkerpsychologie. Vols. 1 and 2. Die Sprache. Leipzig: Engelmann, 1911 and 1912.
107. Zwaardemaker, H., L'analogue graphique de l'écriture analphabétique par signes de Jespersen en phonétique. *Arch. néerl. Physiol.*, 1927, 11, 509–545.

A GLOSSARY OF MOTOR PHONETIC TERMS

ABEYANCE — Said of syllables and syllable factors which will reappear when the proper rate and stress of the syllable train occurs. The syllable pattern is inherent in the breath group though not apparent.

ABDOMINAL ACTION IN SPEECH — The muscles of the abdomen compress the viscera and force up the diaphragm, thus reducing the volume of the chest. The movement of the abdominal muscles makes the stress, grouping of the feet, and breath groups.

ABLAUT — Vowel is changed for morphological purpose—swim, swam, swum; common in Indo-European (and in Semitic languages).

ABUTTING, LINKING, DOUBLING — When the arresting consonant of one syllable occurs close enough to fuse with the releasing consonant of the next syllable, the consonants are said to abut. If the consonants are the same consonant repeated, they are called doubles. Linking is a synonym.

ACCESSORY MOVEMENTS in syllables — The syllable movement is a unit which must be released and arrested either by the intercostals (self-release, self-arrest) or by accessory movements of articulation. Contrasts with auxiliary movements, concurrent movements, concomitant movements which are not essential to the syllable unit.

ACOUSTIC — Used of the physical properties of sound independent of perception. Oscillogram gives a picture of the physical properties of sound from which the auditory properties cannot be reduced.

ACROPHONIC — Used of the early Semitic alphabets which indicated the syllable by the releasing consonant.

ADVENTITIOUS DOUBLES — Doubles which appear mechanically as a result of rate or stress but which are not prescribed. The following releasing consonant is drawn back by the heavy stress into the preceding syllable.

AFFIX — A syllable or syllable factor attached to the basic group. If it precedes it is a prefix, if it follows it is a suffix.

AIR PRESSURE in mouth — Produced by the chest pressure during the consonant occlusion, but it may be modified by the action of the glottis and the changing consonant orifices.

ALPHABET VS SYLLABARY — The characteristic factors distinguished in a given language listed in a conventional order constitute the alphabet. It contrasts with the syllabary in which the list of syllables are distinguished in a given language.

ALLOPHONES — In the phonemic system the variations of the phoneme pattern due to rate vs stress.

AMBISYLLABIC — Belonging to two syllables. Viëtor proposed that a consonant between syllables might belong to both syllables. Experimental evidence shows that this is false.

ANLAUT — (German) Termination of the articulatory movement which introduces the syllable. Bell assumed that the articulations were positions with glides between; Anlaut and Auslaut is the German termination of the "glide".

A O — AIR OUTSIDE — "Air Outside" translates Rousselot's souffle which is recorded with a mouthpiece. The American mouthpiece is ventilated so that there is no excess pressure.

APHASIA (Sub-cortical motor) — Neural lesion which interferes with speech. Rousselot noted a type of lesion which paralyzes the articulatory apparatus but leaves the chest pulse of the syllable.

APPUYANTES, APPUYEE — Romance phonologists noted that the arresting consonant drooped while the releasing consonant persisted. The releasing consonant was said to be appuyée by the arresting appuyante. The arresting consonant was supposed to buttress the releasing consonant and to take the shock.

ARRESTING CONSONANTS — The syllable factor which brings the syllable pulse to a close. Contrasts with the releasing consonant.

ARTICULATE LANGUAGE — Mathematics, music and the exact sciences develop a language which is not uttered. The articulate languages are the languages developed by communication using the speech apparatus.

ARTICULATORY PATTERN — The temporal pattern of the syllable and syllable series—syllables, feet, breath groups.

ARTIFICIAL LARYNX — A reed actuated by the air from the tracheotomy tube; the air pressure and tone are introduced through a tube at the corner of the mouth and modulated by the habitual articulations. A hand bellows may be substituted in the laboratory for the air-pulses from the trachea.

ARTIFICIAL PALATE — A thin plate molded to the shape of the palate. Covered with powder it registers the contact of the tongue in the course of a single articulation.

ASPIRATION — When the air pressure in the mouth is high, the détente of the consonant releases the air with a characterizing audible sound.

ASSIMILATION — Two adjacent sounds modify each other; used especially of abutting consonants.

ASSIMILATION, LAW of — Generalizes the fact that abutting consonants modify each other.

AUDITORY VS ACOUSTIC — The perception of the acoustic patterns depends on the context. The same acoustic pattern may be heard in different ways in different contexts. Different acoustic patterns may be heard as the identical articulation in proper contexts.

AUSLAUT — (German) Termination of the glide which leads from a syllable. Sweet thought of the articulations as fixed positions with glides between them.

AUXILIARY MOVEMENTS — Not essential to the syllable movement but characterize the articulations of both consonants and vowels.

BACK STROKE — A ballistic movement is composed of a beat and back stroke. The back stroke arrests the excursion of the beat stroke and may return the limb to the original position for the next stroke, as in repeated tapping.

BALLISTIC MOVEMENT — A movement started by the momentary impulse of the driving muscle group. During most of the excursion no force is acting on the moving limb: It is carried by momentum. In a tense, controlled movement the muscle groups act continuously on the moving limb. A tracing of the excursion of the limb in time shows uniform speed during the momentum phase. It contrasts with tense, controlled movements.

BEARINGS OF ARTICULATION — The areas which come into contact or approach each other.

BEAT STROKE — A ballistic movement is composed of two phases or strokes. The beat stroke is the result of the contraction of the driving muscle group and delivers the blow.

BISYLLABIC — Pertaining to two syllables. Viëtor popularized the notion that a consonant might belong to two syllables, but experimentation shows that this is impossible.

BLADE OF TONGUE — The median part of the tongue between tip and rear.

BOUNDARY MARKERS (GRENZSIGNALE) — Used by Trubetzkoy to indicate various changes—usually of the phonemes—at various "junctures".

BREATH GROUP — The syllables are grouped by the breathing movements of the abdominal muscles. It is the simplest expiratory movement which groups the intercostal pulses in the chest. The intercostals make the syllable pulses but do not adjust the volume of the chest which is the function of the abdominal expiratory movement.

BREATH PULSE — The syllable is made by pulse of air produced by the intercostals. It is not the result of a steady pressure of air in the chest like the air pressure of the organ.

CENTROID — Scripture's term for a generalization of the concept of prominence. It was determined by stress, pitch, duration, precision of utterance.

CHARACTERIZATION OF FACTORS OF SYLLABLE —

aspirates	linguals (front, back)
aspiration	liquids
continuants	nasals
dentals	occlusives
fricatives	palatals
glottals	semi-vowels
gutterals	sibilants
labials	sonants
labiodentals	surds
laryngal (laryngeal)	tense-lax vowels
lax-tense vowels	

The modification of the syllable factors which is conditioned as the signal or symbol and characterizes the phoneme.

CHEST PULSE — The breath pulse from the chest is produced by the intercostals which do not adjust the chest for loss of volume. The expiratory movement which accomodates to loss of volume occurs in, the abdomen.

CHIUNTANTE — French expression for the modified s-sounds, sh and c.

CLICKS — Consonants produced by negative buccal pressure instead of positive. Hottentot and Zulu abound in such clicks.

CLOSED SYLLABLES — The closed syllable is arrested by a consonant in contrast to the open syllable.

CLUSTER — A common term for a compound

consonant or for abutting consonants. It is unsatisfactory because ambiguous. An adequate notation will distinguish between the compound cluster and the abutting cluster.

COMPOUND CONSONANT — A delimiting syllable factor composed of the movements of two or three consonants. It contrasts with abutting consonants, linkage, in that the abutting consonants each have a function in a different syllable. The proper rate and stress will cause the compound consonant to separate into abutting consonants.

CONSTRICTION OF VOCAL CANAL — Due to articulatory movements of lips, tongue, glottis and jaw. May be complete or partial.

CONSTRUCTIVE DOUBLE — The arresting consonant adds to the duration of the syllable so that the interval necessary for an arresting consonant is equal to that for a double consonant (the releasing doublet does not add to the duration of its syllable).

CONSONANT — In contrast to the vowel which emits the syllable pulse, the consonant delimits the movement of the pulse by constricting the vocal canal. It may release or arrest the syllable pulse. Such a function in the syllable is essential to a consonant. The consonant cannot occur alone.

CONSONANT CHANGE — Includes all consonant shifts and modifications.

CONSONANT MODIFICATION — Changes of rate and stress cause the consonant to change its characterization.

CONSONANT SHIFT — Changes of rate and stress cause the consonant to move from the arresting position in a syllable to the releasing position in the following syllable.

CONTINUANTS — The constriction of the vocal canal by the consonant stroke results in a characteristic partial (leaky) closure. Contrasts with occlusive which involves a complete closure.

DACTYL — Phonetic unit of three syllables grouped round a stressed initial syllable.

DEMARCATION OF SYLLABLE — The accessory movements which release and arrest the syllable mark off the syllable. The demarcation of the syllable is that of a ballistic movement. Cf. a note in music.

DENTAL — English vs Continental — Consonant characterized by the tongue touching the teeth. In the English sounds of this type the tongue does not come to the teeth: they are strictly sub-dentals.

DÉTENTE — The opening of the constriction of the consonant is called the détente. Rousselot made it one of the fundamental phases of an articulation: tension-tenue-detente-arrivée.

DIACHRONOUS CHANGES — Traits and changes which appear during the history of a language contrasted with traits and changes in the contemporary language which are called synchronous, following Soussure.

DIAPHRAGM FOR PHONETICS — Constitutes the floor of the chest cavity. It is forced up by the pressure of the viscera when the abdominal muscles make the movements of expiration of the breath-group.

DIPTHONG — The serial fusion of two (or three) vowels in the one syllable.

DISCRETE SUCCESSION — Law of — At the rate of 14-16 per second it is impossible to distinguish events, and the elements fuse to a single quality.

DOUBLING AND SINGLING — When increasing rate causes the consonants of closed syllables to abut, it is convenient to speak of the series as coming to the doubling phase. Later, when the arresting consonant drops, the series is said to "single".

DROPPING OF CONSONANTS AND SYLLABLES — When the rate increases it may become so rapid that the arresting consonants cannot be pronounced. The rate may eliminate syllables. A dropped phoneme or syllable is in abeyance and with a slower rate will reappear.

ECONOMY, LAW of — The fusion of articulations (movements) and the dropping of articulations (movements), occasioned by changes in rate and stress, are often grouped under a "law of economy of effort".

EINSATZ — German translation of "onset" indicates the releasing factor of a syllable.

ELEMENT — Element is an indeterminate term for a phonetic unit: it refers to the characterized syllable.

ENPHONIC, ENPHONETIC — A sound which is common to two languages, cf. an enharmonic chord in music.

EPENTHÈSE — A consonant is assumed to substitute for a syllable.

EXPIRATION, EXPIRATION FORCE — The muscles of expiration are the gross muscles of the chest and the abdomen. The expiratory force is furnished by the pulses of the intercostals. There is no constant expiratory force.

EXPLOSION — The sudden opening of the releasing consonant was characterized as explosive in contrast to the implosive consonant.

EXTRUDED — *Phonemes and syllables*. Those that are caused to drop out of the series as a result of changes of rate and stress; with proper rate and stress they re-appear.

FACTOR OF SYLLABLE — The syllable is emitted by the vowel and delimited by the intercostals, or by the articulatory movements of the consonants. There are three factors: 1) release, 2) vowel-shape for emission, and 3) arrest. These are the fundamental functions. The factors, when characterized, are the phonemes.

FOOT — The foot is the rhythmic unit group composed of one stressed syllable only in the case of the one-syllable foot; composed of stressed and unstressed syllables in the case of trochees and dactyls, iambs and anapests, and of unstressed and stressed syllables in the case of the iambs and anapests. The foot corresponds to the figure in music, not to the measure.

FORM, FREE FORM — Not a phonological term. Refers to a morphological unit.

FORMANT (Syllable formant) — The element which is essential to the syllable, the core of the syllable. Usually a reference to the vowel.

FORTIS-LENIS — The consonant with a high mouth pressure, usually the surd, is counted fortis, strong. Contrasts with the lenis, usually sonant, weak, with low mouth pressure.

FOURIER'S THEOREM — The mathematical basis for reducing a complex tone to simple (sine) waves which are partials of the basic cycle.

FRICATIVE — A consonant with an incomplete closure during which the escaping air contributes a hissing sound which characterizes the syllable factor.

FRONTIER OF THE SYLLABLE — Phase in which the syllables abut, and in which the syllables are delimited. The sandhi changes occur at the frontier.

FUNCTION (OF FACTOR IN SYLLABLE), (OF SYLLABLE IN FOOT), (OF FOOT IN BREATH GROUP) — The consonants and vowels have definite functions in the syllable. They are not merely in series but have specific parts to play in the syllable movement. The stressed and unstressed syllables play their parts in the foot and in the breath group.

FUSION OF PHONEMES — When the syllable factor is composed of several articulations they are said to fuse.

GLOTTAL — The subglottal cavities and processes are in the trachea and chest. The super-glottal cavities and processes are in the pharynx and mouth.

GLOTTALS — Those consonants which are characterized by the action of the glottis, i.e., the aspirate *h*, and the glottal stop.

GLOTTAL STOP — When the consonant-arrest is due to a sudden closure of stricture of the glottis.

GLOTTIS — The slit between the vocal folds.

GRENZSIGNALE — Trubetzkoy noted that the delimitation of the syllable, foot, and breath group, often involved some distinctive sign. English: "boundary marker".

GUTTERALS — Phonemes characterized by articulations in the back of the oral cavity, in the pharynx and larynx.

HARMONIC ANALYSIS — Reduction of a complex tone to sinusoidal vibrations by computation or by apparatus (Henrici Analyzer).

IAMB — The rhythmic unit composed of a short syllable followed by a stressed syllable.

IAMBIC TELESCOPING — The increase of rate of a syllable train may lead to the elimination of the vowel of the short syllable of the iamb.

IMPLOSION — The arresting consonant, closing the vocal canal, brings the syllable to a stop. The action was contrasted with the explosion. The group of articulations which might be explosive or implosive were called plosives.

INFIX — A significant articulation, usually morphological, is introduced into the syllable rather than between syllables.

INFLECTED CONSONANT CURVES — The curve of pressure in the mouth for an English sonant is affected by the change in the mouth volume during the articulation. The duration distinguishes the form from the bimaximal abutting curve.

INTENSITY IN SPEECH — Basically a matter of increased muscular force. In many cases the acoustic intensity is a fair measure of the muscular force. The muscles involved are the gross musculatures of the chest and the abdomen. The intercostal muscles are reflexly affected, but the sense of intensity is due to the larger speech musculatures.

INTERCOSTALS — The muscles between the ribs which produce the syllable pulses. Although the internal intercostals are counted "expiratory", and the external intercostals are counted "inspiratory", they are not muscles of respiration. The adjustments for volume are made by the gross chest muscles and the abdomen.

INTER-VOCALIC — Consonants "between vowels". The expression does not indicate the syllable to which the consonants belong. Like "cluster", the expression is the indeterminate notation for a group of phonemes.

INTONATION — Significant frequency changes in the course of the breath group.

I.P.A. (INTERNATIONAL PHONETIC ALPHABET) — It undertakes to characterize the articulation independent of meaning. As a notation it does not indicate the syllable or the factors of the syllable. Based on the notion of speech as a series of phonemes, rather than a series of syllables.

JUNCTURE — Indeterminate expression for any connection between: phoneme and phoneme; syllable and syllable; foot and foot; breath group and breath group. It does not distinguish the radical differences involved.

KANA — The Japanese system of syllabic writing, dating from the 8th or 9th century. It is a syllabary of 47 purely phonetic characters.

KYMOGRAM — A tracing recorded by means of a kymograph usually employing the pneumatic method of transmission. In Motor Phonetics, kymograms are obtained of pressure inside the mouth, outside the mouth, from the nose, and from within the chest. Also, kymograms of the contacts of the lips, the tongue with the palate, and the movements of the breathing muscles are recorded. The kymograph has also been used to record action potentials from the breathing muscles.

LABIALS — Consonants made by the stroke of the lips, i.e., the surd and sonant *p* and *b*, and the continuant *m*. Phonemes characterized by various lip articulations constitute the labials.

LABIO/DENTAL — In English the characteristic *f/v* are not made by the lips but by the lower lip and the teeth.

LA LANGUE — F. de Saussure's system of symbols which constitute the language independent of any utterance.

LANGUAGE MECHANISM — The universal speech apparatus is conditioned in each language to a set of definite habits which constitute the language mechanism.

LA PAROLE — Speech as uttered is contrasted with the language as a system in the abstract and independent of utterance. The contrast between *la langue et la parole* is fundamental to Saussure's system.

LARYNGELAS (LARYNGALS) — The articulations which are developed in the pharynx and the larynx.

LARYNGECTOMY — Removal of the larynx, after which the patient breathes through an opening of the trachea just above the sternum.

LARYNX (AND LARYNX MASS) — The vocal folds with their musculatures are mounted within the larynx. The extrinsic musculature of the larynx and of the cartileges above the larynx moves the larynx mass up and down. This movement is important for voicing the consonants and for the pitch of the vowel.

LAX VOWELS — The lax vowel is the syllable movement characterized by arrest by the consonant articulation. Contrasts with the tense vowel when the vowel is arrested by the chest muscles.

LINGUALS — The bearings of the tongue are varied from the tip across the blade to the back tongue area, characterizing the whole series of lingual consonants.

LINKAGE — Abutting consonants are said to be linked.

LIQUID — The consonants *l* and *r* are so characterized in part because they leave the vocal canal fairly open, and along with the nasals, *n, m, -ng*, they may substitute for vowels.

LONG CONSONANTS — Not phonemic in English, French and German.

LONG VOWEL — The long vowel has a specific quality which is characteristic. The long vowel may shorten indefinitely. Contrasted with the short vowel which is not prolongable.

MARKER — The lip and tongue markers are thin, wedge-shaped, resilient pneumatic applicators which respond to the contact between the lips and between the tongue and palate.

MÉTHODE GLOBALE — The treatment of speech in terms of syllables or words rather than individual elements.

MONAD — Brøndol wished to emphasize the self-contained character of a language at any given period.

MORPHOPHONEME — A phoneme which differentiates a linguistic form.

MOUILLÉE — An articulation characterized by a concurrent approach of the tongue blade to the palate is said to be *mouillée*.

MOUTHPIECE — A mask of metal or of rubber is fitted about the lips to register the air pressures just outside the mouth. The mouthpiece must not interfere with action of the muscles and must be ventilated to prevent the piling up of pressure. The French tracings for souffle are taken with such an embouchure, small and without ventilation.

NASAL OLIVES — A borrowed French term for the nasal plugs used to record the air pressure from the nostrils.

NASAL — Sonant articulations may be produced with the nasal pharynx closed off by the velum (sonant stops), or it may be open and the resulting nasal resonance characterizes the vowel or the sonant consonant (sonant continuant).

NEUTRALIZATION — Trubetzkoy based his phonemic system on "opposition", i.e., the differentiation of words by a minimum phonic difference. But it is apparent that a phonic difference like that of voicing may disappear with changes of rate and stress and that such a loss of the distinguishing trait may be called neutralization.

NONSENSE SYLLABLE — Any syllable handled with reference to its phonetic traits and without reference to meaning becomes a nonsense syllable. The term is usually applied to syllables which have no meaning in the language under discussion.

OCCLUDED — A phoneme or a syllable which drops out with a change of rate or stress, but which is not lost to the overall pattern and will re-appear.

OCCLUSIVE — When the closure of the articulation is complete, the consonant is called an occlusive or a stop. In English *p/b, t/d, k/g*.

OFF-PHASE, IN-PHASE — Oscillations of sound, or other repeated movements may occur together so that they are in step, in phase, and reinforce each other, or out of step, off phase, so that they tend to neutralize each other.

ONE-MEMBER — The abutting consonants may be produced by a single member, cf. "hum*b*ug", "u*pp*uppy", or by two members, "flagpole, advent".

ONE-SYLLABLE FOOT — The rhythmic unit of a single foot is very common in English.
"Break, break, break
On thy cold gray stones, O sea."

ONSET — (German Einsatz) Used to characterize the releasing movement of a new syllable.

OPPOSITION — Saussure and Trubetzkoy made the differentiation of words (syllables) by a minimum phonic difference the basis of the system of phonemes. The contrast of a phoneme with all others in the language was called "opposition".

OSCILLOGRAM — Sound waves may be transformed into electric oscillations and recorded photographically; mechanical recording of sound waves by apparatus, etc., Miller's phonodeik. Action currents from muscles are also recorded by the oscillograph. The method is important for studying the action of the intercostals and the muscles of the larynx.

OSCILLOGRAPH — Instrument for recording electrical oscillations used for acoustic recording and for the recording of action currents from contracting muscles.

PALATALS — The various articulations characterized by a stroke to the palate are so termed. Every palatal is also a lingual.

PALPATION, TACTUAL PALPATION OF SPEECH — The deaf-blind depend on the sense of touch to perceive the movements and vibrations of speech. The thumb and fingers are disposed so as to catch the movements of lips, jaw and larynx; the changes in the shape of the floor of the mouth indicate tongue movements. As a method of perception, palpation is superior to lip-reading. It has been used on occasion in the teaching of speech and lip-reading to the deaf.

PARTIAL — One of the simple component vibrations of which a complex tone is composed.

PATTERN DESIGN — Pattern as a structure, independent of specific occurrences, constitutes a "design". Contrasts with pattern event which has repeated occurrences.

PATTERN EVENTS — Patterns as they occur are events; there may be an indefinite number of these events of the same pattern. Contrasts with pattern design which is independent of the occurrences.

PAUSE, SILENCE — Pause is an indeterminate term for any interruption of the oral train. Pause in the sense of a cessation of sound occurs both within and between syllables. The acoustic pattern is made up of a series of sounds and silences.

PHARYNX — The rear cavity in the mouth; for phonetics it is defined by the approach of the back of the tongue toward the palate in the two-cavity vowels.

PHONEME — The sound is recognized as an articulatory symbol with variants and the term phoneme covers the symbol with its variants.

PHONEMIC PHRASE — Just as the phonemicists are forced to recognize the syllable as a suprasegmental unit, so the breath group proves essential to phonemic formulation, and is termed the "phonemic phrase" which is organized by the grouping with stress of the syllable.

PHONEMICS — Trubetzkoy called his system of phonemes, differentiated and classified by "oppositions", "*Phonologie*". The corresponding English term has come to be phonemics.

PHONES — The typical articulations are called phonemes; it is evident that the occurrences of the phoneme present variations. The term "phone" and "allophone" are phonemic terms for these variants.

PHONETIC LAWS — Changes which are invariable, either synchronous or diachronous, are said to be due to a law.

PHONETICS — The treatment of articulations, syllable factors, syllables, feet and breath groups as physiological events which may be used as vocal signals. Contrasts with phonemics which treats the groups of articulations primarily as symbols.

PHONODEIK — A diaphragm, activated by acoustic phenomena, which actuates a mirror for viewing and recording sound oscillations.

PHONOLOGY — The traditional use of the word has been to indicate the history of sounds and the explanation of their changes. Since the contemporary changes become historical changes, and since the contemporary changes are pronounced, recent usage has made phonology discuss the relations and changes of the articulations. Trubetzkoy used the term for the theory of phonemes; in English "phonemics" translates "Phonologie".

PITCH, SCALE — Pitch figures in the phonology of the "tone languages" in that change of pitch differentiates the syllable. Cf. Chinese. Definite arrangements of pitch differences constitute the scales in music. The scales attract the attention of phonologists as differentiating aspects of the musical notes which correspoisd to the syllables. The intervals of the scale might be called tonemes.

PLOSIVES — A group of consonants which are thought of as opening and closing a syllable. They are divided into the explosives and implosives.

PNEUMODEIK — A substitute for the Marey tambour employed in pneumatic recording. It has a metal diaphragm, the characteristics of which are high sensitivity and wide linear range. It is stable and can be calibrated.

POSITION — In the classical metrics, a syllable is said

to be long "by position" if it is followed by abutting consonants. Such linkages are said to "make position"; they contrast with the releasing compound consonant.

POST-VOCALIC — The arresting syllable factor which occurs after the vowel. Contrasts with pre-vocalic, the releasing syllable factor, and with inter-vocalic which is indeterminate as to the syllable in which the consonant(s) occurs.

PRE-VISION, Law of — Coming articulations are anticipated, which modifies the articulations actually in process.

PRE-VOCALIC — The releasing syllable factor which occurs before the vowel of the syllables. Contrasts with post-vocalic, the arresting syllable factor; and with inter-vocalic which is indeterminate as to the syllable in which the consonant(s) occurs.

PROMINENCE — The carrying power was supposed to differentiate the phonemes and so mark the peaks of the syllables. But sonority proved not a physical concept and it was not possible to measure the carrying power. The later practice has been to fall back on the noncommital "prominence" which may be due to stress, sonority, duration, or with Scripture, to precision of utterance.

RADICAL IN SEMITIC LANGUAGE — The typical semitic word is composed of three syllables, characterized by the three releasing consonants which are the stable essentials for the meaning. These are the radicals. The radicals are variously voiced by the inflecting vowels and supplemented by affixes and infixes.

RELAXATION PHASE OF MOVEMENT — The relaxation phase of a movement accounts primarily for the dissipation of momentum. In a tense movement there is also the relaxation of the driving muscles. In a rapid alternating movement the term relaxation does not fit, for the backstroke process both cares for the momentum and returns the limbs.

RELEASING CONSONANT — The syllable factor which initiates the syllable pulse. Contrasts with the arresting consonant.

RESONANCE — Describes the conditions in which the frequency of the generating tone and the natural period of a cavity (resonator) are identical. For the acoustics of the vowel it is significant that resonance requires several cycles in which to develop.

RHYTHM — Not a matter of audition. It is basically a matter of movement and may be silent. Auditory perception is a convenient way of communicating rhythm. The rhythm of speech involves the entire process of grouping and stress. The unit groups, the feet, are the primary rhythmic terms employed in phonetics.

RHYTHMIC UNIT — The rhythmic units are the feet, the one-syllable foot, the iamb, and the anapest, the trochee, the dactyl and the amphibrach. In music, the rhythmic units are the figures.

RIB-CAGE for PHONETICS — In phonetics the rib-cage is raised and lowered by the gross muscles of the chest. The abdominal muscles are attached to the lower edge of the rib-cage. The intercostal contractions produce slight compressions of the rib-cage for the syllable pulses.

RIME — Rime is a phonetic trait dependent on rhythmic grouping. The rime involves two or more occurrences of contrasting syllables. The releasing factors must be unlike, the vowel and arresting factors identical. In feminine rime one or more identical syllables follow the stressed riming syllable. In rhythmic grouping the rime occurs at the end of a phrase and must have the main stress of the phrase.

SANDHI — Phonetic changes resulting from assimilation.

SEGMENTATION — The term given to the process of analyzing, or subdividing articulations, or speech sounds, into consecutive sub-units which are called segments. The process ignores the basic fact that articulations have definite functions within the syllable and as such are "bound" events, and cannot be notated as a simple additive series.

SEMI-VOWELS — A loose term implying that certain sounds—consonants which only slightly constrict the vocal canal, l, r, w, y, and highly constricted vowels, u, i,—are neither consonant nor vowel, but partake the character of both. The classification ignores the fact that its function as a syllable factor determines the nature of the sound, and that it will be a consonant or a vowel, depending upon this function.

SEPTUM (Elastic) — A device employed in connection with the negative pressure recorder to support the negative pressure required to hold the applicator in place and at the same time to permit the recording tambour to operate at atmospheric pressure.

SCHWA — The indefinite, or neutral vowel. Also, a vowel reduced to its simplest quality as the result of rapid rate of utterance or loss of accent.

SIGN DESIGN — The arbitrary, graphic notation of sign event such as the dots and dashes of the Morse Code, or the phonetic alphabet.

SIGN EVENT — A unit of a consecutive series of objective events, such as movements or sounds which may form a variety of temporal patterns, for instance, the clicks of the telegrapher's key, or a train of syllables with their factors in speech.

SONANT — The term used to describe speech sounds, the distinguishing feature of which is the presence of the laryngeal tone during its articulation. It is used especially to distinguish between voiced and voiceless (surd) consonants.

SONORITY — A subjective quality related to loudness used by Sievers to distinguish syllables in which he could observe no stress differences. Sonority syllables (Schallsible) are distinguished from pressure syllables (Drucksilbe).

SOUND SPECTROGRAPH — An acoustic analyzer especially designed to display the frequency components of speech sounds as a function of time (Spectrogram).

SPECTROGRAM — In experimental phonetics a graphic analysis of speech sounds in which the component frequencies and intensities are shown as a function of time.

STANCHION — Apparatus designed to study the details of speech breathing movements. The stanchion prevents gross bodily movements and at the same time supports recording devices which may be applied to any desired body area.

STASIS — A stasis is said to occur when, in a rapid movement sequence, both flexor and extensor muscle groups contract simultaneously. The result is a reduced, irregular excursion, or a complete fixation of the limb.

STRESS — The term is usually applied to the degree of force of syllable utterance. Stress implies both acoustic and physiological intensity.

STRESS ACCENT — Certain syllables within the foot, or the breath group, are uttered with greater force than that given to others which are said to be subordinated to the stressed syllable. Stress accent is a primary factor in speech rhythm.

SURD — The term used to describe speech sounds, a distinguishing feature of which is the absence of the laryngeal tone during its articulation. It is used especially to distinguish between voiceless and voiced (sonant) consonants.

SYLLABARY — A series of written characters each of which represents a distinct syllable, and containing the body of syllables within a given language.

SYLLABIC — The vowel shaping factor as distinguished from the releasing or arresting syllable factors. Also a sound, usually a continuant consonant which may occur as a vowel shape, i.e., the *n* in cotton, or the *l* in little.

SYLLABLE — The smallest, indivisible phonetic unit. Basically, the syllable is a puff of air forced upward through the vocal canal by a compression stroke of the intercostal muscles. It is usually modulated by the action of the vocal folds. It is accompanied by accessory movements (syllable factors) which characterize it. These are the *release* (by the action of either the chest muscles or the releasing consonant), the *vowel shaping* movements of the vocal canal, and the *arrest* (by the action of either chest muscles or the arresting consonant). Four basic syllable types are possible:

1) Chest released, chest arrested, OVO *ah, oh.*
2) Chest released, consonant arrested, OVC, *at, up.*
3) Consonant released, chest arrested, CVO, *for, too.*
4) Consonant released, consonant arrested, CVC, *top, cook.*

SYLLABLE FACTORS — Every syllable has three invariable factors which a) release the pulse either by the action of the chest muscles or by a consonant, b) emit it by a movement which shapes the vocal canal for the vowel and c) arrest it either by the action of the chest muscles or by a consonant. Syllable factors are "bound" events which can occur only in the syllable.

SYLLABLE PULSE — A rapid ballistic movement of the intercostal muscles which moves a puff of air through the vocal canal. The pulse may be released and arrested by the muscles themselves, or by accessory movements of articulation, i.e., releasing and arresting consonants.

SYNCHRONOUS CHANGE — Phonetic changes that occur in speech as a result of the current conditions of utterance, degree of stress, etc. Synchronous changes are reversible.

TABLATURE — One form of early musical notation used signs for the movements of playing the instrument (still used for ukelele, etc.) and is a convenient analogy for the notation of speech in terms of the articulatory movements and positions.

TENSE-LAX CHARACTERIZATION — The tense vowel is the syllable movement characterized by an arrest by the chest muscles. Contrasts with the lax vowel in which the syllable is arrested by the consonant articulation.

TENSION (Tenue détente arrivé of Saussure's syllable) — Rousselot reduced Saussure's scheme for the opening and closing of the syllable to the simplest articulation. As the articulation comes into position (open or closed) the action is called "tension" (later *"arrivée"*). This may be followed by a stable state, the tenue. When the articulation leaves position (open or closed), the action is called "détente". Rousselot did not discuss the inevitable overlaps of the tensions and détentes of successive articulations.

TONE — General term for a sound characterized by a pitch; usually composed of partials with minor noises. Contrasts with noise.

TONEMES — The differentiation of syllables by pitch changes involves a differential called a toneme.

TRACHEA — Windpipe leading from lungs to larynx.

TRACHEOTOMY TUBE — A tube is inserted in the trachea for breathing if the larynx is no longer available.

TRANSCRIPTION — The process of reducing speech to phonetic symbols. Depends largely on the predilections of the transcriber. For careful phonetic analysis such a transcription must be checked and interpreted by kymographic and oscillographic tracings.

TRANSPOSITION — In some cases the changes of phonemes leave the relations much the same. So with the vowel change in English. It can be compared with "transposition" in music, whence the term is borrowed.

TROCHAIC REDUCTION — In rapid utterance the median consonant of the trochee may be reduced or crowded out.

TROCHEE — The unit group of two syllables with stress on the first syllable.

TWO-MEMBER — Abutting consonants are often made by different members, as in fla*gp*ole and bla*ckb*oard. Two-member contrasts with one-member abutting consonants, as in hu*mb*ug and bla*ckg*uard.

TYPE OF UTTERANCE — The rate and stress of utterance determine the type. The nature of the speech traits depends on these conditions of rate and stress. Social conditions determine rate and stress and it is convenient to distinguish three types: 1) slow, careful utterance; 2) varied utterance of everyday speech; and 3) rapid utterance.

VANISH OF VOWEL — In English the long vowels, if they are not brief, end in a second phase, the transitory "vanish" which produces a diphthong. At a rapid rate the vanish disappears and the long vowels become monophthongs.

VELUM — The flexible muscular membrane which closes the nasal cavities from the pharynx.

VIBRATO — Rapid oscillation (4–10 per second) of pitch or intensity. Due to rapid alternating contractions of the muscles.

VOCAL CANAL — The pharynx and buccal cavities shaped by tongue, jaw and lips, constitute the common vocal canal.

VOCALIZATION — Vocalization is a concept of the Semitic orthography in which the syllable is indicated by the releasing consonant which is thought of as vocalized by the vowel. The vowel is counted an attribute of the releasing consonant.

VOICED — The manipulation of the air-pressures above and below the larynx causes the glottis in opposition to sound in voiced consonants (sonants). Contrasts with voiceless, unvoiced (surds).

VOWEL — The characterized syllable factor which emits the syllable pulse, usually with tone from the glottis, is counted the vowel. Contrasts with the consonant which delimits the syllable pulse.

VOWEL CAVATIES — A common classification of the vowels is based on the fact that vowels *u* to *ah* are formed by a single mouth cavity with the single orifice at the lips. The vowels from *ee* to *ah* are formed by two cavities, the rear cavity of the pharynx formed by the tongue and with a coupling orifice between the tongue and the palate, and the front cavity with an orifice at the lips. The relations of these cavities, controlled by the tongue, are reciprocal and there are varying combinations for the same vowel.

WEBER'S LAW — In a field of perception an increase of stimulus to be barely perceptible must always be a constant fraction of the stimulus present. The fraction varies with the sensory modality involved.

WORD — The word when isolated is a group of syllables with specific meaning. The word is not a phonetic unit as is the syllable and breath group.

WORD ACCENT — In many languages the stress pattern of the word is invariable and is observed in the structure of the breath group. This constitutes the (invariable) word accents.

BIBLIOGRAPHY OF PUBLISHED WORKS BY R. H. STETSON[1]

Articles

Hubbard, A. W. and Stetson, R. H. (1938). An experimental analysis of human locomotion. American Journal of Physiology, 124, 300–313.

Hudgins, C. V., Moses, E. R. and Stetson, R. H. (1940). Palatograms change with rate of articulation. Archives Néerlandaises de Phonetique Experimentale., 16, 52–61.

Hudgins, C. V. and Stetson, R. H. (1937). Relative speed of articulatory movements. Archives Néerlandaises de Phonetique Experimentale., 13, 85–94.

Hudgins, C. V. and Stetson, R. H. (1932). A unit for kymograph recording. Science, 76, 59–60.

Hudgins, C. V. and Stetson, R. H. (1935). Voicing of consonants by depression of larynx. Archives Néerlandaises de Phonetique Experimentale., 11, 1–28.

Stetson, R. H. (1937). Can all laryngectomized patients be taught esophageal speech? Transactions of the American Laryngeal Association, 59, 59–71.

Stetson, R. H. (1943). Contributions of teachers of the deaf to the science of phonetics. Volta Review, 45, 19–20.

Stetson, R. H. (1937). Esophageal speech for any laryngectomized patient. Archives of Otolaryngology (Chicago), 26, 132–142.

---

[1]Prepared by John Christopher Reid (B.A., Oberlin College, 1958). This bibliography was selected from the publications of Dr. Raymond H. Stetson (1872–1950), Head of the Department of Psychology, Oberlin College, 1900–1939; Professor Emeritus and Director of the Oscillograph Laboratory, 1939–1950. In addition to the works listed, Dr. Stetson was the author of a mimeographed paper and other articles in the Alumni Magazine of Oberlin College and in School and Society. Reprinted with permission from the Journal of Speech and Hearing Disorders August 1958, Vol. 23, No. 3.

Stetson, R. H. (1923). The hair follicle and the sense of pressure. Psychology Monographs, 32, 1–17.

Stetson, R. H. (1921). Helping students to find themselves. Alumni Magazine of Oberlin College, 17, 86–87.

Stetson, R. H. (1937). Oesophageal speech: methods of instruction after laryngectomy. Archives Néerlandaises de Phonetique Experimentale, 13, 95–110.

Stetson, R. H. (1937). The phoneme and the grapheme. Mélang. Ling. Philol. Off. Van Ginneken, 353–357.

Stetson, R. H. (1920). Physiological aspects of piano-playing. Transactions of Music Teachers National Association, 13, 1–10.

Stetson, R. H. (1897). Piano tone-color from a physical and psychological standpoint. Music, 11, 713–717.

Stetson, R. H. (1929). Practice hints in sight reading. Musician, 34, 31.

Stetson, R. H. (1926). Psychology of reading music at sight. Etude, 44, 255–256.

Stetson, R. H. (1936). The relation of the phoneme and the syllable. Proceedings of the Second International Congress of Phonetic Sciences, 245–252.

Stetson, R. H. (1949). Segmentation. Lingua, 2, 46–53.

Stetson, R. H. (1933). Speech movements in action. Transactions of the American Laryngeal Association, 55, 29–41.

Stetson, R. H. (1945). Speech rehabilitation after laryngectomy. Journal of the Iowa State Medical Society, 35, 433–435.

Stetson, R. H. (1923). Teaching of rhythm. Music Quarterly, 9, 181–190.

Stetson, R. H. (1948). Traits of articulate language. Quarterly Journal of Speech, 34, 191–193.

Stetson, R. H. (1896). Types of imagination. Psychological Review, 3, 398–411.

Stetson, R. H. and Bouman, H. D. (1933). The action

current as a measure of muscle contraction. *Science*, 77, 219–221.

Stetson, R. H. and Dashiell, J. F. (1919). A multiple unit system of maze construction. *Psychological Bulletin*, 16, 223–230.

Stetson, R. H. and Fuller, F. L. (1930). Diphthong formation. *Archives Néerlandaises de Phonetique Experimental*, 5, 31–36.

Stetson, R. H. and Hudgins, C. V. (1930). Functions of the breathing movements in the mechanism of speech. *Archives Néerlandaises de Phonetique Experimental*, 5, 1–30.

Stetson, R. H. and McDill, J. A. (1923). Mechanism of the different types of movement. *Psychological Monographs*, 32, 18–40.

Stetson, R. H. and Throner, G. C. (1936). Training for flexible posture and relaxation movements. *Research Quarterly of the American Physiological Education Association*, 7, 143–150.

Stetson, R. H. and Tuthill, T. E. (1923). Measurement of rhythmic unit-groups at different tempos. *Psychological Monographs*, 32, 41–51.

Young, I. C. and Stetson, R. H. (1930). Analysis of vowels. *Science*, 74, 223.

Books

Stetson, R. H. (1945). *Bases of Phonology*. Oberlin: Oberlin Colege. Reprinted with corrections, 1954.

Stetson, R. H. (1928). Motor phonetics. *Archives Néerlandaises de Phonetique Experimental*, 3, 1–216. Second edition published at Amsterdam: North-Holland Publishing Co. (1951).

Monographs

Stetson, R. H. (1931). Breathing movements in singing. *Archives Néerlandaises de Phonetique Experimental*, 6, 115–164.

Stetson, R. H. (1905). A motor theory of rhythm and discrete succession. *Psychological Review*, 12, 250–270; 293–350.

Stetson, R. H. (1903). Rhythm and rhyme. *Psychological Review Monographs*, 4, 413–466.

Stetson, R. H. and Bouman, H. D. (1935). The coordination of simple skilled movements. *Arch. néerl. Physiol.*, 20, 179–254.

Reviews

Dickinson, E. (1915). *Music and the Higher Education*. Rev. by R. H. Stetson, *Alumni Magazine* of Oberlin College, 12, 45–47.

Lowie, R. H. (1946). *Hidatsa Text*. Rev. by R. H. Stetson, *International Journal of American Linguistics*, 12, 136–138.

Pike, K. L. (1947). *Intonation of American English*. Rev. by R. H. Stetson, *International Journal of American Linguistics*, 13, 189–193.

Pike, K. L. (1945). *Phonetics*. Rev. by R. H. Stetson, *Bases of Phonology*. Oberlin: Oberlin College, 109–112.

Spiller, G. (1905). The problem of emotions. Rev. by R. H. Stetson, *Psychological Bulletin*, 2, 304–305.

Strong, A. L. (1910). *The Psychology of Prayer*. Rev. by R. H. Stetson, *Alumni Magazine* of Oberlin College, 6, 69–70.

Travis, L. E. (1932). *Speech Pathology*. Rev. by R. H. Stetson, *Journal of Social Psychology*, 3, 253–256.

Tsanoff, R. A. (1916). On the psychology of poetic construction. Rev. by R. H. Stetson, *Alumni Magazine* of Oberlin College, 12, 202–203.

AUTHOR INDEX

Aristotle, 119
Beach, 32
Bell, A.G., 62, 63, 128
Bell, A.M., 63, 158
Binet, 71
Bloch, 114, 173, 178, 188
Bloomer, 61
Cledat, 74
Coleman, 119
Crandall, 47, 63
Curry, 63
Devaux-Charbonnel, 62
Dhorme, 156
DiCarlo, 116
Emeneau, 189
Fouche, 159
Fourier, 64
Gemelli, 47, 63, 64, 67
Grandgent, 64
Grammont, 159
Green, 62, 65, 202
Gregoire, 73, 82
Groot, de, 148, 181, 193
Hackett, 188
Harris, S., 177, 188, 189, 191
Haycock, 159
Helmholtz, 35, 47, 63
Henri, 71
Hermann, E., 177
Hermann, 10
Hockett, C. F., 188
Hudgins, 41, 44, 45, 48, 116
Jespersen, 159
Jones, D., 119
Josselyn, 84, 129
Joos, 178, 179
Klestadt, 61
Kopp, 62, 65, 202
Laclotte, 143

Lewis, 167
Marage, 62, 70
Marey, 35, 68
Marichelle, 38, 48, 64, 68, 77, 79, 80, 115, 159
Martinet, 173
Menzerath, 182
Meyer, 129
Miller, D.C., 47, 63
Mitford, 119
Musehold, 74
Navarro Thomás, 194
Negus, 55
Oakley-Coles, 35
Paget, 64
Passy, 67, 71, 114, 146, 148, 160, 173, 194
Perret, 194
Pike, 178
Poirot, 84
Potter, 47, 62, 65, 202
Rosapelly, 35, 44, 46
Rousselot, 3, 31, 35, 44, 46, 53, 61, 62, 63, 70,
    72, 73, 77, 84, 86, 88, 89, 100, 106, 111,
    112, 114, 125, 135, 136, 143, 144, 158, 185,
    193, 194
Russell, G.O., 64, 115
Sapir, 33, 159, 160
Saussure, F. de, 31, 53, 70, 76, 77, 114, 158, 159,
    161, 173, 175, 180, 194
Scripture, 73, 82, 129, 158
Sen, 44
Shahara, 61
Sievers, 31, 60, 62, 69, 82, 84, 114, 159, 193, 194
Sommerfelt, 159
Speiser, 177
Stetson, 25, 26, 34, 44, 45, 48, 52, 83
Stumpf, 35, 47, 63, 181
Swadesh, 116
Sweet, 63, 107, 146, 147, 159, 173
Trager, 114, 175, 188

Trubetzkoy, 29, 35, 159, 160, 161, 173, 178, 180, 181, 182, 183, 184, 186, 188
Twaddell, 170, 171
Velten, 167
Vercelli, 63, 64
Verrier, 68
Wanger, 129
Wundt, 120
Zwaardemaker, 44

SUBJECT INDEX

Abeyance, 96
Accent, apogic, 127
Accented groups, four syllable, 150
   three syllable, 150
   two syllable, 150
Acoustic intensity, tracings of, 202 $f.$
Action currents, records of, 120
Action potentials, oscillograms of, 44
Affiliation of languages, 176
Air column, as intermediary between chest and articulatory muscles, 75–76
   as moving member, 56
Air pressure, behind consonant closure, 31
   manipulation of, 116
Air pressure changes, above the larynx, 46
   from the nose, tracings of, 46
   method of recording, 46
   outside the mouth, 46
   outside the mouth, typical arresting form, 71
Air pressure inside the mouth, doubling form, 88
   fortis and *lenis*, 74
   inflected tracing of, 110, 111
   method of recording, 46
   at rapid rate, 95
   typical arresting form, 70
Akkadian, 155, 176
Alliteration, 117
Allophones, 161
Alphabet, 155 156
   Greek, 116
   Phoenician, 156
   phoneme, 174
   phonetic, 174
   phonetic IPA, 116, 158, 159, 160, 173, 175
   Ras Shamara, 156, 176
   Sanskrit, 116
   Semitic, 116
Amphibrach, transitional form, 130
Aphasia, subcortical, 193

Archiphoneme, 183
Arresting consonant within the foot, 185
   in short syllables, 129
Arresting-releasing consonant fusion, 94
Articulation, maximum rate of, 160
   stereotyped by conditioning, 163
Articulate language, analogies of, 33
   two phases of, 29
Articulatory movements, inclusive character of, 178
   rate of, 62
Articulatory organs, contacts of, 44
Artificial larynx, 26, 28, 37, 38, 40, 62, 63, 64, 74, 119, 153–154, 188
   method of using, 153–154
Artificial palate, 35
   construction of, 45, 46
   with kymograph, 174
   with windows, 39, 45
Aspirated stops, 44
Assimilation, law of, 145
   progressive, 102, 146
   regressive, 102
   at syllable frontier, 184–185
Association of languages, 176
Assonance, 117
Auxiliary movements, analogies of, 75
   consonants delimit chest pulse, 102

Back stroke, 54
   condensation of, 72
Bases of Phonology, 23
Beat stroke, 54
   reduced excursion of, 98
Bellows, chest analogy, 26
   fire, 38
   hand, 26
Bengali dialects, 44
Bi-lingual speaker, 175
Bi-maximal, 88, 95

Boundary markers, 29, 161
  in motor phonetic terms, 192
Breath group, 28
  analogies of, 32–33
  basis of rhythmic organization, 130–131
  dynamic pattern of, 119
  feet prolonged, 137
  foot length of, 137
  four syllables, 122–123, 125–126, 137, 142
  with heavy word stress, 180
  metrical formulations of, 177
  of more than four syllables, 141
  movement of abdominal muscles in, 48
  organization of, 121
  as phase of rhythm, 89–90
  rate of, 56
  shown in chest pressure, 127
  stress of, 56
  three syllables, 126
  two syllables, 126
  with variable word stress, 180
Breathing mechanism in speech, two aspects of, 36–37
Broad transcription, 117
Buccal whisper, 194

Cavity orifice, 81
Cesura, 143
Chanson de Roland, 61
Chest-abdomen musculature, bellows analogy, 55
Chest-arrested syllables, 93, 94
Chest pressure, minimum point of, 70–71
Chest pulse, 27
  from gastric balloon, 56
  maximum rate of, 65
  from trachea, 55, 56, 58, 61, 89, 91, 95, 104, 107, 122–124, 125, 137, 142
Clicks, Zulu, 187
Clicks Suction, 32, ft. note 3
Column of air, false assumptions, 188
Conditioning, auditory signals, 162
  the child to speech symbols, 164
  and the units of speech, 162
Consonants, aspirate, 74
  astride, 89
  auxiliary movements, 58
  as auxiliary movements in syllables, 55, 75, 182
  as boundary markers, 185
  classification of, 116
  gutteral, 74
  implosive, explosive, 53, 70
  internal, 107
  labial occlusives and labial continuants, 116
  length of, 73

  length of compared with other rapid movements, 73
  lengths, doubles, abutting pairs, 87–88
  lengths in increasing rate series, 140
  length as phonemic, 116
  length, physiologic limit of, 87
  length of singles, 88
  lengths in stressed groups, 141
  lingual occlusives and lingual continuants, 73
Consonants, abutting, 53, 84, 116–117, 150, 190
  assimilation of, 102–103, 116
  causes of, 89
  comparison of lengths, 101
  eliminated within foot, 121
  intersyllabic pair, 84
  one member, 95
  two member, 98, 99, 100, 101
  and singles compared, 116–118
  two members overlap, 100, 101
Consonant arresting, 70, 150
  action of, 70
  drops out, 92
  in English, in French, 71
Consonant and chest pulse movements, relations of, 94
Consonants, compound, 84, 105–106, 116, 191
  as arresting, 109, 110
  check list of, 200–201
  or cluster, 68
  development of, 107
  fusion of, 185
  fusion of movements, 145
  intersyllabic group, 106
  as releasing, 109
  separation of, 115
  test of, 111, 116
  as test of phoneme, 111
  types of, 110–111
Consonant contact, tracings of, 45
Consonant constriction, 65
Consonants double, 53, 84, 190
  air pressure curve inside the mouth, 85
  in English, 85
  forms of, 88
  two distinct maxima, 85
Consonant median, reduction of, 132
  causes of, 133
Consonant movement, 27
  momentum of, 71–72
Consonant releasing, 71
  beat and back stroke of, 71
  maximum rate of, 71
  releasing and arresting functions, 116
Consonants, simple, 116

SUBJECT INDEX

Consonant stops and continuants, 116
Consonant strokes, anlaysis of, 72, 73
Consonants syllabic, 66
Consonants surd and sonant, 116
Consonants unvoiced (surd), 74
Consonants voiced (sonant), 74
Consonants voiced and unvoiced, 62
Consonant, vowel, confusion of, 66
Consonants and vowels, fusion of, 65–66, 82
    distinction based on function in syllable, 114
    distinguished, 69
Constrictions, graded series of, 183
Constructive doubles, 150
Continuant consonants listed, 183
    in English, 183
Contraction, 138
Contrast, double with arresting consonant, 104
Contrasts between double and single consonant, 196–199
Coordination of articulatory apparatus and chest movement, 76
Coptic, history of, 176
Corpus of syllables, analysis of, 174
Coupled resonators, 115
Cryptographer, 30
Cue, auditory, 31
    kinesthetic, 31
    visual, 31
Cuneiform, 116
Cycles, typical, 63

Dactyl, 121, 125
Dark "e", 114
Deaf, teaching speech to, 158
Diachronous change, 69, 148
Diffusion, regional, 177
Dipthongization of vowels and stress syllables, 173
Dipthongize, 66, 68, 89
Dipthongs, 69, 191
    serial fusion, 116
Discontinuities, between consonants, 93–94
    between syllables, 93–94
    between vowel and consonant, 81
    between vowel and vowel, 81
Distribution of consonant lengths, 139
    of syllable rates, 139, 141
Division of syllables, changes in, 141–142
Doubles, adventitious, 123, 127, 131, 133, 137–138, 140–141
    adventitious between feet, 137
    developed by increasing speed of utterance, 149
    formation of, 126
    induced by increasing rate, 93
Doubling and singling in grouping of syllables, 126

Doubling stage, 89–90
Doubling in stressed syllables, 127
Economy, law of, 145
Electrodes, placement of, 42
Elision of syllables, 135
    in four syllable group, 137
Epenthèse, 135
Expiratory force, measurement of, 120

Factors, intra-syllablic, 195
Feet, types of, 120
Finnish, 68
Foot, 28
    abdominal pulse, 28, 42
    one-syllable, 121
    smallest unit group, 28
Fusion, law of, 145

Gastric balloon, 40
Glottal, 116
Glottal stop, 185, 187, 190
Grenzsignale, 161
Gutteral, 116

Hand-writing, changes in, at rapid rate, 95
Hottentot, clicks, 177
    language of, 28
Hurrian, 155, 176
Hybrid consonant, 131

Iamb, 121
    telescoping of, 135
    and trochee, duration of, 134
Iambic group, length of, 131
Iambic telescoping, 132, 139, 143
Idiograms, 155
    Chinese, 116
Implosion-explosion, 194
Inclusive units, 178
Increasing rate as method, 85
Interference and absorption, 47
Intersyllabic, interval, 88, 115
    space, 126
Intonation, 29, 191
    pattern of, 29
    as phonemic, 117
Isochrony, 68

Jaw, movement of, 46–47
Jaw movements, mark series of syllables, 69
    maximum rate, 46
    method of recording, 47
    primary function of, 69
Junction, implosive, explosive, 70

Juncture, apparent boundaries, 177
   close, 192
   close, open, 195
   open, 173
   as part of movement coordination, 184
   as pause, 195
   reciprocal relations of types, 177
   summary of, 185
   within syllables, 184

Kana, 116
Kota, 189, 190
Kymographic and palatographic, methods combined, 45
Kymographic recording, methods of, 48, 65
Kymographic tracings, processing of, 48, 49

Labial, 116
  -dental, 116
La langue, series of stable phonemes, 160
  la parole, fundamental division, 180
  la parole, distinguished, 159, 162
La parole, unstable articulations in speech, 160
Languages, American-Indian, 177
  with fixed stress, 177
  Japanese, 187
  mechanism, 29, 30
  non-literate, 173
  open-syllable type, 177
  rich in compound consonants, 186–187
  South Sea Island, 187
  teaching, methods of, 168
  tone, 26
  types of, 180
Langue et la parole, 35
Laryngectomized subjects, 37–38
Larynx, action of, 44
  function in speech, 55
  vertical movement of, 44
Lingual-front, 116
  -velar, 116
Lip marker, 35
Lip and tongue marker, construction of, 44
Lists of, nonsense syllables discussed in text, 151
  words and phrases discussed in text, 151

Median consonant, reduction of, 127
Mid-sag, pressure change, 70–71
Modulation, zones of, 47, 81
Modulation bars, 64
  influence of consonants on, 64
Modulation of larynx tone, 64
Momentum, 54
Morphophonemes, 161
  defined, 189
  in motor phonetic terms, 190
Motor phonetics, defined, 30 31
  and visible speech, 78, 202 *f.*
Movement, analysis applied to speech, 54–55
  Ballistic, 29, 32, 54–55
  classification of, 54
  controlled, 32, 54
  coordination, two-member type, 179
  definition of, 193
  of fixation, 53
  their initiation, culmination, termination, 32
  maximum rate of, 54
Movements, bound, 185
  conditions by other movements, 186
  mutually exclusive, 187
Movement units, of speech, 30
  involving speech, 180
Muscles, abdominal, 56–57
Muscle groups, antagonistic, 54
Muscles, rectus abdominus, 42–43
Muscles, intercostals, 26, 43, 55
  external, 57
  internal, 57
Music, analogy of junctures, 185

Narrow transcription, 117
Nasal olives, 46
Negative pressure applicator, 40
  area for placement of, 40
Negative pressure recorder, 40 *f.*
Negative pressure tracings, 42, 120
  of feet and breath group, 44
Neural speculation, 179
Neuremes, 161
Neutralization, of phonemes, 184
Non-aspirated stops, 44
Non-syllabic, 26

Occlusive consonants listed, 183
Occlusives in English, 183
Old Testament, 176
Orthography, approximately phonetic, 173
  English, 82
  traditional, 173
Oscillography record, 23, 181
Oscillography tracings, 42, 49, 65
Overlap, consonants and vowels, 70

Palatogram, 68
Parallelism in languages, 177
Patter, 91, 95, 121, 126
Pause, intersyllabic, 66
  intersyllabic interval, 128
Pauses, insubordination of, 142

SUBJECT INDEX

Phoneme, 28, 30
   as a class, 30
   classification of, 114
   components of, 189
   different languages, 176
   at a differential, 188
   distinguished by phonic differences, 160
   distribution of, 191
   enphonic, 175
   influencing factors, 174
   language to language, 175
   in motor phonetic terms, components of, 189
   as segmental, 189
   as a syllable factor, 188
   symbol of speech signal, 181
   Trubetzkoy's differentiations of, 181
   universal, 35
Phoneme, segmental, 161
Phonemics, American, 188
Phonemic classification, basis for, 183
Phonemic signs, bound character of, 178
Phonetic analysis, two approaches to, 35
Phonetic changes, 53
   defined, 30–31
   historical experimental, 35
   and phonemics, contrast of, 30
   physiological, 35
Phonetic units, inclusive function of, 178
Phonic difference versus linguistic meaning, 174
   minimum, 174
Phonology, 29, 35
   Greek, 156–157
Phrase, 28
Physiological apparatus for speech, 171
Piano playing, maximum rate of, 179
Pitch, change in speech, 119
   as factor in accent, 119
Pitch accent, 147
Pneumodeik, 41, 48
Polygraph, 48, 49
Position, analysis of, 186
   refers to function of element in the syllable, 186
Posture, 55
Prescribed consonants modified, 141
Pressure build-up behind consonants, 46
Pressure, sub-glottal, 38
Prevision, law of, 144
Prominence, 114, 159, 195
Pronunciation, American, 141
   English, 141
Prosodic features, 190
   in motor phonetic terms, 190
Prosodic unit, 181
Prosodemes, 138

Rate, of doubling and singling, 92
   at which doubling begins, 92
   effect of on syllables with arresting consonants, 126
   effect of on syllables with releasing consonants, 126
   factor in grouping, 126
   influence on doubling, 91
   of rhythmic series, 126
   syllable division in, 126
Rate of utterance, 125 126
   as determined by doubling and singling, 140–141
   effects upon vowels, 143
   sudden increase in, 95
Reciprocal influence of sounds, 144
Recorder, action potential, 38, 39
   jaw, 39
   larynx, 39
Recording system, pneumatic, 48
Reduction of language to phoneme, 173
   of syllables, general rule of, 137–138
Relaxation, oscillator, 47
   phase, 55
Releasing-arresting, function of, 188
Releasing consonant as dominant member, 145
Resonance bars, 48, 81–82
Restoration of prescribed consonant, 96
Reversion, to original form, 71, 98
   of prescribed form, 141
Rhythm, 119
Rhythmic grouping, 147
   organization, 190
   pattern in French, 147
   patterns in English and German, 148
Rime, 117
   conditions of, 117

Sandhi, 196–197
Sanskrit, grammarians, 176
   phonology, 156
Schwa, 114
Segmentation, 178
   difficulties of, 178
Semi-vowels, 66, 74, 114
Septum, elastic, 41
Shibbleth, 176
Sign design, 169–170
Signal-events, 163, 171
   signs of, 163
Signals, articulatory, 30, 169, 170
   train of, 163
Sonant, surd phase of, 89
Sonority, basis for the syllable, 114
   concept, 177
   differences of, 159

Sonority, basis for the syllable (*continued*)
   syllable, 159, 160, 191
Sounds, overlapping of, 53
Sound types, as members of a phonemic class, 189
   in motor phonetic terms, 189
Spectogram, 79
Spectograph and kymograph combined, 202
Speech intensities, 120
Speech muscles, two fundamental groups, 55–56
Speech apparatus, 29
Stanchion, 35, 44
Stasis, following beat stroke, 95, 115
Stetson, W.H.
   biographical sketch of by L.D. Hartson, 1–8
   education of, 1–2
   idiosyncracies of, 7–8
   interests of, 3–4
   research of, 4–5
   works of, 2–3, 5–7
Stetson, W.H., recollections of
   by R. Galambos, 9–11
   by J.M. Pickett, 15–21
      characteristic attitudes of, 16
      laboratory studies, 19–21
      legacy of, 21
      phonetic theories of, 16–19
      students of, 19
   by R. Sperry, 12–14
Stress, 26
   agogic, apogogic, 129
   as culmination of movement, 119
   effects on long vowels, 127
   effect on rate, 89
   effects on short vowels, 127
   effect on syllable factors, 89
   in English and German, 102
   as factor in phonetic change, 89
   fixed, 127
   -heavy word, 115, 184
   influence of in phonetic change, 89
   -phrase, 29
   prescribed, determines types of feet, 138
   primary and secondary, 125
   and rate in languages, 62
   -sentence, 26, 29
   in trochees, and iambs, 121
Stress accent, 147
Stress-word, 26, 29
   effect upon syllable duration, 68
   as optional, 117
   as phonemic, 117
Suprasegmental features, 190
Surd consonant between vowels, 135
Syllabary, 155
   Babylonian, 157
   cuneiform, 155, 176

   Cypriote, 177
   Japanese, 116, 160
   Semitic, 156
   Sumarian, 176
Syllable, back stroke, 32
   as ballistic movement, 54
   beat stroke, 32
   changing rate of, 65, 66
   characteristics of, 58
   chest arresting, 32, ft. note 2
   chest released, 32, ft. note 2
   consonant arresting, 32, ft. note 2
   consonant released, 32, ft. note 2
   corpus of, in Greek, 157
   delimited by consonant, 114
   demarcation of, 193
   division of, 193
   duration of, 61
   fundamental phonetic unit, 53
   Greek, four types, 157
   long and short in breath groups, 127
   maximum rate of, 61
   movement of, 53
   number in a given language, 173
   with one-member abutting pairs, 149
   with two-member abutting pairs, 149
   prevailing forms in English and German, 82
   types of, 27
   types of as determined by consonants, 74
   unit in rhythm, 102
   as unitary signals of speech, 160
   unstressed, 68
Syllable arrest, as combined consonant and chest action, 75
Syllable closed, duration of, 82
Syllable division, between double consonants, 84–85
   and double consonant relation of, 195
Syllable factors, 26, 28, 30, 61, 154
   arresting, 28
   aspects of, 28, 188
   functions of, 32, ft. note 2
   rate of, 62
   releasing, 28
   vowel shaping, 27–28
Syllable forming sonant, 53
Syllable length, limited by consonant arrest, 82
   in different languages, 147
Syllable pressure, 193, 194, 195
Syllable pulse, 27
   four methods recording, 36
Syllable, sonority, 193, 194
Syllabic, 26, 61
   consonants, 114
Sumarian, syllable factors in, 155
   system of representing syllables, 155

SUBJECT INDEX

Symbols, phonemic, 30
   schematized, 170
   for syllabic factors, 170
   systems of, 116–117
Synchronous change, 31, 148

Talking dog, 165
Tambour and boss, 42–43
Tambour recording, 40
Teaching reading, method of, 170
Teledeltos paper, 49
Tension tenue detente, of Rousselot, 65, 70, 84
Time-line, 49
Tonemes, 162
Tongue marker, 36
Tracheotomized subjects, 39, 40
Tracheotomy tube, 37–38
Traits of syllables and of breath groups correlated, 174
Trochaic group, length of, 313–132
Trochaic reduction, 138, 139, 143
Trochee, 121, 125
   reduction of, 131–132
Truncation of arresting consonants, 127
Two syllable groups, types of, 130

Umlaut, not serial fusion, 116
Unconditioned stimulus, 164
Unit-groups, 119
Unvoiced consonants, listed, 183
Utterance, rate of, 89, 90
   rate of as cause for phonetic change, 90
   slow type of, 65

Valve action, 26
Varying rates, effect of, 186–187
Visible speech, 65, 66, 79, 145
   patterns of, 69, 202
Vocal canal, shaping of, 27
   shaped by continuant consonant, 114
Vocal folds, action of, 63
   not essential to syllable, 61
Vocalization of releasing surd, 92
Voiced consonants listed, 183
Voicing, mechanism of, 144
Voicing of consonants, buccal pressure in, 74
   chest pressure in, 74
Vowel, acoustic quality of, 115
   analysis, Fourier's, Vercelli's, 47
   audibility of, 67
   cardinal, 68
   cardinal in English, 115
   classification of, 114, 115
   classification of cavity and orifice, 114, 115
   classification by position of tongue, 114, 115
   continental, 115
   dipthongized, 115
   duration, 67
   formant, 47
   French, 68
   Harmonic analysis of, 63
   harmony, 118
   in heavy stressed syllables, 115
   length, 67
   length as phonemic, 115
   long, 61, 62, 69
   long and short in trochee, 134
   moving pictures of, 69
   physiological traits of, 69
   prominence of, 61
   range of positions, 115
   segmentation of, 47
   shape as position, 115
   steady state, 47, 64
   system, 68
   tense and lax, 67, 115, 127
   two cavity, 64
   two series of, 181–182
   versus consonant, the fundamental distinction, 181
   as vocal canal shape, 53
   X-ray, 64
   whispered, 63, 115
Vowel analysis, phase relations, 63
Vowel-consonant, the basic disjunction in phonology, 182
Vowel-consonant, contrast, 190
Vowel cycles, interference patterns, 68, 115, 127–128
   modification of, 143
   in pronunciation, 62
Vowel recording, methods of, 46 47
   artificial palate, acoustic, X-ray, wedges between teeth, 47
Vowels, unstressed, 115
   reduced to schwa, 173
Vulgar Latin, 148

Whispered syllables, 66, 71
Whistle-aspirated, 66
White noise, 64, 66
Word, identity of, 127
   stability of, 176
Word accent, nature of, 119
Word stress, in breath groups, types of, 180
   fixed, 130
   in Hebrew, 143
   in syllabic grouping, 126–127
   in Teutonic languages, 146

Yokuts language, 177

Zulu, 177